DR WARWICK CARTER MB. BS. FRACGP.

the COMPLETE HOME GUIDE *to* MEDICATION

A practical guide to prescription
& non-prescription drugs

• Also Covers Ointments and Creams
• Interactions with Other Drugs
• Usage • Side Effects
• Warnings

This book is intended as a reference volume only, not as a manual for self treatment. If you suspect that you have a medical problem, please seek competent medical care. The information here is designed to help you make informed choices about your health. It is not intended as a substitute for any treatment prescribed by your doctor.

Published by
Hinkler Books Pty Ltd
17-23 Redwood Drive
Dingley Victoria 3172 Australia
www.hinklerbooks.com

ISBN: 1 86515 381 8

Copyright © Warwick Carter 2001

First printed 2001, reprinted 2002

Printed and bound in Australia

CONTENTS

Preface

All medications on the market have been extensively tested for effectiveness and lack of serious side effects. Never the less, every medication has potential problems, interactions, adverse reactions and correct methods of use. For these reasons it is important for everyone who takes any medication that they know as much as possible about its uses and actions.

This book is designed to educate users of medication in simple language about the medications they are taking. If you have any concerns, discuss them further with your doctor or pharmacist.

Every entry has a standard format, and entries are extensively cross referenced. Every prescription medication available in the country (with the exception of general anaesthetics and some injections used in operating theatres and for exotic cancer treatments) is explained, as well as many non-prescription pharmacy only medicines.

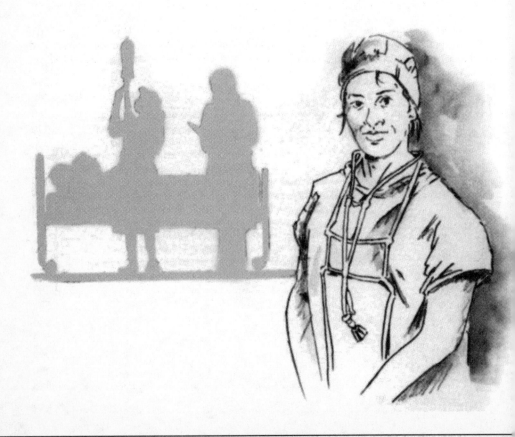

The terminology of medications can be confusing. Every medication has at least three names - a chemical name which is normally only used by scientists, a generic (common) name which is specific to that medication, and a trade name (or several trade names) which is given to the medication by the various manufacturers. For example:-

Chemical name : Acetyl salicylic acid

Generic name: Aspirin

Trade names: Angettes, Caprin, Disprin etc.

Every medication also belongs to a class of similar medications (some belong to two or more classes). Aspirin belongs to the Analgesic, Salicylate and Non-steroidal Anti-inflammatory (NSAID) classes. Common drug classes are listed with the drug generic names in the main part of the book.

The main entries are either under the medication's generic name or its drug class. It will depend on the complexity of the listing if all medications in one drug class can be listed together (eg: all Proton Pump Inhibitors are listed together) or separately (eg: the various forms of Penicillin are listed separately). These entries are listed in alphabetical order in the body of the book and are cross- referenced between generic drug name and drug class so that looking up either will lead you to the required entry.

If you wish to find a medication by its trade name, consult the index where you will be directed to the appropriate entry.

If you wish to find different medications that treat the same condition (eg: epilepsy), look up one medication that treats the condition, see which drug class it is in (eg: Anticonvulsant), and under that drug class you will find listed other medications that will treat that condition.

Some illegal drugs (Cocaine, Marijuana and Heroin) are also covered in this book.

Understanding the medications they are using by referring to this book will help patients cope with their condition, and enable them to understand why their doctor has chosen a particular course of action.

Dr. Warwick Carter MB.BS., FRACGP, FAMA.

August 2000

Format

Generic Name or DRUG GROUP NAME

(Alternative Name)

TRADE NAMES, or TRADE and GENERIC NAMES:

Trade Names of medication listed above, or **Trade Name** followed by generic names within a drug group. The specific ingredient that is being discussed in this entry is underlined when there is any possibility of confusion.

DRUG CLASS

Class of drug to which medication belongs. Only common drug classes are mentioned, as not all medications can be put into a drug class that has any meaning outside university laboratories.

USES

The conditions that can be treated by the medication.

DOSAGE

 The way in which the medication should be taken.
Normal adult dose shown.

PRECAUTIONS

The precautions that a doctor or pharmacist should warn a patient about if taking this medication, including its use in pregnancy (with pregnancy risk categorisation in brackets after the word "pregnancy" - see below), breast feeding and children.

 Do not take if:

- suffering from certain conditions
- under other circumstances

FORMS

The ways in which the medication is presented eg: capsules, mixture, injection (colour and storage precautions in brackets).

Aerosol Spray

Atomiser spray
Inhaler

Capsule
Rotacap

Cream, Gel
Lotion
Ointment, Paste

Drops

Elixer, Liquid
Gargle, Mixture

Lozenge
Pessary, Supository

Nasal spray

Paint
Tincture

Powder

Ampoule
Intravenous injection
Syringe, Injection,
Infusion

Flimtabs
Tablets

Syrup

1 Teaspoon = 5 ml

1 Desertspoon = 10 ml

1 Tablespoon = 15 ml

SIDE EFFECTS

Common: Unwanted problems that many patients may experience.

Unusual: Less common problems that fewer than 3% of patients may experience.

Severe but rare (stop medication, consult doctor): Rare and serious complications.

INTERACTIONS

Other drugs:

- Drug name that may interact with medication. This interaction may affect the medication unfavourably, increase or decrease its action or side effects, or increase or decrease its excretion from the body. Some interactions may improve the effects of the drug. Discuss any possible interaction with your doctor or pharmacist.

Other substances:

- Reactions with substances such as alcohol, caffeine, foods,exercise etc.

PRESCRIPTION

Whether a prescription is required for the medication.

PERMITTED IN SPORT

Can the medication be taken legally while competing in high standards of sport.

OVERDOSE

The effects of an overdose, and the first aid treatment of an overdose. See section on "Overdose" and "Poisoning" in Introduction for further information.

OTHER INFORMATION

Other relevant and interesting information about the medication, including problems with addiction and long term use.

See also Other Related Medication

DRUG GROUP NAME

(Explanation of drug group action)

See Generic Name(s)

Generic Name

See DRUG GROUP NAME

Pregnancy Risk Categorisation

The following system is used in this book. The risk category is shown in the **PRECAUTIONS** section of most entries in brackets after the word "pregnancy". The definitions of the categories are:-

A	No proven direct or indirect harmful effects to the foetus.
B1	Studies in animals have shown no evidence of increased foetal damage.
B2	Studies in animals are inadequate, but available data shows no evidence of increased foetal damage.
B3	Studies in animals have shown evidence of increased foetal damage, but the significance of this in humans is uncertain.
C	May cause harmful effects to the foetus but not malformations. These effects may be reversible.
D	Cause an increased incidence of foetal malformations, other irreversible damage and/or adverse pharmacological effects on the foetus.
X	High risk of permanent damage to the foetus. Should not be used if pregnancy is even a possibility.

Safe Storage of Medication

Accidental overdoses of medications, even common ones like paracetamol (eg: Calpol) can kill children. Many tablets and capsules are brightly coloured and naturally attractive to little people who want to find out what they are like.

A safe storage area for all medications is absolutely essential. A high, locked cupboard with a child proof latch is best.

Home Medicine Chest

A comprehensive home medical chest should contain the following items:

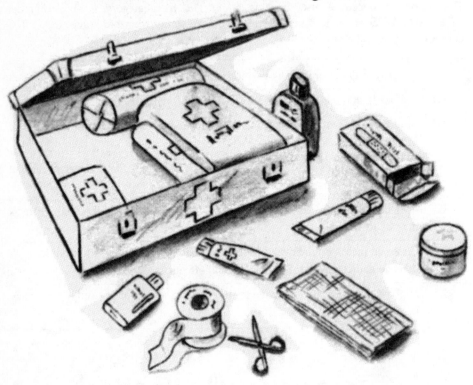

Soluble Aspirin Tablets
Paracetamol Tablets
Paracetamol Liquid
Charcoal Tablets or Solution
(for overdose)
Lotion for bites and stings.
Anti-itch cream.
Antiseptic cream.
Antiseptic Concentrated Liquid
Pseudoephedrine Tablets and/or Liquid
(for nasal congestion)
Decongestant Nose Drops
Menthol Inhalant.

Cough Syrup
Antiseptic Ear Drops
Antiseptic Eye Drops
Sunscreen Lotion or Cream.
Splinter Forceps
Triangular Bandage (sling).
Adhesive Dressing (various sizes)
Elastic Bandages (wide)
Cotton Gauze (NOT cotton wool)
Adhesive Tape

EMERGENCIES

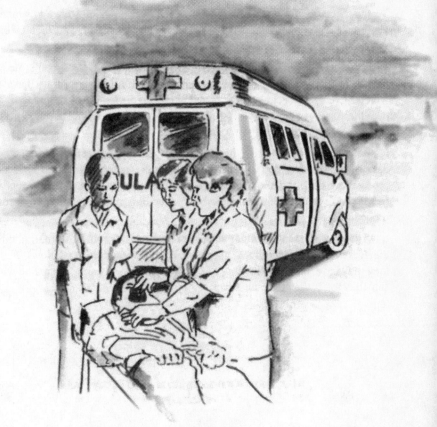

Allergy Reaction

An allergy is excess sensitivity to a substance that produces a reaction in the body.

Allergies may occur on exposure to almost any type of chemical. As well as medications, animal hair, dust, milk, eggs, pollen, fish, fruit, insect bites, moulds and parasites are just a few of the thousands of possible allergic substances.

An allergen is a substance (such as a medication) that causes an allergic reaction. When the body first encounters an allergen, the defence mechanisms of the body are triggered, but there is usually no detectable effect. On the second and subsequent occasions of exposure to the allergen, the defence mechanism over reacts, causing effects that may be merely a nuisance, or severe and life threatening (see Anaphylactic Reaction below), in different areas of the body.

In an allergic reaction, a substance called histamine is released. It causes rapid swelling of the tissue, which in the nose or lungs then secretes copious amounts of watery phlegm, and becomes intensely itchy.

The body gradually breaks down the histamine itself, and the reaction disappears, but this process can be speeded up by the use of anti-histamine drugs that are taken by mouth or injection to destroy the histamine that is causing the allergy reaction.

In an emergency, anyone exposed to a medication or substance to which they have an allergic reaction should be given antihistamines by mouth and then taken to a doctor. Antihistamines are available without prescription from chemists.

Tests may be performed to determine whether or not you are allergic to a particular medication, but because there are so many possibilities, you must have some idea of which medication is causing the problem before the tests are commenced. The tests may take the form of skin pricks with a number of suspected substances, or blood tests that can detect the bodies reaction to an allergen.

If someone is found to be highly allergic to a specific substance, they can be desensitised so that they do not react as strongly, or sometimes do not react at all. This process is often long and involved, and unfortunately does not always work, but many people have had life threatening and disabling allergies cured or reduced by this procedure.

Allergies are usually annoying rather than serious, but in a small number of people, they may become a life threatening anaphylactic reaction (see below). Those who know they may have a life threatening allergy should always carry adrenaline with them, to be self-injected if they have an attack.

Anaphylactic Reaction

An anaphylactic reaction is an immediate, severe, life-threatening allergic reaction. Death may occur within minutes if medical help is not immediately available.

The patient becomes rapidly sweaty, develops widespread pins and needles, swelling develops in one or more parts of the body (possibly including the tongue and throat), starts wheezing, becomes blue around the lips, may become incontinent of urine, loses consciousness, convulses and stops breathing.

Swelling of the tongue and throat alone may be enough to cause death if air is unable to pass into the lungs. The terrified victim suffocates.

First aid can give only limited assistance. The patient must be placed on their back with the neck extended to give the best possible airway, and mouth to mouth resuscitation, and external cardiac massage may be necessary.

Medical treatment must be sought urgently, as an injection of drugs such as adrenaline, aminophylline, hydrocortisone or an antihistamine will reverse the allergic reaction rapidly, and save the patient's life.

Patients who are aware that they may have an anaphylactic reaction usually carry an injectable form of adrenaline with them at all times to be used in an emergency.

Insect stings (eg: bees, hornets, wasps and ants) and injected drugs are the most likely substances to produce acute anaphylaxis. It is rare for inhaled, touched or eaten substances to cause this reaction.

Choking

If a piece of food or other foreign body is caught in the windpipe, the person may die from asphyxiation in a few minutes. It is essential to dislodge the blockage as rapidly as possible.

In a child, turn him upside down, and while holding him by the feet, bang firmly on the back.

In an older child or adult, with the patient sitting or standing, place your arms around them from behind, and cross your wrists over the breast bone. Firmly compress the chest by pressure on the breast bone to force the air out of the lungs, and hopefully the foreign body out of the windpipe.

Alternatively, lie the patient in the coma position on their side on the floor, give several sharp blows between the shoulder blades, and then if necessary, give several firm quick pushes on the side of the chest wall below the arm pit.

If unsuccessful, lie the victim on a table or bed, with the body above the waist hanging over the edge, and bang on the back several times before repeating the chest compression. These manoeuvres are successful in the vast majority of cases.

If you fail to dislodge the food blocking the windpipe, and the patient is turning blue, mouth to mouth resuscitation should be started, in an attempt to force some air past the blockage and into the lungs.

Diarrhoea

Diarrhoea has causes that vary from the serious (cancer, ulcerative colitis), to the annoying (food poisoning, drug reactions), but the most common type of diarrhoea is that caused by a viral infection of the gut.

A virus may infect your bowel to cause diarrhoea, in the same way that another may cause a cold by infecting your nose and throat. The virus particles enter the gut on food or droplets of breath, they are swallowed, and immediately start multiplying into incredibly large numbers. Billions upon trillions of them will eventually be present.

Once in the stomach in these vast numbers, viruses irritate the tissue around them. This in turn causes the lining of the gut to secrete large amounts of fluid, and it also interferes with the normal absorption of food from the intestine, so anything eaten passes straight through.

The third effect is an irritation of the gut, causing it to go into repeated spasms. This causes severe, colic-like pain, and anything that is inside the gut is pushed out through the nearest appropriate orifice (mouth or anus) by these strong contractions.

The upper part of the gut is normally attacked first, causing six to twelve hours of vomiting. This settles as the virus moves down the intestine, and the lower gut becomes inflamed, causing diarrhoea that may last from one to three days.

Because the infection is caused by a virus, antibiotics have no effect on the disease - they may in fact, make the diarrhoea worse.

It is not desirable in most circumstances to use drugs to stop the diarrhoea either, as all this does is hold the virus in the body, and allow it to reproduce further. The body is cleaning the infection from the gastrointestinal system with the diarrhoea, and within reason, it is best to allow this process to proceed.

The treatment of viral gastroenteritis is therefore primarily rest and diet. Fluids and food should be taken in small amounts frequently, not large amounts occasionally.

For the first 24 hours, only clear fluids should be taken by mouth. Commercial preparations that contain salts and sugars are ideal, but clear soups, cordial and very dilute cordials with a pinch of salt added may also be used as a short term substitute. Freezing the liquid and allowing the child to lick the resultant block is an excellent way to get fluids into a vomiting child.

Plain water should not be drunk, as the body requires the salts and sugars for the absorption of fluids from the gut.

On the second and subsequent days, food should be gradually introduced. Cereals, bread, rice and dry biscuits are the first foods to be tried, and if they cause no problems, boiled vegetables, fruit and white meat can be added.

It is important to avoid all dairy products, eggs, fatty and fried foods until you are completely better.

Only if the vomiting lasts more than twelve hours, or the diarrhoea is excessively severe or prolonged, is further medical attention and medication required.

Extra care must be observed with young children, as severe diarrhoea may cause dehydration in less than a day.

Overdose

Excessive doses of medication can be taken by accident (eg: children finding a bottle of pills, confused elderly people) or deliberately (eg: suicide attempt). The appropriate first aid by the person discovering the overdose may be lifesaving.

Some medications are far more dangerous than others when taken in excess. These relative dangers are discussed in the "Overdose" section in the section on each medication in the main part of this book.

For virtually all medication overdosages, the first aid treatment is to administer charcoal to neutralise the medication. Activated charcoal solutions are readily available from chemists without a prescription, and should be included in any home medicine chest.

If activated charcoal is not available, and there will be some delay in obtaining medical attention it is preferable to induce vomiting rather than allow the medication to be absorbed. Vomiting should NOT be induced if the patient is unconscious or otherwise liable to inhale any vomitus.

Activated charcoal should be given at any time after the overdose being taken. Induction of vomiting is most beneficial within 30 minutes of the overdose being taken, but even up to two hours later it may be beneficial. Many medications cause vomiting as part of their overdose effects, but by this time, the drug has already been absorbed and the vomiting is unlikely to reduce the effects of the drug significantly.

Vomiting can be induced by giving Ipecacuanha syrup and water, by giving soapy water to drink, by applying pressure to the upper belly or by putting a finger down the back of the persons throat (be careful not to be bitten, particularly if patient likely to convulse). The patient should be lying on their side with the neck extended, or sitting up and leaning over to avoid inhaling vomitus.

Carers should seek medical advice as soon as possible, and sometimes urgent medical attention must be obtained.

Advice is available from your own general practitioner or local hospital.

See also "Poisoning" below.

Poisoning

Innumerable substances in our environment can poison the human body. A brief summary of common poisons and their treatment follows, but if in doubt, contact your general practitioner or local hospital.

CHEMICAL/DRUG	EFFECT OF POISON	FIRST AID TREATMENT
Alkalis (household bleaches)	Burning, vomiting, shock, difficult breathing.	Dilute with milk, allow vomiting, give vinegar.
Aspirin (Disprin, Caprin etc.)	Rapid breathing, brain disturbance, coma, kidney failure.	Give activated charcoal or induce vomiting.
Barbiturates	Drowsiness, confusion, coma, breathing difficulty.	Give activated charcoal or induce vomiting, black coffee, assist breathing.
Codeine (in pain killers, cough mixtures, antidiarrhoeals)	Constipation, reduced breathing, stupor, coma, heart attack.	Give activated charcoal or induce, assist breathing.
Digoxin (Lanoxin)	Vomiting, irregular pulse, heart failure.	Dilute with milk or water then give activated charcoal or induce vomiting.
Insecticides	Vomiting, diarrhoea, difficult breathing, convulsions.	Dilute with large amount of milk, give activated charcoal or induce vomiting, assist breathing.
Lysol and creosote	Burning of throat, vomiting, shock, breathing difficulty.	Dilute with large amount of milk. **Do NOT induce vomiting.**
Mushrooms	Varies depending on type.	Dilute with water, give activated charcoal or induce vomiting, assist breathing.
Narcotics (Morphine, heroin)	Headache, nausea, excitement, weak pulse, shock, coma.	Give activated charcoal or induce vomiting if narcotic swallowed, assist breathing.
Paracetamol (Alvedon, Calpon, Medinol etc.)	Vomiting, low blood pressure, liver damage, death [>50 tabs].	Give activated charcoal or induce vomiting.
Petroleum products (petrol, kerosene, etc.)	Liver damage, lung damage.	**Do NOT induce vomiting,** dilute with milk.
Tranquillisers (Phenothiazines)	Drowsiness, low blood pressure, rapid pulse, convulsions, coma.	Give activated charcoal or induce vomiting.
Tricyclic antidepressants (Sinequan, Tofranil, Prothiaden, Allegron etc.).	Coma, muscle spasm, convulsions, death.	Give activated charcoal or induce vomiting, assist breathing.

Vomiting

The stomach, and sometimes the upper part of the small gut, will go into spasm and discharge their contents via the gullet and mouth for a very wide variety of reasons. Some causes of vomiting are common and innocuous, but others may indicate serious disease.

By far the most common reason to vomit is a toxin irritating the gut. This is food poisoning, and a contaminated prawn, sausage or other foodstuff is usually responsible. The vomiting occurs 2 to 8 hours after eating the food, and is usually sudden, violent and short-lived. It is unusual for the problem to persist for more than a few hours, and is only occasionally accompanied by diarrhoea.

Gastroenteritis is the other very common cause of vomiting. In this, a virus enters the stomach, causing it to become inflamed. In this state it secretes excess amounts of digestive juices and can go into spasm very easily, particularly if any further food is eaten. Initially the upper part of the gut is affected, and as the virus moves down through the alimentary canal, the large bowel is involved. When the gut goes into spasm, its contents is expelled causing vomiting and/or diarrhoea, and may be associated with painful abdominal cramps.

The virus can easily spread from one person to another, and so one member of the family after another may become infected. Spread is avoided by hand washing, especially after toilet and before eating. Fortunately, the disease is self limiting, and a strict diet for a few days is all that is normally required for treatment.

Nausea (the feeling that you want to be sick) and vomiting often accompany migraine type headaches. Some patients find that their migraine actually eases after vomiting.

Overindulgence in food and alcohol is another common cause of this distressing condition. Even today, sympathy for a self induced condition is not often forthcoming, but 2000 years ago, the Romans sometimes left a feast to vomit so that they could consume even greater amounts of the delicacies being offered.

Other people who may induce vomiting in themselves are those suffering from bulimia and anorexia nervosa. They have a compulsive desire to be thin, and may appear to eat normally, but later regurgitate their food. They steadily loose weight, and may become extremely ill as a result.

Vomiting after a head injury is a sign that there may be some brain damage. One or two vomits are not unusual, but if it becomes prolonged, urgent medical attention should be sought.

Sinusitis and colds may be associated with nausea and vomiting because of the large amounts of infected phlegm that are swallowed. Medications are available to dry up the phlegm and control the sinus infection.

Many rarer diseases from meningitis and stomach cancer to liver disease and pregnancy may be associated with vomiting. If you suffer from this condition, and it does not settle rapidly, have the cause diagnosed and treated by your family doctor.

Abacavir

TRADE NAME

Ziagen.

DRUG CLASS

Antiviral.

USES

Treatment of AIDS and HIV infection.

DOSAGE

 One tablet or 15mLs. solution twice a day.

FORMS

Tablet (300mg.), solution.

PRECAUTIONS

Intolerance to fructose in solution.

SIDE EFFECTS

Common: Liver damage, diarrhoea, tiredness.

INTERACTIONS

None significant known at this time.

PRESCRIPTION

Yes.

PERMITTED IN SPORT

Yes.

OVERDOSE

Effects not known.

OTHER INFORMATION

Released in 1999 as one of numerous medications that may be beneficial in slowing the progress of AIDS.

Abciximab

TRADE NAME

Reopro.

DRUG CLASS

Anticoagulant.

USES

Prevents blood clots during heart and artery surgery.

DOSAGE

 Given by injection via a drip only.

FORMS

Injection vial.

PRECAUTIONS

Used only under strict supervision in hospital. May cause abnormal and excessive bleeding.

SIDE EFFECTS

Common: Unwanted bleeding.

Unusual: Development of antibodies to the medication.

INTERACTIONS

None serious.

PRESCRIPTION

Yes.

PERMITTED IN SPORT

Yes.

OVERDOSE

May cause excessive bleeding.

OTHER INFORMATION

Prevents complications of surgery on heart and arteries.

Acamprosate

TRADE NAME

Campral EC.

USES

Reduces desire for alcohol in alcoholics.

DOSAGE

 One or two tablets three times a day.

FORMS

Tablets of 333mg.

PRECAUTIONS

Reduce dose in elderly and small body weight patients.

Use with caution in pregnancy (B2) and breast feeding.

Not to be used until completely withdrawn from alcohol.

 Do not take if:

- suffering from severe kidney disease, severe liver disease.

SIDE EFFECTS

Common: Diarrhoea.

Unusual: Itch, red skin, reduced libido.

INTERACTIONS

Other drugs:

- Psychotropic drugs.

PRESCRIPTION

Yes.

PERMITTED IN SPORT

Yes.

OVERDOSE

Serious effects unlikely.

OTHER INFORMATION

Introduced in 1999.

See also Disulfiram, Naltrexone.

Acarbose

TRADE NAME

Glucobay.

DRUG CLASS

Hypoglycaemic.

USES

Maturity onset diabetes type 2.

DOSAGE

 50 to 200 mg two to three times a day.

PRECAUTIONS

Use with caution in pregnancy (B3) breast feeding and children. Regular blood tests to check sugar levels and liver function.

FORMS

Tablets.

SIDE EFFECTS

Common: Low blood sugar, nausea, diarrhoea.

Unusual: Liver abnormalities.

INTERACTIONS

Other drugs:

• Other hypoglycaemics (medications that lower blood sugar levels), neomycin, cholestyramine.

PRESCRIPTION

Yes.

PERMITTED IN SPORT

Yes.

OVERDOSE

May cause coma due to excessively low blood sugar levels. Give activated activated charcoal or induce vomiting if medication taken recently. Seek medical assistance.

ACE INHIBITORS

(Angiotensin Converting Enzyme Inhibitors).

TRADE and GENERIC NAMES

Accupro (Quinapril).

Accuretic (Quinapril, Hydrochlorthiazide).

Acepril, Capoten (Captopril).

Capozide (Captopril, Hydrochlorthiazide).

Carace, Zestril (Lisinopril).

Carace Plus, Zestoretic (Lisinopril, Hydrochlorthiazide).

Coversyl (Perindopril).

Gopten, Odrik (Trandolapril).

Innovace (Enalapril).

Innozide (Enalapril, Hydrochlorthiazide).

Perdix (Moexipril).

Staril (Fosinopril).

Tanatril (Imidapril).

Tarka (Trandolapril, Verapamil).

Triapin, Triapin Mite (Ramipril, Felodipine).

Tritace (Ramipril).

Vascace (Ciliazapril).

DRUG CLASS

Antihypertensive.

USES

High blood pressure, heart failure, improves survival after heart attack.

DOSAGE

 Different forms are longer acting than others. Follow doctors instructions. Dosage varies from one capsule or tablet a day, to two capsules or tablets three times a day. Do not vary dosage without medical advice.

FORMS

Tablets, capsules, injection and mixture.

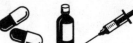

PRECAUTIONS

Should not be used in pregnancy (D). Should be used only if specifically medically indicated and with caution in children and while breast feeding.

Do not take if:

• suffering from severe kidney disease, reduced blood supply to brain or taking immunosuppressive drugs.

SIDE EFFECTS

Common: Dry cough, swelling of ankles and other tissue, rash.

Unusual: Stomach upsets, abnormal taste.

Severe but rare (stop medication, consult doctor): Abnormal bleeding.

INTERACTIONS

Other drugs:

• Interacts with Diuretics, and some arthritis drugs, but often carefully used with these drugs.

• Reacts with Lithium, potassium increasing drugs, Tetracycline, Vasodilators.

PRESCRIPTION

Yes.

PERMITTED IN SPORT

Yes.

OVERDOSE

May cause low blood pressure. First aid involves giving activated charcoal or induction of vomiting and seeking medical attention.

OTHER INFORMATION

Relatively new group of drugs that are rapidly becoming the first choice in the treatment of high blood pressure and heart failure. First released early 1980,s, but many new forms coming onto the market in the mid 1990,s. Angiotensin is a hormone that naturally increases blood pressure. ACE Inhibitors reduce the amount of angiotensin produced in the body to reduce blood pressure.

See also Angiotensin II Receptor Antagonists

Acebutolol
See BETA BLOCKERS

Aceclofenac
See NSAID

Acemetacin
See NSAID

Acetazolamide

TRADE NAME

Diamox

USES

Glaucoma, retention of fluid, swelling, petit mal and some other forms of epilepsy.

DOSAGE

Complex. Depends on condition being treated, its severity and weight of patient. Must be individually determined for each patient by doctor.

FORMS

Tablets (white) of 250mg.

PRECAUTIONS

Not to be used in pregnancy (B3). Use with caution in breast feeding and children.

Care must be used in long term use.

Regular blood tests to check blood chemistry advisable.

Use with caution in emphysema.

Do not exceed recommended dose.

Do not take if:

- suffering from disorders of blood chemistry, liver disease. kidney disease, adrenal gland disease.

SIDE EFFECTS

Common: Pins and needles, frequent passing of urine, loss of appetite.

Unusual: Biochemical imbalances in blood.

INTERACTIONS

Other drugs:

- Aspirin, Hypoglycaemics, Anticoagulants, Phenytoin, Digoxin.

PRESCRIPTION

Yes.

PERMITTED IN SPORT

No.

OVERDOSE

Significant abnormalities in blood chemistry may occur. Give activated charcoal or induce vomiting if medication taken recently. Seek medical assistance.

OTHER INFORMATION

In glaucoma, usually taken in combination with eye drops.

Acetic acid

TRADE NAME

Aci-Jel, EarCalm
Otomize (with Dexamethasone, Neomycin).

USES

Ear drops - EarCalm removes water from ears to prevent swimmers ear - Otomize treats swimmers ear Gel - restores vaginal acidity.

DOSAGE

Ear drops - 4 to 6 drops in each ear after swimming. Gel - 1 applicator full of gel twice a day.

FORMS

Ear drops, vaginal gel.

PRECAUTIONS

Ear drops - safe in pregnancy.
Gel - not for use in pregnancy.

Do not use ear drops if:-

- suffering from ear infection, ear discharge, blocked ear canals, perforated ear drum.
- grommets inserted.

SIDE EFFECTS

Ear drops - ear canal irritation
Gel - minimal.

INTERACTIONS

None.

PRESCRIPTION

Aci-Jel, EarCalm - No.
Otomize - Yes.

PERMITTED IN SPORT

Yes.

OVERDOSE

Not likely to be harmful if swallowed.

Acetominophen

See Paracetamol.

Acetylcholine chloride

TRADE NAME

Miochol (with Mannitol).

DRUG CLASS

Miotic.

USES

Rapid contraction of the pupil in the eye.

DOSAGE

 As determined by doctor.

FORMS

Eye drops.

PRECAUTIONS

Use with caution in pregnancy (B2).

Drops must be prepare immediately before use.

SIDE EFFECTS

Reduced vision in dull light.

INTERACTIONS

None significant.

PRESCRIPTION

Yes.

PERMITTED IN SPORT

Yes.

OVERDOSE

Unlikely to have adverse effects if swallowed.

OTHER INFORMATION

Used only by ophthalmologists (eye doctors) in their rooms or hospital.

See also Carbachol.

Acetylcysteine

TRADE NAME

Parvolex
Ilube (with Hypromellose).

USES

Injection: Paracetamol overdose.
Eye drops: Dry eyes with excess mucus.

DOSAGE

 Eye drops: One or two drops, three or four times a day
Injection: As determined by doctor.

FORMS

Eye drops, injection.

PRECAUTIONS

Use with caution in pregnancy (B2), worsening asthma.

 Do not take if:

- suffering from severe liver or kidney disease.
- wearing soft contact lenses

SIDE EFFECTS

Common: Minimal

Unusual: Asthma.

INTERACTIONS

None significant.

PRESCRIPTION

Yes.

PERMITTED IN SPORT

Yes.

OTHER INFORMATION

Should be used within 10 hours of paracetamol overdose. Minimal benefit after 15 hours.

Acetylsalicylic Acid

See Aspirin.

Aciclovir

TRADE NAME

Zovirax.

DRUG CLASS

Antiviral.

USES

Treatment of genital herpes, shingles, cold sores, chickenpox and herpes eye infections.

DOSAGE

 Tablets: 200mg to 800mg every four to eight hours
Cream: Apply five times a day starting as soon as possible after onset of symptoms.

Eye ointment: Insert five times a day for 14 days.

FORMS

Tablets of 200mg., 400mg. and 800mg.; suspension; injection; eye ointment; skin cream.

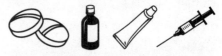

PRECAUTIONS

Use in pregnancy (B3) and breast feeding only when medically essential. May be used in children.

Lower doses necessary in elderly.

Use tablets with caution in serious kidney disease, dehydration, brain disorders.

SIDE EFFECTS

Common: Minimal.

Unusual: Tablets - Nausea, vomiting, headache.

INTERACTIONS

Other drugs:

• Probenecid, Diuretics (fluid tablets), Interferon, Methotrexate.

PRESCRIPTION

Yes.

PERMITTED IN SPORT

Yes.

OVERDOSE

Exacerbation of side effects likely.

OTHER INFORMATION

Very safe and effective medication that has a very high success rate in treating Herpes infections. Chickenpox and shingles are caused by Herpes zoster, and cold sores and genital herpes by Herpes simplex. It is vital that any patient who suspects they have shingles must see their doctor immediately as Aciclovir only works if started within 72 hours of onset of rash. Chickenpox and cold sores are normally only treated under special circumstances as the medication is quite expensive. Eye infections with Herpes may cause blindness if not treated rapidly and effectively. Cream effective against cold sores only if started as soon as symptoms appear.

ACIDS

See Lactic acid, Salicylic acid (SALICYLATES).

Acipimox

TRADE NAME

Olbetam.

DRUG CLASS

Hypolipidaemic.

USES

Some types of high blood cholesterol and triglycerides.

DOSAGE

 Maximum of 1200mg. a day divided into two or three doses.

FORMS

Capsule.

PRECAUTIONS

Do not use in pregnancy (B2) and breast feeding.

Regular blood tests to check liver and kidney function and blood fat levels recommended.

Use with caution with low blood pressure and poor liver or kidney function.

 Do not take if:

• suffering from peptic ulcer, stomach upsets, recent heart attack, severe kidney disease, diabetes, gout, heart disease, gall bladder disease, glaucoma, tendency to bleed easily.

SIDE EFFECTS

Common: Rashes, red skin, stomach upsets, nervousness, headache, tiredness.

Unusual: Dry skin, skin pigmentation.

Severe but rare (stop medication, consult doctor): Yellow skin.

INTERACTIONS

Other drugs:

• Drugs used to treat high blood pressure.

• Steroids, Hallucinogens, Reserpine, Chlordiazepoxide.

PRESCRIPTION

Yes.

PERMITTED IN SPORT

Yes.

OVERDOSE

Causes flushing, itch, vomiting, diarrhoea, heartburn, belly cramps, fainting. Induce vomiting if tablets taken recently. Seek medical assistance.

OTHER INFORMATION

Derived from nicotinic acid.

See also Nicotinic Acid

Acitretin

TRADE NAME

Neotigason

DRUG CLASS

Keratolytic.

USES

Severe psoriasis.

DOSAGE

 Determined individually for each patient. 25 to 50mg a day.

FORMS

Capsules of 10mg and 25mg.

PRECAUTIONS

Absolutely forbidden in pregnancy (X). Use with caution in children and adolescents. Use with great caution in liver and kidney disease.

SIDE EFFECTS

Common: Dry skin, itchy skin, rashes, fragile skin.

Unusual: Kidney and liver abnormalities, eye irritation, increased blood fat and cholesterol levels, bone and brain growths.

Severe but rare (stop medication, consult doctor): Rare and serious complications.

INTERACTIONS

Other drugs:

• Mini-contraceptive pill, tetracycline antibiotics, phenytoin.

Other substances:

• Vitamin A, alcohol.

PRESCRIPTION

Yes. Hospitals only.

PERMITTED IN SPORT

Yes.

OVERDOSE

May cause headache, vomiting, flushing, mouth soreness and dryness, abdominal pain, flushing and incoordination. Seek medical assistance.

OTHER INFORMATION

First introduced in 1997 to replace Etretinate. A very potent and potentially dangerous drug, but if used correctly can dramatically and often permanently cure severe chronic psoriasis. Use in pregnancy will always cause severe damage to foetus. Vitamin A derivative.

Acrivastine

See ANTIHISTAMINES, NON-SEDATING.

Actinomycin D

(Dactinomycin).

TRADE NAME

Cosmegen.

DRUG CLASS

Cytotoxic.

USES

Cancer of the kidney (Wilm's tumour), brain, testes, uterus and bone.

DOSAGE

 By drip into vein as determined for each patient by doctor.

FORMS

Injection.

PRECAUTIONS

Not to be used in pregnancy (D), breast feeding or infants.

Use with caution in children.

Use with caution if having radiotherapy.

Do not allow solution to touch skin - extremely corrosive. Ensure there is no leakage from drip into tissues outside vein.

Regular blood tests essential to check function of liver, kidney, bone marrow and blood cells.

 ### Do not take if:

• suffering from chickenpox or shingles.

SIDE EFFECTS

Common: Skin rashes, nausea, vomiting, tiredness, muscle pain, fever, anal pain, belly pain, loss of appetite.

Unusual: Liver damage, anaemia.

INTERACTIONS

None significant.

PRESCRIPTION

Yes.

PERMITTED IN SPORT

Yes.

OVERDOSE

Very serious. Only given under strict medical supervision.

Activated Charcoal

See Charcoal.

Adapalene

TRADE NAME

Differin.

USES

Severe acne.

DOSAGE

 Apply thinly once a day at bedtime to clean dry skin.

FORMS

Gel, cream

PRECAUTIONS

Do not use if pregnant (D). Use with caution in children and breast feeding. Avoid eyes, lips, mouth, nostrils.

Do not apply to broken skin, moist skin, moist tissues, eczema, dermatitis.

Avoid sun exposure.

 ### Do not take if:

• suffering from certain conditions.

• under other circumstances.

SIDE EFFECTS

Common: Red skin, dry skin.

Unusual: Itch, burning, scaly skin.

INTERACTIONS

Other drugs:

• Retinoids, astringents, drying agents.

Other substances:

• Abrasive cleansers.

PRESCRIPTION

Yes.

PERMITTED IN SPORT

Yes.

OVERDOSE

Wash affected area thoroughly.

Adenosine

TRADE NAME

Adenocor.

DRUG CLASS

Antiarrhythmic.

USES

Control of some types of irregular heart beat starting in the upper chambers of the heart (the atria).

Dilates arteries of heart to allow adequate x-ray pictures to be taken.

DOSAGE

 Given rapidly by injection into a vein.

FORMS

Injection.

PRECAUTIONS

Use with caution in pregnancy (B2), children and breast feeding.

Must only be used if type of irregular heart rhythm has been definitely established.

SIDE EFFECTS

Common: Flushed face, headache.

Unusual: Shortness of breath, pressure in chest, light headedness, nausea, very slow heart rate.

INTERACTIONS

Other drugs:

• Carbamazepine, xanthines, dipyridamole.

PRESCRIPTION

Yes.

PERMITTED IN SPORT

Yes.

OVERDOSE

Serious. Always given under close medical supervision.

Adrenaline

TRADE NAME

Epipen, Eppy, Simplene Ganda (with Guanethidine)
Often combined with various local anaesthetics (eg: Lignocaine).

DRUG CLASS

Vasoconstrictor, Mydriatic.

USES

Constriction of blood vessels to prolong effect of medication (eg: local anaesthetics).

Control of very severe allergy reactions and asthma.

Dilates the size of the pupil in eye surgery and examination.

Treatment of certain type of glaucoma (chronic simple glaucoma).

Emergency treatment of some forms of heart disease.

DOSAGE

 Eye drops: One drop in affected eye once or twice a day.

Injection: Self inject for severe allergic reaction.

FORMS

Injection, injection pen, eye drops.

PRECAUTIONS

May be used in pregnancy, breast feeding and children.

Eye drops should not be used for prolonged periods.

Injections only used by doctors in emergency situations.

Never inject into ear, fingers, toes or penis.

Never inject into artery or vein.

Use with caution if suffering from overactive thyroid gland, heart disease, high blood pressure, psychiatric conditions or diabetes.

SIDE EFFECTS

Common: Eye drops: Eye pain, headache, brow ache, red eye. Injection: Rapid heart rate, reduced circulation at site of injection, difficulty in breathing, dizziness, weakness, tremor, headache, irritability, anxiety, fear.

INTERACTIONS

Other drugs:

• Injection may interact with Tricyclic antidepressants, Thyroxine and some Antihistamines.

Other substances:

• Do not use alcohol or caffeine, or undertake vigorous exercise.

PRESCRIPTION

Yes

PERMITTED IN SPORT

Eye drops: Yes
Injection: No

OVERDOSE

Eye drops: Flush eye with water.

Injection: Very serious. May result in stroke, heart attack and death. Extremely urgent medical attention required to administer counter acting drugs.

OTHER INFORMATION

Widely used to prolong effect of local anaesthetics and reduce bleeding at operation site. Effective in extreme cases of severe allergy to reduce effects of swelling.

See also Isoprenaline.

Alclometasone

TRADE NAME

Modrasone.

DRUG CLASS

Corticosteroid.

USES

Eczema, dermatitis.

DOSAGE

 Apply thinly two or three times a day.

FORMS

Cream, ointment

PRECAUTIONS

Should be used with caution in pregnancy and breast feeding. Safe for use in children. Avoid eyes.

Use for shortest period of time possible.

 Do not use if:

- suffering from any form of skin infection, skin ulcers, acne or cracked lips.

SIDE EFFECTS

Minimal.

INTERACTIONS

None significant

PRESCRIPTION

Yes.

PERMITTED IN SPORT

Yes.

OTHER INFORMATION

Extremely effective and useful medication, particularly on the face, on delicate skin and in children. Lowest dose and shortest possible course should be used. Not addictive. Introduced late 1980s.

Alcohol

See Ethanol.

Alendronate

TRADE NAME

Fosamax.

DRUG CLASS

Bisphosphonate.

USES

Osteoporosis, Paget's disease.

DOSAGE

 Complex. Take one tablet a day 30 minutes before eating or drinking after waking in morning. Remain erect until after eating.

FORMS

Tablets of 5mg and 10mg.

PRECAUTIONS

Use with great caution in pregnancy (B3), breast feeding and children.

Use with caution with recent peptic ulcer and kidney damage.

Calcium and vitamin D levels must be monitored.

 Do not take if:

- suffering from peptic ulcer.
- under other circumstances.

SIDE EFFECTS

Common: Nausea, vomiting, indigestion.

Unusual: Ulceration of oesophagus and stomach, mouth ulcers, peptic ulcers, muscle pain, headaches.

Severe but rare (stop medication, consult doctor): Vomiting blood, black motions.

INTERACTIONS

Other drugs:

• Calcium supplements, antacids, biphosphonates, aspirin. May affect almost any medication taken by mouth.

PRESCRIPTION

Yes.

PERMITTED IN SPORT

Yes.

OVERDOSE

Very low blood levels of calcium may occur. This may interfere with the function of nerves and other tissues. Other symptoms may include indigestion and vomiting. Induce vomiting if medication taken recently, or drink large amounts of milk.

OTHER INFORMATION

Potent and effective medication for osteoporosis introduced in 1996.

Alfacalcidol

TRADE NAME

AlfaD, One-Alpha.

USES

Severe body calcium chemistry diseases involving the parathyroid glands and/or kidneys (eg. renal osteodystrophy), rickets, osteomalacia.

DOSAGE

 As determined by doctor.

FORMS

Capsules, mixture.

PRECAUTIONS

Not for use in pregnancy and breast feeding.

Blood tests required regularly to monitor calcium levels.

 Do not take if:

• suffering from kidney failure.

• under other circumstances

INTERACTIONS

Other drugs:

• Barbiturates, Anticonvulsants, Danazol, Digoxin, Antacids, Thiazide diuretics, Sucralfate, Colestipol, Cholestyramine.

Other substances:

• Mineral oils.

PRESCRIPTION

Yes.

PERMITTED IN SPORT

Yes.

OVERDOSE

Serious. Seek urgent medical attention.

Alfentanil

TRADE NAME

Rapifen.

DRUG CLASS

Narcotic.

USES

Pain relief while under anaesthesia.

DOSAGE

 Calculated by anaesthetist for each individual patient.

FORMS

Injection.

PRECAUTIONS

Must not be used in pregnancy (C) or children under 12 years.

Use with caution in head injuries, obesity and elderly.

 Do not take if:

- suffering from liver failure, underactive thyroid gland.

SIDE EFFECTS

Unusual: Reduced ability to breathe, muscle rigidity, slow heart rate, low blood pressure, throat spasm.

INTERACTIONS

Other drugs:

- Some anaesthetics, erythromycin, cimetidine, MAOI, medications that depress brain function.

PRESCRIPTION

Yes. Controlled drug.

PERMITTED IN SPORT

No.

Alfuzosin

TRADE NAME

Xantral.

USES

Enlarged prostate gland.

DOSAGE

 One tablet three times a day after meals.

FORMS

Tablet.

PRECAUTIONS

Not for use in pregnancy, breast feeding and children.

Use with caution in heart, kidney and liver disease.

Blood pressure should be checked regularly.

 Do not take if:

- suffering from prostate cancer, low blood pressure or significant liver disease.
- angina or chest pain occurs.
- if having a general anaesthetic.

SIDE EFFECTS

Common: Dizziness, giddiness, headache, nausea, diarrhoea.

Unusual: Low blood pressure, fainting, tiredness, rapid heart rate, palpitations, rash, itch, flushes, swelling of feet and hands.

Severe but rare (stop medication, consult doctor): Angina. (chest pain).

INTERACTIONS

Other drugs:

- Medications that lower blood pressure, other medications that reduce prostate gland size.

PRESCRIPTION

Yes

PERMITTED IN SPORT

Yes

OVERDOSE

Serious. May cause diarrhoea, vomiting, difficulty in breathing, weakness, low blood pressure, slow heart rate and heart attack. Seek urgent medical attention.

Alginic acid

See ANTACIDS

ALKYLATERS

See CANCER TREATING DRUGS

Allantoin

TRADE and GENERIC NAMES

Available only in combination with other medications.

Actinac (with Chloramphenicol, Hydrocortisone, Sulphur and other ingredients)

Alphosyl HC (with Tar, Hydrocortisone).

Alphosyl (with Tar).

USES

Repairs damaged skin, minor burns, grazes, acne, psoriasis.

DOSAGE

 Apply several times a day.

FORMS

Powder, cream, ointment, lotion.

PRECAUTIONS

Safe to use in pregnancy, breast feeding and children.

Avoid eye contact.

SIDE EFFECTS

Minimal

INTERACTIONS

None significant.

PRESCRIPTION

Alphosyl - No
Others - Yes

PERMITTED IN SPORT

Yes

Allergen extracts

TRADE NAME

Allergens against a wide range of plants, foods, animals, moulds, insects etc. available.

DRUG CLASS

Antiallergen.

USES

Reduction of allergy reaction to specific substances.

DOSAGE

 Complex. Series of injections over many months in very slowly increasing concentrations and doses as determined by doctor.

FORMS

Injection.

SIDE EFFECTS

Common: Local redness of skin at site of injection.

Unusual: Widespread redness and itching of skin around site of injection.

Severe but rare: Generalised severe anaphylactic (allergy) reaction that may be life threatening unless treated promptly.

INTERACTIONS

None.

PRESCRIPTION

Yes.

PERMITTED IN SPORT

Yes.

OVERDOSE

Very severe, life threatening anaphylactic (allergy) reaction may occur. Adrenaline should be injected subcutaneously every few minutes to counteract anaphylaxis. Doctor may need to give oxygen and cardiopulmonary resuscitation.

PRECAUTIONS

Patient must wait in surgery for 30 minutes after injection given in case of serious allergy reaction.

Injection must be given subcutaneously (just under the skin) and not into muscle or a vein.

Should not be used in pregnancy, but unlikely to be serious consequences if administered inadvertently.

 Do not take if:

- allergy reaction at time of planned injection.

Allopurinol

TRADE NAME

Zyloric.

DRUG CLASS

Uricosuric...

USES

Prevention of gout and its complications.

DOSAGE

 One or two tablets once a day.

FORMS

Tablets of 100mg. and 300mg.

PRECAUTIONS

Use with caution in pregnancy (B2) and breast feeding. Not for use in children.

Use with caution in kidney and liver disease.

SIDE EFFECTS

Common: Minimal.

Unusual: Fever, arthritis, nausea.

Severe but rare (stop medication, consult doctor): Rash.

INTERACTIONS

Other drugs:

- Azathioprine, Mercaptopurine, Sulfinpyrazone, Probenecid, Aspirin.

Other substances:

- Alcohol may aggravate gout.

PRESCRIPTION

Yes.

PERMITTED IN SPORT

Yes.

OVERDOSE

May cause vomiting, diarrhoea and dizziness.

OTHER INFORMATION

Widely used, very safe and effective medication for the prevention of gout. Does not cause dependence or addiction.

ALPHA BLOCKERS

(Control blood pressure)

See Doxazosin, Indoramin, Labetalol, Prazosin, Tamsulosin, Thymoxamine.

Alpha tocopherols

See Tocopherols.

Alprazolam

See ANXIOLYTICS.

Alprostadil

(Prostaglandin E1).

TRADE NAMES

Caverject, Muse, Prostin VR, Viridal.

USES

Prostin VR - to keep arteries open in newborn babies with heart defects.

Others - inability to obtain an erection in the male penis.

DOSAGE

 Caverject, Viridal - inject into shaft of penis as directed by doctor.
Muse - insert pellet with applicator into urethral opening at end of penis.
Prostin - as determined by doctor.

FORMS

Injection, pellet.

PRECAUTIONS

Do not use for erection if:

• suffering from blood borne diseases.

• partner pregnant.

• suffering from curvature or deformity of penis.

• penile implant inserted.

SIDE EFFECTS

Common: Pain during injection and erection, bruising.

Unusual: Prolonged erection, scarring and curvature of penis.

INTERACTIONS

Other drugs:

• Warfarin, heparin.

Other substances:

• Reactions with substances such as alcohol, caffeine, foods, exercise etc.

PRESCRIPTION

Yes.

PERMITTED IN SPORT

Yes.

OVERDOSE

Prolonged painful erection, diarrhoea, depression, rapid breathing. Medical attention essential for any penile erection lasting longer than 4 hours.

OTHER INFORMATION

Injection introduced in 1996 as a safe and effective form of treatment for impotence. Muse introduced in 1998 as an alternative to injected form.

See also Sildenafil.

Alteplase

See FIBRINOLYTICS.

Altretamine

(Hexamethylmelamine).

TRADE NAME

Hexalen.

DRUG CLASS

Antineoplastic.

USES

Advanced cancer of the ovary.

DOSAGE

 As determined by doctor.

FORMS

Capsules of 50mg.

PRECAUTIONS

Regular blood tests essential. Regular checks on nerve function required. Not to be used in pregnancy (D) or breast feeding.

 Do not take if:

- suffering from bone marrow or nerve disease.

SIDE EFFECTS

Common: Abnormal stimulation or loss of function of nerves, nausea, vomiting.

Unusual: Bone marrow damage, kidney damage.

INTERACTIONS

Other drugs:

- Monoamine oxidase inhibitors (used for severe depression), cimetidine, pyridoxine.

PRESCRIPTION

Yes.

PERMITTED IN SPORT

Yes.

OVERDOSE

Serious damage to bone marrow, nerves and kidneys possible.

OTHER INFORMATION

Introduced in 1998 for use when other treatments have failed.

Aluminium chloride

TRADE NAME

Anhydrol Forte, Driclor.

USES

Excessive sweating from arm pits, hands and feet.

DOSAGE

 Apply nightly initially, reducing to once or twice a week depending on response.

FORMS

Solution.

PRECAUTIONS

Safe to use in pregnancy, breast feeding and children over six years.

Avoid contact with eyes.

Do not use on broken or damaged skin.

Do not shave arm pit within 24 hours of use.

Do not bathe immediately before use.

SIDE EFFECTS

None significant.

INTERACTIONS

None.

PRESCRIPTION

No.

PERMITTED IN SPORT

Yes.

OVERDOSE

Seek medical attention if swallowed.

OTHER INFORMATION

One of the more useful treatments for the distressing condition of hyperhidrosis (excess sweating).

Aluminium oxide

See KERATOLYTICS.

Aluminium salts

See ANTACIDS.

Alverine Citrate

TRADE NAME

Spasmonal, Spasmonal Forte Spasmonal Fibre (with Sterculia).

DRUG CLASS

Antispasmodic.

USES

Irritable bowel syndrome, bowel spasms.

DOSAGE

 Capsules: One or two, two or three times a day
Fibre: One or two heaped teaspoons once or twice a day.

FORMS

Capsules, granules.

PRECAUTIONS

Ensure adequate fluid intake with fibre. Use with caution in pregnancy. Safe in breast feeding.

 Do not take if:

- obstructed bowel, bowel cancer.

SIDE EFFECTS

Common: Mild feeling of belly distension.

INTERACTIONS

May interfere with the absorption of many medications.

PRESCRIPTION

No.

PERMITTED IN SPORT

Yes.

OVERDOSE

Take additional water. Belly discomfort and passing excess wind only effects.

Amantadine

TRADE NAME

Lysovir, Symmetrel.

DRUG CLASS

Antiparkinsonian.

USES

Parkinson's disease, prevention of influenza type A.

DOSAGE

 Parkinson's disease: Increase slowly over several weeks under doctor's instructions
Influenza A prevention: One capsule twice a day.

FORMS

Capsule of 100mg.

PRECAUTIONS

Use in pregnancy (B3) only if medically essential. Use in breast feeding with considerable caution. Not for use in children under 9 years.

Use with caution in glaucoma, enlarged prostate gland, confused or psychiatrically disturbed patients, heart failure, low blood pressure, liver and kidney disease.

Do not stop suddenly, but reduce dose slowly.

Lower dose required in elderly.

SIDE EFFECTS

Common: Indigestion, excitement, dizziness, poor concentration, dry mouth, blurred vision, constipation, anxiety, confusion, swelling of ankles and feet.

Unusual: Tremor, headache, slurred speech, incoordination, sleeplessness, palpitations, difficulty in passing urine.

Severe but rare (stop medication, consult doctor): Unable to pass urine, convulsions, irrational behaviour.

INTERACTIONS

Other drugs:

• Other antiparkinsonians, L-Dopa.

Other substances:

• Reacts adversely with alcohol and caffeine.

PRESCRIPTION

Yes.

PERMITTED IN SPORT

Yes.

OVERDOSE

May cause confusion, hallucinations, delirium, rapid heart rate, rapid breathing, vomiting, dry mouth and retention of urine. Deaths have not been reported. Induce vomiting if medication taken recently. Seek medical attention.

OTHER INFORMATION

Widely used for decades to help Parkinsonism, but has the additional benefit of protecting against one form (the less common form) of influenza, which may be useful during an epidemic.

Amethocaine

See ANAESTHETICS, LOCAL.

Amifostine

TRADE NAME

Ethyol.

USES

Decreases damage to white blood cells and kidneys in patients having chemotherapy for cancer.

DOSAGE

 Complex. As determined for each patient by doctor.

FORMS

Injection.

PRECAUTIONS

Use with caution in pregnancy (B3), elderly and children.

Blood pressure and blood calcium levels must be checked regularly.

Use with caution in kidney, liver, heart and brain disease.

SIDE EFFECTS

Common: Low blood pressure, nausea, vomiting, flushing, chills, dizziness, tiredness.

Unusual: Hiccups, sneezing.

INTERACTIONS

Other drugs:

• Drugs that lower blood pressure and blood calcium levels.

PRESCRIPTION

Yes.

PERMITTED IN SPORT

Yes.

Amikacin

TRADE NAME

Amikin.

DRUG CLASS

Aminoglycoside antibiotic.

USES

Short term treatment of serious infections.

DOSAGE

 As determined by doctor.

FORMS

Injection.

PRECAUTIONS

Must not be used in pregnancy (D). Use with caution in elderly, children and during breast feeding.

Not designed for long term use as it may accumulate in body.

Adequate fluid intake essential.

 Do not take if:
• suffering from severe kidney disease.

SIDE EFFECTS

Unusual: Adverse effects on ears, kidneys and brain.

INTERACTIONS

Other drugs:

• Other antibiotics, fluid removing medications (diuretics), anaesthetics and muscle relaxants.

PRESCRIPTION

Yes.

PERMITTED IN SPORT

Yes.

OVERDOSE

Causes ringing in ears, dizziness, deafness which may be permanent, rash, fever, headache, pins and needles sensation and kidney failure. Seek urgent medical attention so that blood dialysis can be performed.

Amiloride

TRADE and GENERIC NAMES

Only available in Britain in combination with diuretics (fluid removers).

Amil-Co, Moducren, Moduret, Moduretic (with Hydrochlorthiazide).

Burinex A (with Bumetanide)

Fru-Co, Frumil, Lasoride (with Frusemide)

Kalten (with Atenolol and Hydrochlorthiazide).

Navispare (with Cyclopenthiazine).

DRUG CLASS

Potassium sparing diuretic.

USES

High blood pressure, conserving potassium within body, excess fluid in body.

DOSAGE

 One to four tablets in morning.

FORMS

Tablets.

PRECAUTIONS

Should only be used in pregnancy (C) and breast feeding if medically essential. Should not be used in children. Should be used with caution in diabetes or liver disease.

 Do not take if:
- suffering from kidney disease.

SIDE EFFECTS

Common: Minimal.

Unusual: Nausea, loss of appetite, belly discomfort, rash, excess wind.

INTERACTIONS

Other drugs:
- Lithium.
- Do not use with potassium supplements or Triamterene.

PRESCRIPTION

Yes.

PERMITTED IN SPORT

No.

OVERDOSE

Dehydration may occur. Induce vomiting if tablets taken recently. Give extra fluids.

See also TRIAMTERENE.

Aminobenzoic Acid

See Potassium p-Aminobenzoate.

Aminoglutethamide

TRADE NAME

Orimeten.

USES

Breast cancer, Cushing's syndrome.

DOSAGE

 Must be individualised for each patient by doctor depending on disease.

FORMS

Tablets (white) of 250mg.

PRECAUTIONS

Must not be used in pregnancy (D) unless the mother's life is at risk. Breast feeding must be ceased before use. May be used with caution in children.

Regular checking of blood pressure essential.

Regular blood tests to check thyroid gland and blood chemistry essential.

 Do not take if:

• suffering from porphyria.

SIDE EFFECTS

Common: Tiredness, incoordination, dizziness, rash, nausea.

Unusual: Confusion, vomiting, fever.

INTERACTIONS

Other drugs:

• Dexamethasone, Anticoagulants, Hypoglycaemics.

PRESCRIPTION

Yes.

OVERDOSE

May cause incoordination, sedation, difficulty in breathing and coma. Death unlikely. Induce vomiting if medication taken recently. Seek urgent medical assistance.

AMINOGLYCOSIDES

(Type of antibiotic)

See Amikacin, Gentamicin, Neomycin, Tobramycin.

Aminophylline

TRADE NAME

Phyllocontin.

DRUG CLASS

Bronchodilator.

USES

Asthma, emphysema, chronic bronchitis.

DOSAGE

 One or two tablets twelve hourly.

FORMS

Tablets of 100mg. (orange), 225mg. (cream), and 350mg. (yellow).

PRECAUTIONS

Safe to use in pregnancy (A), breast feeding and children.

Use with caution in infants.

Use with caution in heart disease, stomach ulcers, heartburn, kidney disease and liver disease.

Lower doses necessary in elderly and lighter patients.

Higher doses may be necessary in smokers.

Blood tests to monitor drug levels may be necessary.

SIDE EFFECTS

Common: Nausea, vomiting, belly discomfort, rapid heart rate, tremor, palpitations.

Unusual: Irregular heart rate, convulsions, angina.

INTERACTIONS

Other drugs:

• Cimetidine, Erythromycin.

Other substances:

• Reacts with alcohol, caffeine and nicotine.

PRESCRIPTION

No.

PERMITTED IN SPORT

Yes.

OVERDOSE

Serious. May cause vomiting, headache, irritability, rapid heart rate, confusion, fever, delirium and convulsions. Seek urgent medical assistance.

OTHER INFORMATION

An early treatment for asthma that is still very useful. Dose must be finely adjusted to give adequate clinical response while avoiding side effects.

See also Theophylline.

Amiodarone

TRADE NAME

Cordarone X.

DRUG CLASS

Antiarrhythmic.

USES

Severe rapid irregular heart beat.

DOSAGE

 One tablet, one to three times a day.

FORMS

Tablet of 100mg. and 200mg., injection.

PRECAUTIONS

Should not be used in pregnancy (C) unless medically essential. Not to be used in breast feeding or children.

Regular cardiograph (ECG) and blood test monitoring may be required.

Should be used with caution in heart failure and liver disease.

 Do not take if:

• suffering from slow heart rate, thyroid disease or iodine sensitivity.

SIDE EFFECTS

Common: Serious heart irregularities, slow heart rate, sensitivity to sunburn increased, nausea .

Unusual: Grey skin pigmentation, rashes, vomiting, loss of appetite, metallic taste, constipation, tremor, sleeplessness, headache, dizziness, anxiety, shortness of breath.

Severe but rare (stop medication, consult doctor): Angina, weight loss, restlessness.

INTERACTIONS

Other drugs:

• Beta blockers, Calcium Channel Blockers, Digoxin, Anticoagulants.

• Other drugs for treatment of irregular heartbeat.

Other substances:

• Alcohol use should be restricted.

• Smoking should be ceased.

• Caffeine intake should be restricted.

PRESCRIPTION

Yes.

PERMITTED IN SPORT

Yes.

OVERDOSE

Exaggerated side effects only response. If tablets taken recently, give activated charcoal or induce vomiting. Seek medical advice.

OTHER INFORMATION

Medication reserved for the most serious forms of heart arrhythmia.

Amisulpride

TRADE NAME

Solian.

DRUG CLASS

Antipsychotic.

USES

Some types of schizophrenia.

DOSAGE

 400mg. to 1200mg. a day in divided doses.

FORMS

Tablets of 50mg. and 200mg.

PRECAUTIONS

Not to be used in pregnancy (D), breast feeding or children.

Use with caution in kidney disease, epilepsy, Parkinson's disease and the elderly..

 Do not take if:

• suffering from certain types of cancer (prolactin dependent tumours), and phaeochromocytoma (tumour of adrenal glands).

SIDE EFFECTS

Common: Sleeplessness, anxiety, agitation, tiredness, nausea, diarrhoea, weight gain.

Unusual: Abnormal muscle movements, incoordination.

Severe but rare (stop medication, consult doctor): Low blood pressure, slow heart rate, allergy reactions, high fevers.

INTERACTIONS

Other drugs:

• Other medications that reduce brain activity (sedatives etc.) and lower blood pressure (antihypertensives).

PRESCRIPTION

Yes

PERMITTED IN SPORT

Yes

OVERDOSE

Serious. If tablets taken recently, give activated charcoal or induce vomiting. Seek urgent medical advice.

Amitriptylene

See TRICYCLICS.

Amlodipine

See **CALCIUM CHANNEL BLOCKERS.**

Ammonium chloride

TRADE NAMES

Found in numerous over the counter cough mixtures and bladder infection treatments.

DRUG CLASS

Urinary acidifier, cough suppressant.

USES

Maintains acid urine, increases urine production, eases coughs.

DOSAGE

 Take every four hours.

FORMS

Tablets, mixture.

PRECAUTIONS

Safe for use in pregnancy (A), breast feeding and children. Blood tests to check level of potassium recommended if used long term.

 Do not take if:

• suffering from kidney or liver disease.

SIDE EFFECTS

Common: Nausea.

Unusual: Vomiting, belly pains, low blood potassium.

INTERACTIONS

None significant

PRESCRIPTION

No

PERMITTED IN SPORT

Yes

OVERDOSE

Exacerbation of side effects likely.

Amorolfine

TRADE NAME

Loceryl

DRUG CLASS

Antifungal

USES

Fungal infections of the nails.

DOSAGE

 Apply lacquer to affected nails once or twice a week. Apply cream to skin once a day in evening.

FORMS

Nail lacquer, cream.

PRECAUTIONS

Should not be used in pregnancy (B3). Use with caution in children. Do not apply to skin.

SIDE EFFECTS

Common: Temporary burning sensation, itching.

Unusual: Redness, nail discolouration, scaling of nail.

INTERACTIONS

Nil

PRESCRIPTION

Yes

PERMITTED IN SPORT

Yes

OVERDOSE

Serious effects if swallowed. Seek urgent medical attention.

OTHER INFORMATION

Introduced in 1996 as a very effective way of treating severe fungal infections of nails that caused disfigurement.

Amoxapine

See **TRICYCLIC ANTIDEPRESSANTS**

Amoxycillin

TRADE NAME

Amoram, Amoxil.

Augmentin (with Clavulanic acid).

Heliclear (with Lansoprazole and Clarithromycin).

DRUG CLASS

Penicillin antibiotic.

USES

Treatment of infections caused by susceptible bacteria.

Heliclear used to destroy Helicobacter pylori, a bacteria that may be responsible for peptic ulcers.

DOSAGE

 Most forms - One or two capsules every eight hours before food. Heliclear - Complex dosage schedule of multiple capsules taken three times a day. Course (usually 5 to 7 days) should be completed.

FORMS

Capsules, mixture (store in door of refrigerator), injection.

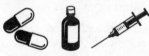

PRECAUTIONS

Safe in pregnancy (A), children and breast feeding.

Use with caution in kidney failure and leukaemia.

 Do not take if:

- allergic to Penicillin
- suffering from glandular fever

SIDE EFFECTS

Common: Mild diarrhoea, nausea, vomiting.

Unusual: Genital itch or rash, headache, dizziness, hot flushes, tiredness.

Severe but rare (stop medication, consult doctor): Itchy rash, hives, severe diarrhoea, jaundice, muscle pains, throat tightness.

INTERACTIONS

Other drugs:

- Allopurinol.

Other substances:

- Alcohol should be avoided.
- May cause false positive results for glucose in urine.

PRESCRIPTION

Yes.

PERMITTED IN SPORT

Yes.

OVERDOSE

Not life threatening unless allergic to penicillin. Vomiting and diarrhoea likely.

OTHER INFORMATION

One of the most commonly used antibiotics. Does not cause dependence or addiction.

AMPHETAMINES

See Dexamphetamine

Amphoterecin

TRADE NAME

Abelcet, Ambisome, Amphocil, Fungilin, Fungizone.

DRUG CLASS

Antifungal.

USES

Injection: Severe internal fungal infections.
Other forms: Fungal infections of gut and mouth.

DOSAGE

 Suspension: 1mL four times a day with meals.
Lozenges and tablets: One four times a day.

FORMS

Lozenges, suspension, tablets, injection.

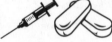

PRECAUTIONS

Must be used with caution in pregnancy (B2). May be used in breast feeding and children.

Use medication without a break for full course or until infection resolves.

SIDE EFFECTS

Suspension, tablets and lozenges - nil. Injection - causes significant and varied effects in most patients.

INTERACTIONS

Other drugs:

• Flucytosine.

PRESCRIPTION

Yes.

PERMITTED IN SPORT

Yes.

OVERDOSE

Unlikely to be serious.

OTHER INFORMATION

Amphoterecin is very well tolerated and effective when taken by mouth as it is not absorbed from the gut, but when given by injection for severe life threatening fungal infections it can cause significant side effects which must be balanced against the severity of the infection.

Ampicillin

TRADE NAME

Penbritin.

Magnapen (with Flucloxacillin).

DRUG CLASS

Penicillin antibiotic.

USES

Treatment of infections caused by susceptible bacteria.

DOSAGE

One or two capsules every eight hours before food. Course (usually 7 days) should be completed.

FORMS

Capsule, injection.

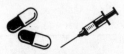

PRECAUTIONS

Safe in pregnancy (A), children and breast feeding.

Use with caution in leukaemia.

Do not take if:

- allergic to Penicillin.
- suffering from glandular fever.

SIDE EFFECTS

Common: Mild diarrhoea, nausea, vomiting.

Unusual: Headache, dizziness, black tongue, tiredness.

Severe but rare (stop medication, consult doctor): Itchy rash, hives, severe diarrhoea, yellow skin (jaundice), throat tightness.

INTERACTIONS

Other drugs:

- Allopurinol.

Other substances:

- Alcohol should be avoided.
- May cause false positive results for glucose in urine.

PRESCRIPTION

Yes

PERMITTED IN SPORT

Yes

OVERDOSE

Vomiting and diarrhoea only likely effects.

OTHER INFORMATION

Widely used in the 1970s, but has been superseded in most cases by Amoxycillin. Does not cause dependence or addiction.

Amsacrine

TRADE NAME

Amsidine.

DRUG CLASS

Antineoplastic.

USES

Leukaemia not responding to other treatment.

PRECAUTIONS

Must not be used in pregnancy (D) or breast feeding.

Must be given by a drip into a centrally located vein.

Regular blood tests to monitor blood cells necessary.

Use with caution in heart disease.

Adequate fluids must be given through drip or by mouth.

Do not take if:

- suffering from bone marrow depression or significant infection.

DOSAGE

 As determined by doctor.

FORMS

Intravenous infusion.

SIDE EFFECTS

Common: Multiple including diarrhoea, vomiting, mouth ulcers, hair loss and heart rhythm irregularities.

Unusual: Liver and kidney damage, rash.

Severe but rare (stop medication, consult doctor): Brain function disturbances.

INTERACTIONS

None significant.

PRESCRIPTION

Yes

PERMITTED IN SPORT

Yes

OVERDOSE

Very serious. Seek urgent medical attention.

OTHER INFORMATION

Introduced in 1998 for very serious forms of leukaemia.

See also CANCER TREATING DRUGS.

Amylmetacresol

TRADE NAME

Found in some over the counter throat lozenges.

DRUG CLASS

Antiseptic.

USES

Minor mouth and throat infections.

DOSAGE

 One lozenge dissolved in mouth every two or three hours.

FORMS

Lozenges.

PRECAUTIONS

Safe in pregnancy and children.

 Do not take if:
• suffering from diabetes.

SIDE EFFECTS

Nil.

INTERACTIONS

Nil.

PRESCRIPTION

No.

PERMITTED IN SPORT

Yes.

OVERDOSE

Diarrhoea only likely result.

Amylobarbitone

See BARBITURATES

ANABOLIC STEROIDS

(Repair and build tissue).

See Nandrolone, Stanozolol.

ANAESTHETICS, LOCAL

TRADE and GENERIC NAMES

AAA Spray (Benzocaine).

Ametop (Amethocaine).

Betnovate Rectal (Lignocaine, Betamethasone, Phenylephrine).

Bradosol Plus (Lignocaine, Domiphen bromide).

Calgel (Lignocaine, Cetylpyridinium chloride).

Citanest (Prilocaine).

Depo-Medrone with Lidocaine (Lignocaine with Methylprednisolone).

EMLA (Lignocaine, Prilocaine).

Hemocane (Lignocaine, Zinc oxide, Bismuth oxide, Benzoic acid, Cinnamic acid).

Instillagel (Lignocaine, Chlorhexidine and other ingredients).

Intralgin (Benzocaine, Salicylamide).

Lidocaine, Xylocaine, Xylocard (Lignocaine with or without Adrenaline).

Marcain (Bupivacaine).

Merocaine (Benzocaine, Cetylpyridinium).

Minims Lignocaine and Fluorescein (Lignocaine, Fluorescein dye).

Minims Local Anaesthetic (Amethocaine, or Lignocaine, or Oxybuprocaine or Proxymetacaine).

Minims Proxymetacaine and Fluorescein (Proxymetacaine, Fluorescein dye).

Naropin (Ropivacaine).

Perianal (Lignocaine, Hydrocortisone).

Proctosedyl (Cinchocaine, Hydrocortisone).

Scheriproct (Cinchocaine, Prednisolone).

Tyrozets (Benzocaine, Tyrothricin).

Ultraproct (Cinchocaine, corticosteroids and other ingredients).

Uniroid HC (Cinchocaine, Hydrocortisone).

Xyloproct (Lignocaine, Aluminium acetate, Zinc oxide, Hydrocortisone).

NB:Generic medications with the suffix "-caine" and underlined are local anaesthetics.

USES

Relief of superficial pain of skin, mouth, lips, vagina, penis, anus and other areas. Lignocaine injection may relieve migraine and irregular heart beat.

DOSAGE

Skin preparations: Apply three to four times a day.
Mouth and lip preparations: Apply or use every two to four hours.
Anal and vaginal preparations: Apply or use three or four times a day. Eye drops and injections used by doctors only.

PRECAUTIONS

Safe in pregnancy (A), breast feeding and children.

Use skin preparations with care on thin skin, genitals, broken skin, eczema or infected skin.

Elderly may need lower doses.

Special precautions apply to eye preparations and injections. Eye must be protected after use.

Drops should not be used for prolonged period.

Area injected must be protected from inadvertent injury.

Advise doctor before injection if:-

• suffering from heart disease, over active thyroid gland.

FORMS

Cream, eye drop, gel, injection, lozenge, ointment, paint, paste, patch, spray, suppository.

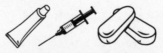

SIDE EFFECTS

Common: Injections - nervousness, dizziness, blurred vision, tremor, drowsiness, ringing in ears, numbness, nausea, vomiting, low blood pressure, slow heart rate. Eye preparations - eye irritation, stinging. Other preparations - Adverse reactions rare.

Unusual: Injections - Convulsions, allergy.

Severe but rare: Injection - Unconsciousness, cessation of breathing.

INTERACTIONS

Other drugs:

• Creams - Other local anaesthetics, Sulfonamides.

• Injection - Drugs acting on heart, Cimetidine, Anticonvulsants.

PRESCRIPTION

Most creams, ointments, gels, lozenges etc.: No
Eye drops, patches, anal preparations, injections: Yes

PERMITTED IN SPORT

Yes

OVERDOSE

No serious effects except from injection. Effects of injection overdose are very serious and include irregular heart beat, cessation of breathing, heart attack and death.

OTHER INFORMATION

All local anaesthetics are derived from cocaine, but are not addictive. Widely used in many forms for relief of pain and discomfort, and generally very safe. Poorly absorbed through skin, but well absorbed through mucous membranes of mouth, anus, vagina etc.

See also Cocaine

ANALGESICS

(Relieve pain)

See Aspirin, Benorylate, Buprenorphine, Capsaicin, Codeine, Dextromoramide, Dextropropoxyphene, Dihydrocodeine, Fentanyl, Heroin, Meptazinol, Methadone, Morphine, Nefopam, NSAID, Oxycodone, Paracetamol, Pentazocine, Pethidine, SALICYLATES

Anastrozole

TRADE NAME

Arimidex

DRUG CLASS

Antineoplastic.

USES

Treatment of advanced breast cancer.

DOSAGE

 One tablet a day.

FORMS

Tablet of 1mg.

PRECAUTIONS

Must not be used in pregnancy (C), breast feeding or children.

Caution with use before the menopause, liver and kidney disease.

SIDE EFFECTS

Common: Hot flushes, dry vagina, nausea, thinning of hair.

Unusual: Vaginal bleeding, tiredness, headache, rash, vomiting, diarrhoea, increase in blood cholesterol.

Severe but rare (stop medication, consult doctor): Liver or kidney failure.

INTERACTIONS

Other drugs:

• Oestrogen.

PRESCRIPTION

Yes

PERMITTED IN SPORT

Yes

OVERDOSE

Very serious. Seek urgent medical attention. Induce vomiting or administer activated charcoal.

OTHER INFORMATION

Introduced in 1996. Acts to destroy oestrogen producing cells in the body.

ANGIOTENSIN CONVERTING ENZYME INHIBITORS

See ACE Inhibitors

ANGIOTENSIN II RECEPTOR ANTAGONISTS

TRADE and GENERIC NAMES

Amias (Candesartan).

Aprovel (Irbesartan).

Cozaar (Losartan).

Cozaar-Comp (<u>Losartan</u>, Hydrochlorthiazide).

Diovan (Valsartan).

Micardis (Telmisartan).

Teveten (Eprosartan).

DRUG CLASS

Antihypertensives

USES

High blood pressure (hypertension), congestive heart failure.

DOSAGE

 Usually one tablet a day, but may be increased to two a day.

FORMS

Tablets.

PRECAUTIONS

Not to be used in pregnancy (D) or breast feeding. No trials on use in children have been performed.

Use with caution in heart failure, primary hyperaldosteronism, dehydration, heart valve disease and kidney transplant.

 Do not take if:

• Severe kidney, liver or bile duct disease.

SIDE EFFECTS

Common: Minimal.

Unusual: Diarrhoea, back and muscle pain.

Severe but rare (stop medication, consult doctor): Liver damage.

INTERACTIONS

Other drugs:

• Potassium supplements.

PRESCRIPTION

Yes

PERMITTED IN SPORT

Yes

OVERDOSE

Low blood pressure most likely effect. Take activated charcoal to reduce absorption. Seek medical attention.

OTHER INFORMATION

Very similar in action to ACE Inhibitors (see separate entry) but with fewer side effects. Some forms combined with a thiazide diuretic (fluid tablet - hydrochlorthiazide) to increase effectiveness. Only released on to market between 1998 and 2000.

See also ACE Inhibitors

ANTACIDS

TRADE and GENERIC NAMES

Algicon, Maalox, Mucogel (Aluminium hydroxide, Magnesium salts).

Alu-Cap (Aluminium hydroxide).

Asilone (Aluminium hydroxide, Magnesium salts, Dimethicone).

Gastrocote (Alginic acid, Aluminium hydroxide, Sodium bicarbonate).

Gaviscon Advance (Alginates, Potassium bicarbonate).

Gaviscon Infant (Alginates).

Gaviscon Liquid (Alginic acid, Calcium carbonate, Bicarbonates).

Gaviscon Tablets (Alginic acid, Aluminium hydroxide, Magnesium salts, Bicarbonates).

Kolanticon (Aluminium hydroxide, Dimethicone, Dicyclomine)

Mucaine (Aluminium salts, Magnesium salts, Oxethazine).

Peptac (Sodium bicarbonate, Calcium carbonate, Alginates)

Pyrogastrone (Alginic acid, Carbenoxolone, Aluminium hydroxide, Magnesium salts, Bicarbonates)

Topal (Aluminium hydroxide, Magnesium salts, Alginic acid).

USES

Heartburn, acid reflux, peptic ulcer, gastritis, hiatus hernia, reduce stomach acid, diarrhoea.

DOSAGE

 Multiple presentations. Follow instructions on packaging, or from doctor or pharmacist. Take immediately before meals or one hour after meals.

FORMS

Mixture, tablets, capsules, granules, powder, chewable tablets.

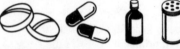

PRECAUTIONS

Safe in pregnancy (A), children and breast feeding.

Care required in patients with kidney disease, bleeding from stomach, irregular bowels.

Should not be taken for prolonged period without medical advice.

 Do not take if:

- suffering from severe belly pain.
- you have recently had kidney or bladder stones.

SIDE EFFECTS

Common: Mild.

Unusual: Constipation, loss of appetite

Severe but rare (stop medication, consult doctor): Severe abdominal pain, muscle weakness, bone pain.

INTERACTIONS

Other drugs:

- Tetracycline antibiotics, Beta blockers, Digoxin

Other substances:

- Food and alcohol reduce antacid effect.

PRESCRIPTION

No

PERMITTED IN SPORT

Yes

OVERDOSE

Very unlikely to be life threatening but may cause weakness, dizziness, tiredness and confusion.

OTHER INFORMATION

Widely used preparations for minor stomach upsets. Many different brands with minor variations in constituents.

Antazoline

TRADE NAME

Otrivine-Anthistin (with Xylometazoline).

DRUG CLASS

Vasoconstrictor.

USES

Allergic conjunctivitis, inflamed eyes.

DOSAGE

 One or two drops in eye three or four times a day.

FORMS

Eye drops.

PRECAUTIONS

May be used in pregnancy and breast feeding. Use with caution in children.

Not to be used for more than two weeks without medical review.

 Do not take if:

- suffering from glaucoma.

SIDE EFFECTS

Common: Stinging on inserting drops.

INTERACTIONS

None significant.

PRESCRIPTION

No

PERMITTED IN SPORT

Yes

OTHER INFORMATION

Widely used and effective treatment for tired, itchy, watery, red eyes. If symptoms do not settle rapidly, seek medical advice.

ANTHELMINTICS

(Treat worm infections of gut and tissue)

See Mebendazole, Niclosamide, Piperazine, Thiabendazole

Anthraquinone glycosides

TRADE NAME

Pyralvex (with salicylic acid)

DRUG CLASS

Antiseptic

USES

Mouth ulcers and inflammation.

DOSAGE

Apply three or four times daily. Do not eat or drink for 15 minutes afterwards.

FORMS

Paint.

PRECAUTIONS

Safe in pregnancy and children.

SIDE EFFECTS

Minimal.

INTERACTIONS

Nil.

PRESCRIPTION

No.

PERMITTED IN SPORT

Yes.

OVERDOSE

Diarrhoea and vomiting only likely effects.

ANTIALLERGEN

(Reduce allergy reactions).

See Allergen extracts.

ANTIANGINALS

(Relieve or prevent angina heart pain).

See BETA BLOCKERS, CALCIUM CHANNEL BLOCKERS, Glyceryl trinitrate, Isosorbide, Nicorandil.

ANTIARRHYTHMICS

(Correct irregular heart rhythm).

See Adenosine, Amiodarone, Bretyllium, Disopyramide, Flecainide, Lignocaine, Mexiletine, Procainamide, Propafenone, Quinidine, Sotalol, Verapamil

ANTIBIOTICS

(Treat bacterial infections)

See Amoxycillin, Ampicillin, Azithromycin, Aztreonam, Bacitracin, Benzyl penicillin, CEPHALOSPORINS, Chloramphenicol, Chlortetracycline, Cilastatin and Imipenem, Cinoxacin, Ciprofloxacin, Clarithromycin, Clavulanic acid, Clindamycin, Demeclocycline, Doxycycline, Erythromycin, Flucloxacillin, Framycetin, Fusafungine, Gentamicin, Gramicidin, Levofloxacin, Lomefloxacin, Meropenem, Metronidazole, Minocycline, Mupirocin, Nalidixic acid, Neomycin, Netimicin, Nitrofurantoin, Norfloxacin, Ofloxacin, Penicillin G, Piperacillin, Pivmecillinam, Polymyxin B, Potassium hydroxyquinolone, Silver sulfadiazine, Sodium fusidate, Sulfametopyrazine, Sulfamethoxazole, Sulfasalazine, SULPHONAMIDES, Tazobactam, Tetracycline, Ticarcillin, Tinidazole, Tobramycin, Trimethoprim, Tyrothricin, Vancomycin.

ANTICANCER DRUGS

See CANCER TREATING DRUGS.

ANTICHOLINERGICS

(Drying agents, relieve spasm, dilate pupil).

See Atropine, Dicyclomine, Homatropine methylbromide, Hyoscine, Ipratropium, MYDRIATICS, Oxitropium, Oxybutynin, Propiverine, Tolterodine.

ANTICHOLINESTERASES

See Distigmine, Pyridostigmine, Rivastigmine.

ANTICOAGULANTS

(Stop blood clotting)

See Abciximab, Aspirin, Clopidogrel, Dalteparin, Dipyridamole, Enoxaparin, Heparin, Nicoumalone, Phenindione, Ticlopidine, Warfarin.

ANTICONVULSANTS

(Stop or prevent fitting)

See BARBITURATES, Carbamazepine, Clonazepam, Ethosuximide, Gabapentin, Lamotrigine, Phenytoin, Piracetam, Primidone, Sodium valproate, Topiramate, Valproic acid, Vigabatrin.

ANTIDEPRESSANTS

(Improve depressed mood)

See Citalopram, Fluoxetine, Fluvoxamine, MAOI, Mirtazapine, Moclobemide, Nefazodone, Paroxetine, Sertraline, Trazodone, TRICYCLICS, Tryptophan, Venlafaxine.

ANTIDIARRHOEALS

(Stop diarrhoea)

See Atropine, Codeine, Diphenoxylate, Kaolin, Loperamide, Pectin.

Antidiuretic hormone

See Vasopressin.

ANTIDIURETICS

(Reduce production of urine by kidneys)

See Desmopressin acetate, Vasopressin.

ANTIDOTES

(Counteract poison or overdose)

See Charcoal, Methionine, Naloxone.

ANTIEMETICS

(Stop vomiting).

See ANTIHISTAMINES - SEDATING, Cyclizine, Domperidone, Granisetron, Hyoscine, Metoclopramide, Ondansetron, PHENOTHIAZINES.

ANTIFUNGALS

(Treat fungal infections)

See Amorolfine, Amphoterecin, Atovaquone, Fluconazole, Flucytosine, Griseofulvin, IMIDAZOLES, Iodine, Itraconazole, Ketoconazole, Nystatin, Potassium hydroxyquinolone, Selenium sulfide, Sulconazole, Terbinafine, Tolnaftate, Undecenoic acid.

ANTIHISTAMINES, NON-SEDATING

TRADE and GENERIC NAMES

Claratyn (Loratadine).

Semprex (Acrivastine).

Telfast (Fexofenadine).

USES

Allergy reactions, hay fever, urticaria (hives).

PRECAUTIONS

Should be used with caution in pregnancy . Should not be used in breast feeding.

 Do not take if:
- suffering from severe liver disease

DOSAGE

 Claratyn, Telfast - Once a day.
Semprex - Three times a day.

FORMS

Capsules, tablets and mixture.

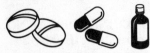

SIDE EFFECTS

Common: Nil.

Unusual: Increase in appetite, fainting, dry mouth, gastric upset, blurred vision, muscle pains, tremor, sweating, rash.

INTERACTIONS

None significant.

PRESCRIPTION

Yes.

PERMITTED IN SPORT

Yes.

OVERDOSE

Mild effects only. Possible heart beat irregularities. First aid involves induction of vomiting and then observing in hospital for a day.

OTHER INFORMATION

Antihistamines are divided into two broad groups - those that cause sedation and those that do not. In an allergy reaction, a substance called histamine is released from special cells (mast cells) to cause swelling, itching and increase in secretions. Antihistamines counteract this reaction. The non-sedating antihistamines will not have any effect on excessive secretions from causes other than allergy (eg: they have no effect on runny noses caused by the common cold).

ANTIHISTAMINES, SEDATING

TRADE and GENERIC NAMES

Atarax, Ucerax (<u>Hydroxyzine Embonate</u>).

Avomine, Phenergan (<u>Promethazine</u>).

Dimotane (<u>Brompheniramine</u>).

Dimotane Plus (<u>Brompheniramine</u>, Phenylephrine).

Galpseud Plus (<u>Chlorpheniramine</u>, Pseudoephedrine).

Haymine (<u>Chlorpheniramine</u>, Ephedrine).

Mistamine, Mizollen (<u>Mizolastine</u>).

Optilsat Drops (<u>Azelastine</u>).

Optimine (<u>Azatadine</u>).

Pamergan P100 (<u>Promethazine</u>, Pethidine).

Periactin (<u>Cyproheptadine</u>)

Piriject, Piriton (<u>Chlorpheniramine</u>)

Primalan (Mequitazine).

Sudafed Plus (**Triprolidine**, Pseudoephedrine).

Tavegil (<u>Clemastine</u>).

Vallergan (<u>Trimeprazine</u>).

Xepin (<u>Doxepin</u>).

Zirtek (<u>Cetirizine</u>).

NB: Antihistamines are <u>underlined</u>.

Sedating antihistamines may be found in many other over the counter cold and cough remedies that are distributed locally.

USES

Allergies (eg: hay fever, hives, urticaria), drug allergies, drying of secretions, itchy skin.

PLUS

Pheniramine & Promethazine: Nausea, vomiting, motion sickness, Meniere's disease.

Hydroxyzine embonate: Anxiety

Cyproheptadine: Prevention of migraine

Promethazine & Trimeprazine: Sedation

DOSAGE

 Follow directions on packaging. Some antihistamines are far longer acting than others. Dose will vary from once a day to four times a day.

FORMS

Tablets, capsules, mixture, cream, injection, eye drops.

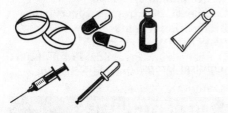

PRECAUTIONS

Promethazine and Trimeprazine should only be used in pregnancy (C) and breast feeding on medical advice.

Azatadine should be used with caution in pregnancy (B2) and breast feeding.

All other sedating antihistamines are safe in pregnancy (A) and breast feeding. All are safe in children over two years. Seek medical advice if using in younger children.

All should be used with caution in patients with liver disease, heart disease, glaucoma, chronic lung disease, enlarged prostate or severe peptic ulcer.

 ### Do not take if:

- operating machinery or undertaking tasks that require concentration and coordination.

- Drinking alcohol.

SIDE EFFECTS

Common: Skin preparations - Sensitivity reactions with repeated use. Other forms - Drowsiness, dry mouth, constipation, restlessness in children, incoordination, blurred vision.

Unusual: Upper belly discomfort, loss of appetite, nausea, diarrhoea, irritability.

Severe but rare (stop medication, consult doctor): Unusual bleeding.

INTERACTIONS

Other drugs:

- May interfere with Anti-coagulants, MAOI (mono-amine oxidase inhibitors), Sedatives and relaxants.

- Skin preparations have no significant interactions.

Other substances:

- Do not use alcohol with sedating antihistamines.

PRESCRIPTION

Varies depending on form and product.

PERMITTED IN SPORT

Yes

OVERDOSE

May result in convulsions, hallucinations, delirium, anxiety, muscle spasms, rapid heart rate, flushing, dry skin, dry mouth and coma. First aid involved inducing vomiting and seeking urgent medical attention.

OTHER INFORMATION

Antihistamines are widely used to dry the excessive secretions of hay fever and common colds. Taken in the correct dosage, they are very safe, but care must be taken with drowsiness.

Antihistamines are divided into two broad groups - those that cause sedation and those that do not. In an allergy reaction, a substance called histamine is released from special cells (mast cells) to cause swelling, itching and increase in secretions. Antihistamines counteract this reaction. The non-sedating antihistamines will not have any effect on excessive secretions from causes other than allergy (eg: they have no effect on runny noses caused by the common cold). Sedating antihistamines are available in a huge range of cold and flu remedies. They are added to pain killers to relax muscles and tension.

See also Cinnarizine, Cyclizine, Emedastine, Ketotifen, Levocabastine, Metoclopramide, Prochlorperazine.

ANTIHYPERTENSIVES

(Treat high blood pressure)

See ACE INHIBITORS, ANGIOTENSIN II RECEPTOR ANTAGONISTS, BETA BLOCKERS, CALCIUM CHANNEL BLOCKERS, Clonidine, Diazoxide, Hydralazine, Indapamide, Labetalol, Methyldopa, Minoxidil, Moxonidine, Prazosin, THIAZIDE DIURETICS.

ANTIMALARIALS

(Treat and prevent malaria)

See Atovaquone, Chloroquine, Dapsone, Doxycycline, Hydroxychloroquine, Mefloquine, Proguanil, Pyrimethamine, Quinine bisulphate.

ANTIMETABOLITES

See CANCER TREATING DRUGS.

ANTIMIGRAINE

(Prevent and treat migraine)

See ANALGESICS, BETA BLOCKERS, Clonidine, Dihydroergotamine, Ergotamine, Methysergide, NSAIDs, Pizotifen, Rizatripan, Sumatriptan.

ANTINEOPLASTICS

See CANCER TREATING DRUGS.

ANTIPARASITICS

(Kill skin parasites).

See Benzyl benzoate, Crotamiton, Permethrin.

ANTIPARKINSONIANS

(Treat Parkinson,disease)

See Amantadine, Apomorphine, Benzhexol, Benztropine, Biperiden, Bromocriptine, Entacapone, LEVODOPA COMPOUNDS, Orphenadrine, Pergolide, Pramipexole, Procyclidine, Ropinirole, Selegiline.

ANTIPSYCHOTICS

(Control psychiatric conditions)

See Amisulpride, Benperidine, Droperidol, Flupenthixol, Haloperidol, Lithium Carbonate, Loxapine, Olanzapine, PHENOTHIAZINES, Pimozide, Quetiapine, Risperidone, Sulpiride, Thiothixene, Zotepine, Zuclopenthixol.

ANTIPYRETICS

(Reduce fevers)

See Aspirin, Paracetamol.

ANTIRHEUMATICS

(Treat rheumatic conditions)

See Chloroquine, CORTICOSTEROIDS, GOLD, Hydroxychloroquine, Methotrexate, NSAIDs, Penicillamine, Sulfasalazine.

ANTISEPTIC, URINARY

(Prevents urine infections).

See Hexamine hippurate.

ANTISEPTICS

(Prevent infection).

See Anthraquinone, Azelaic acid, Benzalkonium chloride, Cetrimide, Cetylpyridinium, Chlorhexidine, Chloroxylenol, Clioquinol, Crotamiton, Dequalinium chloride, Hexachlorophane, Hexetedine, Hydrogen peroxide, Iodine, Povidone-Iodine, Pyrithione zinc, Sodium perborate.

ANTISPASMODICS

(Relieve smooth muscle spasm)

See Alverine citrate, Atropine, Dicyclomine, Flavoxate, Hyoscine, Mebeverine, Peppermint Oil.

ANTITHYROIDS

(Reduce activity of thyroid gland).

See Carbimazole.

ANTIVENOMS

TRADE NAME

Antivenoms against numerous snakes, spiders and ticks are available.

USES

Treatment of bites by specific toxic animal.

DOSAGE

 As determined by doctor depending on patient,condition and weight.

FORMS

Injection.

PRECAUTIONS

May be used in pregnancy, breast feeding and children if medically indicated.

All patients must be carefully monitored and any signs of allergy reaction treated early.

Use with caution in asthma, eczema and previous history of allergy.

Use with caution if antivenom used previously.

SIDE EFFECTS

Common: Minimal.

Unusual: Allergy reaction, generalised illness.

INTERACTIONS

None significant.

PRESCRIPTION

Yes.

PERMITTED IN SPORT

Yes.

OVERDOSE

May cause serious allergy reaction.

OTHER INFORMATION

Life saving, but must be given as soon as possible after any bite.

Most venoms are large compounds and spread very slowly from the site of the bite. The spread of venom can be prevented by applying a firm bandage (not too tight to cut off circulation) while arranging urgent medical care. Keep any dressing or material contaminated by the venom as it can be used to identify the type of animal responsible.

ANTIVIRALS

(Treat viral infections)

See Abacavir, Aciclovir, Amantadine, Didanosine, Efavirenz, Ganciclovir, Idoxuridine, Indinavir, Lamivudine, Nevirapine, Penciclovir, Ritonavir, Saquinavir, Stavudine, Tribavirin, Valaciclovir, Zanamivir, Zidovudine

ANXIOLYTICS

(Relieve anxiety and muscle spasm).

TRADE and GENERIC NAMES

Oxazepam (Oxazepam).

Diazemuls, Diazepam, Stesolid, Valclair, Valium (Diazepam).

Ativan (Lorazepam).

Clobazam, Frisium (Clobazam).

Lexotan (Bromazepam).

Tranxene (Clorazepate).

Xanax (Alprazolam).

DRUG CLASS

Benzodiazepine.

USE S

Short term relief of anxiety, relief of muscle spasm (Diazepam), withdrawal from alcohol dependence, pre-operative sedation, uncontrolled epileptic fit (Diazepam injection).

DOSAGE

 One to four tablets a day in one or more doses Some preparations are longer acting (eg: Clorazepate) than others and should only be used once a day. Do not exceed dose directed by doctor.

FORMS

Tablets, capsules, injection.

PRECAUTIONS

Should be used with caution in pregnancy (C), but not at all if delivery of infant imminent as it may decrease desire to breathe in newborn infant. Should be used with caution in breast feeding. Not for use in children.

Lower dose required in elderly.

Should be used intermittently and not constantly as dependency may develop.

Use with caution in glaucoma, myasthenia gravis, heart disease, kidney or liver disease, psychiatric conditions, schizophrenia, depression and epilepsy.

 Do not take if:

- suffering from severe lung disease, confusion.

- tendency to addiction or dependence.

- operating machinery, driving a vehicle or undertaking tasks that require concentration and alertness.

SIDE EFFECTS

Common: Reduced alertness, dependence.

Unusual: Incoordination, tremor, confusion, increased risk of falls in elderly, rash, low blood pressure, nausea, muscle weakness,

Severe but rare (stop medication, consult doctor): Jaundice (yellow skin).

INTERACTIONS

Other drugs:

- Sedatives, other Anxiolytics, Disulfiram, Cimetidine, Anticonvulsants, Anticholinergics.

Other substances:

- Reacts with alcohol to cause sedation and confusion.

PRESCRIPTION

Yes.

PERMITTED IN SPORT

Most sports: Yes Some sports: No (eg. archery, shooting). Check with organising committee of sport involved.

OVERDOSE

Seldom life threatening. May cause drowsiness, confusion and coma. Induce vomiting if tablets taken recently. Seek medical assistance.

OTHER INFORMATION

Widely used, and very safe if used correctly. Dependency becoming a significant problem, particularly in elderly, due to overuse. First introduced in 1960s, but newer forms still being introduced in 1990s.

See also Buspirone, Chlordiazepoxide, Meprobamate.

Apormorphine hydrochloride

TRADE NAME

Britaject.

DRUG CLASS

Antiparkinsonian.

USES

Severe Parkinson's disease.

DOSAGE

 As determined by doctor for each individual patient.

FORMS

Injection.

PRECAUTIONS

Use with great caution in pregnancy (B3), during breast feeding and in elderly.

 Do not take if:

- suffering from dementia and some psychiatric disorders, liver disease, kidney disease, angina and other unstable heart diseases, poor blood circulation to brain or poor brain function.

- sensitive to morphine or levodopa.

SIDE EFFECTS

Common: Nausea, diarrhoea, drowsiness.

Unusual: Vomiting, nodule at injection site, allergy reaction.

INTERACTIONS

Other drugs:

- Some drugs affecting brain function.

PRESCRIPTION

Yes.

PERMITTED IN SPORT

Yes.

Apraclonidine

TRADE NAME

Iopidine.

USES

Certain forms of severe glaucoma.

DOSAGE

 One drop to affected eye three times a day. Apply pressure to tear duct at inside corner of eye following application.

FORMS

Eye drops.

PRECAUTIONS

Use with caution in pregnancy (B3), children and breast feeding.

Do not use for more than 60 days.

Use with caution in high blood pressure, severe heart disease, depression, liver disease, kidney disease.

SIDE EFFECTS

Common: Eye irritation.

Unusual: Excessive response.

INTERACTIONS

Other drugs:

• MAOI, sympathomimetics, tricyclic antidepressants, beta-blockers, digoxin, clonidine, antihypertensives, brain depressants.

PRESCRIPTION

Yes.

PERMITTED IN SPORT

Yes.

Aprotinin

TRADE NAME

Trasylol.

DRUG CLASS

Fibrinolytic.

USES

Prevention of excessive blood loss during heart surgery, and after serious injury.

DOSAGE

 As determined by doctor for individual patient. Test dose must be given initially.

FORMS

Injection.

PRECAUTIONS

Relatively safe in pregnancy (B1) and children.

May cause severe allergy reaction if used a second time.

SIDE EFFECTS

Common: Excessive sensitivity.

INTERACTIONS

Other drugs:

• Thrombolytics.

PRESCRIPTION

Yes.

PERMITTED IN SPORT

Yes.

OVERDOSE

Very serious. Always given under strict medical supervision.

Arachis Oil

TRADE NAME

Fletcher's Oil, Oilatum Cream Cerumol Ear Drops (with Chlorbutol, Paradichlorobenzene).

Polytar (with Coal tar and other ingredients).

Used as an ingredient in numerous locally produced over the counter preparations.

USES

Softens ear wax, faeces and dry skin.

DOSAGE

 Ear drops - two drops daily for three days. Liquid - use as shampoo once or twice a week Cream - use once or twice daily as moisturiser Enema - use 100 to 130 mLs. once only.

FORMS

Ear drops, soap bar, solution, liquid, enema.

PRECAUTIONS

Safe in pregnancy and breast feeding.

No significant precautions.

SIDE EFFECTS

None significant.

INTERACTIONS

None significant.

PRESCRIPTION

No.

PERMITTED IN SPORT

Yes.

OVERDOSE

Diarrhoea only likely effect if swallowed.

Ascorbic acid

(Vitamin C).

TRADE and GENERIC NAMES

A large number of preparations include Ascorbic acid (Vitamin C) alone or in combination with other medications.

DRUG CLASS

Vitamin.

USES

Scurvy, vitamin deficiency, convalescence.

DOSAGE

 Recommended daily allowance: Males - 40mg., Females 30mg.

FORMS

Tablets, capsules, mixture, drops, injection.

  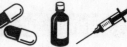

PRECAUTIONS

Safe in pregnancy, breast feeding and children.

Do not take in high doses or for prolonged periods of time.

Use with caution in kidney disease.

SIDE EFFECTS

Common: Minimal.

Unusual: Kidney stones if taken in excessive doses.

INTERACTIONS

None significant.

PRESCRIPTION

No.

PERMITTED IN SPORT

Yes

OVERDOSE

May cause kidney damage if taken in high doses long term.

OTHER INFORMATION

Ascorbic acid is a water soluble vitamin found in citrus fruit, tomatoes and greens. Its level in food is reduced by mincing, grating and contact with copper utensils. It is essential for the formation and maintenance of bone, cartilage and teeth. Remember, vitamins are merely chemicals that are essential for the functioning of the body, and if taken to excess, act as a drug. There is unfortunately, no evidence that it helps the common cold.

Aspirin

(Acetylsalicylic Acid)

TRADE NAME

Angettes, Caprin, Disprin CV, Nu-seals, PostMI Equagesic (with Ethoheptazine, Meprobamate).

Imazin XL (with Isosorbide mononitrate).

Migramax (Lysine aspirin with Metoclopramide).

Radian B (with Menthol, Camphor, Methyl salicylate).

DRUG CLASS

Analgesic (pain killer), NSAID (anti-inflammatory), Anticoagulant (stops blood clotting), Antipyretic (reduces fever).

USES

Relief of pain, reduction of fever, reduction of inflammation, prevention of blood clots and strokes.

DOSAGE

 Prevention of blood clots and strokes: 75mg to 150mg once a day.

Other uses: 600mg (usually two tablets) every four hours. Maximum 4500mg a day.

FORMS

Tablets, capsules, liniment.

PRECAUTIONS

Aspirin should not be used in pregnancy (C) unless medically essential. Should be used with caution in breast feeding and children. Not for use in infants, or children under 15 years with a fever.

 Do not take if:

- suffering from bleeding disorders, peptic ulcer, fluid retention.

- surgery planned in next few days, or recent surgery performed.

SIDE EFFECTS

Common: Gut irritation, heartburn, nausea.

Unusual: Vomiting, blood in faeces, rash, aggravation of asthma, hay fever, ringing in ears.

Severe but rare (stop medication, consult doctor): Unusual bleeding, asthma.

INTERACTIONS

Other drugs:

- Anticoagulants, NSAIDs, Phenytoin, Allopurinol, Sodium valproate, Sulfonamides, Methotrexate, Spironolactone.

Other substances:

• Reacts adversely with alcohol.

PRESCRIPTION

No

PERMITTED IN SPORT

Yes

OVERDOSE

Adult lethal dose is over 25000mg. (about 85 tablets). Symptoms include dizziness, ear noises, deafness, sweating, nausea, vomiting, headache, confusion, fever, rapid breathing, restlessness and coma. If tablets swallowed recently, induce vomiting. Seek medical assistance.

OTHER INFORMATION

First synthesised in 1989, Asprin is now one of the oldest and most widely used medications in the world

Atenolol

See BETA BLOCKERS

Atobisan

TRADE NAME

Tractocile

USES

Delays onset of labour of childbirth when immediate delivery of the infant is not desired due to prematurity.

DOSAGE

 As determined by the doctor.

FORMS

Injection.

PRECAUTIONS

Not for use in pregnancy before 24 weeks or over 33 weeks. Not for use in breast feeding, children or males.

Use with caution in premature rupture of the membranes.

Use with caution in kidney and liver disease. Use with caution on second and subsequent occasions.

Careful monitoring of both mother and infant essential during use.

 Do not take if:

• infant is showing signs of distress, retarded growth.

• suffering from eclampsia, bleeding from the vagina, infection of the uterus or placental abnormality.

SIDE EFFECTS

Common: Nausea, headache, dizziness.

Unusual: Vomiting, hot flushes, rapid heart rate, excess blood sugar level, low blood pressure, reaction at injection site.

Severe but rare (stop medication, consult doctor): Distress of foetus, bleeding from mother.

INTERACTIONS

Other drugs:

• Not known.

PRESCRIPTION

Yes

OTHER INFORMATION

Introduced in 2000 to prevent premature labour.

See also Ritodrine

Atorvastatin

TRADE NAME

Lipitor.

DRUG CLASS

Hypolipidaemic.

USES

Lowers blood cholesterol level.

DOSAGE

 10mg. to 40mg. once a day.

FORMS

Tablets (white) of 10mg., 20mg. and 40mg.

PRECAUTIONS

Not to be used in pregnancy, breast feeding or children.

Use with caution in liver and kidney disease.

Regular blood tests to check cholesterol level and liver function advisable.

 ## Do not take if:

- suffering from active liver disease.

- previous adverse effects (eg: muscle pain or weakness) experienced from other medication used to lower cholesterol.

SIDE EFFECTS

Common: Altered bowel habits (diarrhoea or constipation), indigestion, heartburn, nausea, headache.

Unusual: Belly pain, sleeplessness, rash, itch.

Severe but rare (stop medication, consult doctor): Swelling of face or lips, muscle pain, tingling in hands and feet.

INTERACTIONS

Other drugs:

- Digoxin, Erythromycin, Rifampicin, Phenytoin, Oral Contraceptives, Immunosuppressives, Antifungals, other medications used to lower cholesterol levels.

Other substances:

- Alcohol.

PRESCRIPTION

Yes.

PERMITTED IN SPORT

Yes.

OVERDOSE

Liver and muscle damage possible. Induce vomiting or give activated activated charcoal if taken recently. Seek medical assistance.

OTHER INFORMATION

Introduced in 1998 as an improved version of similar drugs. Much more effective in lowering cholesterol levels in blood, and has fewer side effects than other hypolipidaemics. Designed for long term use as it controls high cholesterol but does not cure the problem. Stopping the medication without advice from a doctor may lead to a rapid increase in cholesterol to the pretreatment level. High cholesterol levels increase the risk of heart attack and stroke.

See also HYPOLIPIDAEMICS.

Atovaquone

TRADE NAME

Wellvone.

Malarone (with Proguanil).

DRUG CLASS

Antifungal and antimalarial.

USES

Wellvone - treatment of specific fungal infections caused by Pneumocystis carinii in AIDS patients.

Malarone - treatment of malaria.

DOSAGE

 Wellvone - 5mls. twice a day. Malarone - once a day with food.

FORMS

Wellvone - suspension.

Malarone - tablets - pink.

PRECAUTIONS

Use with caution in pregnancy (B2), breast feeding and children.

Use with caution in patients with lung and intestinal diseases.

Malarone - use with caution if malaria affects brain and other complicated cases.

SIDE EFFECTS

Common: Loss of appetite, diarrhoea, nausea, rash, headache, belly pain

Unusual: Vomiting, fever, sleeplessness, dizziness, muscle pains.

INTERACTIONS

Other drugs:

• Metoclopramide, rifampicicn, paracetamol, benzodiazepines, aciclovir, morphine, pethidine, codeine, cephalosporins, antidiarrhoeals, laxatives, many other drugs.

PRESCRIPTION

Yes.

PERMITTED IN SPORT

Yes.

OVERDOSE

Severe intestinal effects. Seek urgent medical treatment. Vomiting will probably occur spontaneously.

OTHER INFORMATION

Wellvone introduced in 1997 for treatment of severe complication of AIDS infection. Malarone introduced in 1999.

Atropine

TRADE NAME

Minims Atropine Isopto Atropine (with Hypromellose).

Lomotil (with Diphenoxylate hydrochloride).

Tropergen (with Diphenoxylate).

DRUG CLASS

Mydriatic, Anticholinergic.

USES

Tablets: Diarrhoea , intestinal cramps, drying of secretions. Eye drops: Enlargement of pupil. Injection: Drying of secretions and saliva.

DOSAGE

 Depends on usage. Follow directions on pack or doctor's advice.

Lomotil: One or two tablets four times a day as required for diarrhoea.

FORMS

Tablets, eye drops, injection.

PRECAUTIONS

Safe in pregnancy and children.

Injection and tablets should be used with caution in elderly or debilitated patients.

Do not take if:

- as eye drops if suffering from glaucoma.
- in other forms if suffering from rapid heart rate, heart failure, lung failure or over active thyroid gland.

SIDE EFFECTS

Common: Dry mouth, dilated pupils, dry eyes, difficulty in passing urine, rapid heart rate.

Unusual: Flushing, palpitations, constipation, dry skin, rash, drowsiness, vomiting, mood changes.

INTERACTIONS

Other drugs:

- Additive effect with antihistamines, phenothiazines, and tricyclic antidepressants.

PRESCRIPTION

Yes.

PERMITTED IN SPORT

Yes.

OVERDOSE

May be very serious, depending upon dose and form. Seek urgent medical advice.

OTHER INFORMATION

Widely used for over a century to dry secretions before an operation, to dilate the pupil to aid examination of the eye, and to ease intestinal cramps and diarrhoea. Occurs naturally in certain herbal extracts.

Auranofin
See GOLD.

Aurothiomalate
See GOLD.

Azapropazone
See NSAID.

Azatadine
See ANTIHISTAMINES, SEDATING.

Azathioprine (AZT)

TRADE NAME

Imuran.

DRUG CLASS

Immunomodifier.

USES

Prevents rejection of transplanted organ, autoimmune diseases.

DOSAGE

Complex. Must be determined individually for each patient by doctor.

FORMS

Tablets of 25mg. (orange) and 50mg. (yellow).

PRECAUTIONS

Not to be used in pregnancy (D) unless mother's life at risk. Breast feeding must be ceased before use. May be used with caution in children.

Regular blood tests to monitor response essential.

Use with caution in liver and kidney disease.

Do not take if:

- undertaking dental procedures without consulting doctor.
- having live virus vaccine (eg: Sabin for polio).

SIDE EFFECTS

Very complex. Wide range of side effects may occur, and must be discussed with doctor before use of medication. Report any unusual effects to doctor.

INTERACTIONS

Other drugs:

- Allopurinol, Oxypurinol, Thiopurinol, cancer treating medications, Captopril, many others.

Other substances:

- Reacts with alcohol.

PRESCRIPTION

Yes.

PERMITTED IN SPORT

Yes.

OVERDOSE

May cause damage to immune system which leads to multiple infections, ulceration of mouth and throat, bruising and bleeding. Seek medical assistance.

OTHER INFORMATION

Potent medication that must be finely balanced to prevent rejection of donated organ but allow protection of body against infection.

Azelaic acid

See KERATOLYTICS.

Azelastine

See ANTIHISTAMINES, SEDATING.

Azithromycin

TRADE NAME

Zithromax.

DRUG CLASS

Macrolide antibiotic.

USES

Infections caused by susceptible bacteria (eg: bronchitis, sinusitis, throat infection).

DOSAGE

 Once a day, away from meals.

FORMS

Capsules (white) of 250mg.

PRECAUTIONS

Use in pregnancy (B3) only if medically necessary. Use with caution in breast feeding and children.

Lower doses necessary in elderly and debilitated.

Use with caution in liver and kidney disease.

SIDE EFFECTS

Common: Nausea, diarrhoea, belly pains.

Unusual: Vomiting, palpitations, dizziness, vaginal thrush, rash, headache.

INTERACTIONS

Other drugs:

• Theophylline, Terfenadine, Astemizole, Antacids, Cyclosporin, Digoxin.

PRESCRIPTION

Yes.

PERMITTED IN SPORT

Yes.

OVERDOSE

Exacerbation of side effects likely. Induce vomiting if medication taken recently. Seek medical assistance.

OTHER INFORMATION

Introduced 1995 to treat difficult infections.

AZT

See Azathioprine.

Aztreonam

TRADE NAME

Azactam.

DRUG CLASS

Antibiotic.

USES

Severe bacterial infections.

DOSAGE

 As determined by doctor for each individual patient.

FORMS

Injection.

PRECAUTIONS

Relatively safe in pregnancy (B1), breast feeding and children.

Use caution in use with severe kidney and liver disease.

Use caution in use with premature infants and elderly.

Must be used with caution in gynaecological infections.

SIDE EFFECTS

Common: Minimal.

Unusual: Development of resistant infections.

Severe but rare (stop medication, consult doctor): Bowel inflammation (pseudomembranous colitis).

INTERACTIONS

Other drugs:

• Frusemide.

PRESCRIPTION

Yes.

PERMITTED IN SPORT

Yes.

OVERDOSE

Always given by infusion or injection under strict medical supervision.

OTHER INFORMATION

Only used after other antibiotics have been proved to be ineffective.

Bacitracin

TRADE NAMES

Available only in combination with other medications.

Cicatrin (with Neomycin).

Polyfax (with Polymyxin B).

DRUG CLASS

Antibiotic.

USES

Skin infections.

DOSAGE

 Apply three or four times a day.

FORMS

Cream, ointment, powder.

PRECAUTIONS

Used on the skin, safe in pregnancy, breast feeding and children.

Do not use on large areas that are weeping or lacking in good quality skin.

Not designed for long term use.

SIDE EFFECTS

Common: Skin irritation.

INTERACTIONS

None significant

PRESCRIPTION

Yes

PERMITTED IN SPORT

Yes

Baclofen

TRADE NAMES:

Clofen, Lioresal.

DRUG CLASS:

Muscle relaxant.

USES:

Muscle spasm in multiple sclerosis, muscle spasm in spinal injury, muscle spasm in cerebral palsy, bladder spasm.

DOSAGE:

 5mg. to 25mg. three times a day.

PRECAUTIONS:

Use in pregnancy (B3) only if medically essential. Use with caution in breast feeding and children.

Use with caution in psychiatric disorders, peptic ulcer, heart disease, stroke, lung disease, liver or kidney disease, diabetes, difficulty in passing urine.

Lower doses required in elderly.

Do not stop suddenly, but reduce dosage slowly.

 Do not take if:-

• suffering from epilepsy or brain injury.

FORMS:

Tablets of 10mg. (white).
Injection for use in spinal cord.

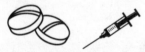

SIDE EFFECTS:

Common: Dose related. Sedation, drowsiness, nausea

Unusual: Dry mouth, vomiting, confusion, dizziness, headache, sleeplessness, mood changes.

Severe but rare (stop medication, consult doctor): Convulsions.

INTERACTIONS:

Other drugs:

• Tricyclics, Sedatives, medications for lowering blood pressure, Levodopa, Diazepam.

Other substances:

• Reacts with alcohol to increase sedation.

PRESCRIPTION:

Yes

PERMITTED IN SPORT:

Yes

OVERDOSE:

Drowsiness, difficulty in breathing, confusion, hallucinations, slow heart rate, coma and rarely death may occur. Administer or induce vomiting if medication taken recently and patient alert. Seek urgent medical attention.

OTHER INFORMATION:

Used successfully in a number of difficult conditions that cause distressing muscle spasms.

Balsalazide

TRADE NAME

Colazide

DRUG CLASS

Salicylate.

USES

Treatment and prevention of ulcerative colitis.

DOSAGE

Treatment: three capsules three times a day with food.
Prevention: two capsules twice a day with food.

FORMS

Capsule of 750mg. (beige).

PRECAUTIONS

Not to be used in pregnancy (D), breast feeding or children.

Use with caution in asthma, bleeding disorders, peptic ulcer or stomach inflammation, mild kidney or liver disease.

Regular blood and urine tests necessary during treatment.

 Do not take if:

• suffering from significant liver or kidney disease.

• allergic to salicylates (eg. aspirin).

SIDE EFFECTS

Common: Headache, nausea, diarrhoea.

Unusual: Belly pain, gall stone formation.

Severe but rare (stop medication, consult doctor): Abnormal bleeding, bruising, sore throat, excessive tiredness.

INTERACTIONS

Other drugs:

• Digoxin, methotrexate.

PRESCRIPTION

Yes

PERMITTED IN SPORT

Yes

OVERDOSE

Symptoms include dizziness, ear noises, deafness, sweating, nausea, vomiting, headache, confusion, fever, rapid breathing, restlessness and coma. If tablets swallowed recently, induce vomiting. Seek medical assistance.

Bambuterol

See BETA -2 AGONISTS

BARBITURATES

TRADE and GENERIC NAMES

Amytal, Sodium Amytal (Amylobarbitone).

Phenobarb (Phenobarbitone).

Prominal (Methylphenobarbitone).

Seconal (Quinalbarbitone).

Soneryl (Butobarbitone).

Tuinal (Amylobarbitone and Quinalbarbitone).

DRUG CLASS

Sedative/Hypnotic, Anticonvulsant.

USES

Sedation, insomnia (sleeplessness), epilepsy (Phenobarbitone).

DOSAGE

 One or two tablets one to three times a day.

FORMS

Tablets, injection.

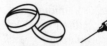

PRECAUTIONS

Should not be taken in pregnancy (D), particularly early pregnancy, unless medically essential (eg: for uncontrolled epilepsy). May be used in breast feeding and children.

Lower doses required in elderly.

Should not be stopped suddenly if used for long period constantly, but dose should be reduced gradually. Use intermittently if possible.

 Do not take if:

• suffering from poor lung function, porphyria, severe liver or kidney disease, uncontrolled pain.

• likely to develop a drug dependency.

• history of alcohol or drug abuse.

• operating machinery, driving a vehicle, or undertaking tasks that require concentration and alertness.

SIDE EFFECTS

Common: Drowsiness, incoordination, slow breathing, hangover sensation, slow heart rate, low blood pressure, nausea, diarrhoea, dependence on drug.

Unusual: Memory defects, dizziness, paradoxical excitement, nightmares, hallucinations, constipation, vomiting, headache.

Severe but rare (stop medication, consult doctor): Loss of consciousness.

INTERACTIONS

Other drugs:

• Griseofulvin, Folic acid, Pethidine, Morphine, Phenytoin, Rifampicin, Oral contraceptives, Chlorpromazine, Tricyclic antidepressants, Coumarin, Antihistamines, MAOI.

Other substances:

• Reacts with alcohol to cause sedation.

PRESCRIPTION

Yes

PERMITTED IN SPORT

Yes

OVERDOSE

Very serious. Low blood pressure, coma, cessation of breathing and death may occur. Induce vomiting if tablets taken recently. Seek urgent medical assistance.

OTHER INFORMATION

Used for many decades to sedate, calm and ease sleeplessness. Dependency problem limits its use today mainly to the control of some forms of epilepsy.

BCG (Tuberculosis) vaccine

TRADE NAME

BCG Vaccine.

DRUG CLASS

Vaccine

USES

Prevention of tuberculosis (TB).

DOSAGE

Single vaccination (skin scratch, not injection).

FORMS

Ampoule.

PRECAUTIONS

Vaccination during pregnancy (B2) is not recommended, but unintentional or necessary vaccination is unlikely to have any adverse effects. May be used safely in breast feeding, children and infants.

Prevent vaccination fluid from being inhaled.

Use with caution near any skin disorder.

 Do not take if:

• suffering from significant illness or reduced immunity.

SIDE EFFECTS

Common: Skin irritation at site of vaccination.

INTERACTIONS

Other drugs:

• Other vaccines.

PRESCRIPTION

Yes

PERMITTED IN SPORT

Yes

OTHER INFORMATION

Routine use is restricted to immigrants. Widely used in poorer countries.

Becaplermin

TRADE NAME

Regranex.

USES

Healing diabetic skin ulcers.

DOSAGE

 Remove surface debris from ulcer. Apply a thin layer of gel across whole ulcer area once a day and cover with a moist saline dressing. Treatment may be necessary for several months.

FORMS

Gel.

PRECAUTIONS

Not for use in pregnancy, breast feeding and children.

Ensure adequate blood supply to area before use.

 Do not take if:

- suffering from skin cancer at or near ulcer site.

- underlying skin or bone infection or malignancy.

SIDE EFFECTS

Common: Infection, redness of skin, pain.

Unusual: Blistering skin reaction.

Severe but rare (stop medication, consult doctor): Swelling of tissue.

INTERACTIONS

Other drugs:

- Other creams, ointments and gels on same area.

PRESCRIPTION

Yes

PERMITTED IN SPORT

Yes

OVERDOSE

Redness, blistering and swelling of skin only likely effect if excess applied. Seek medical attention if swallowed.

OTHER INFORMATION

Recently introduced as a new form of treatment for difficult diabetic skin ulcers.

Beclomethasone dipropionate

TRADE NAME

Aerobec, Asmabec, Beclazone, Becloforte, Becodisks, Beconase, Becotide, Filair, Nasobec, Propaderm, Qvar, Zonivent.

Ventide (with Salbutamol).

DRUG CLASS

Corticosteroid

USES

Prevention of asthma, prevention of hay fever, severe dermatitis, psoriasis.

PRECAUTIONS

Use with caution in pregnancy (B3), breast feeding and children.

Use with caution in lung, nose or throat infection and tuberculosis.

Lung function should be checked regularly to ensure adequate dose is received.

 Do not take if:

- cream if suffering from fungal skin infection.

DOSAGE

 Asthma: One or two inhalations, two to four times a day
Nasal spray: One spray in each nostril twice a day
Cream (Propaderm): Use sparingly once or twice a day.

FORMS

Inhaler, rotacaps , nebuliser solution, nasal spray, cream.

SIDE EFFECTS

Common: Fungal (thrush) infections of mouth, sore throat and mouth, dry mouth.

Unusual: Hoarseness, unusual bleeding and bruising, slowed growth.

INTERACTIONS

None significant

PRESCRIPTION

Yes

PERMITTED IN SPORT

Yes

OVERDOSE

Unlikely to have any serious effects.

OTHER INFORMATION

Beclomethasone is the main medication used to prevent asthma and is designed for long term use. Very safe and effective. Does not cause dependence or addiction. Qvar is in the form of microfine aerosol that penetrates further into the lungs, so lower doses can be used.

See also Budesonide, Fluticasone.

Bendrofluazide

See THIAZIDE DIURETICS

Benorylate

TRADE NAME

Benoral.

DRUG CLASS

Analgesic.

USES

Relieves mild to moderate pain and reduces fever.

DOSAGE

 Two tablets or 5mls. three times a day.

FORMS

Tablets 750mg. (white), mixture.

SIDE EFFECTS

Common: Minimal.

Unusual: Nausea, rash.

INTERACTIONS

Other drugs:

• Anticoagulants, Metoclopramide, Propantheline, Antidepressants, Narcotics, Anticonvulsants.

PRESCRIPTION

No

PRECAUTIONS

Safe in pregnancy (A), breast feeding, children and infants over one month of age.

Use with caution in severe liver and kidney disease.

PERMITTED IN SPORT

Yes

OVERDOSE

Serious. Symptoms may include vomiting, belly pain and sweating. Delayed effect can be serious liver damage that may cause liver failure, jaundice and death. Administer activated charcoal or induce vomiting if medication taken recently. Seek urgent medical attention.

Benoxinate

See Oxybuprocaine in ANAESTHETICS, LOCAL

Benperidol

TRADE NAME

Anquil.

DRUG CLASS

Antipsychotic.

USES

Control of deviant and anti-social sexual behaviour.

DOSAGE

 One to six tablets a day.

PRECAUTIONS

Use with caution in pregnancy and breast feeding. Not for use in children.

Use with caution in liver and kidney disease, and epilepsy.

Regular blood tests for liver function and blood cell counts necessary during treatment.

 Do not take if:

• suffering from significant brain function abnormalities, Parkinson's disease, reduced alertness, depression.

• comatose.

FORMS

Tablets of 0.25mg. (white).

SIDE EFFECTS

Common: Restlessness, tremor, rigidity, dry mouth, stuffy nose, weight gain, drowsiness, tiredness, fatigue.

Unusual: Difficulty in passing urine, rapid heart rate, constipation, blurring of vision, low blood pressure, spasms muscles (particularly eye and neck), impotence, breast milk production, cessation of menstrual periods, skin reactions.

Severe but rare (stop medication, consult doctor): Low body temperature, jaundice (yellow skin), abnormal blood cells, convulsions, abnormal heart rhythm.

INTERACTIONS

Other drugs:

• Sedatives, pain relievers (Analgesics), Antihypertensives, Antidepressants, Anticonvulsants, Diabetic medication, Levodopa, Anticoagulants.

Other substances:

• Alcohol.

PRESCRIPTION

Yes

PERMITTED IN SPORT

Yes

OVERDOSE

Very serious. Symptoms include drowsiness, confusion, restlessness, rapid heart rate, tremor, convulsions, difficulty in breathing and swallowing, coma and death. Administer activated charcoal or induce vomiting if taken recently and patient alert. Seek urgent medical attention.

See also PHENOTHIAZINES

Benserazide

See LEVODOPA COMPOUNDS

Benzalkonium chloride

TRADE and GENERIC NAMES

Bradosol Conotrane (with Dimethicone).

Dermol (with Paraffin, Chlorhexidine and other ingredients).

Drapolene (with Cetrimide).

Emulsiderm (with Paraffin and other ingredients).

Ionil T (with Coal Tar and Salicylic acid).

Oilatum Plus (with Triclosan and Paraffin).

Timodine (with Nystatin, Hydrocortisone and Dimethicone).

DRUG CLASS

Antiseptic

USES

Minor skin and mouth infections.

DOSAGE

 Apply several times a day as required.

FORMS

Cream, liquid, ointment, shampoo.

PRECAUTIONS

Safe to use in pregnancy, breast feeding and children.

Not to be swallowed. Causes eye irritation.

SIDE EFFECTS

Minimal

INTERACTIONS

None significant

PRESCRIPTION

No

PERMITTED IN SPORT

Yes

OVERDOSE

Nausea, stomach cramps and diarrhoea may occur.

OTHER INFORMATION

Safe and effective antiseptic that is widely used.

Benzhexol

TRADE NAME

Broflex.

DRUG CLASS

Antiparkinsonian.

USES

Parkinson's disease, some other movement disorders.

DOSAGE

 Slowly increase dosage under medical supervision until adequate response obtained.

FORMS

Syrup.

SIDE EFFECTS

Common: Dry mouth, blurred vision, nausea, dizziness.

Unusual: Salivary gland disease, rash, constipation, hallucinations, confusion.

INTERACTIONS

None significant

PRESCRIPTION

Yes

PERMITTED IN SPORT

Yes

PRECAUTIONS

Use with caution in pregnancy (B1) and breast feeding.

Use with caution in heart disease, kidney or liver disease, high blood pressure, enlarged prostate gland.

Use with caution in elderly.

 Do not take if:

- suffering from glaucoma

Benzocaine

See ANAESTHETIC, LOCAL

BENZODIAZEPINES

(Relieve anxiety and muscle spasm)

See ANXIOLYTICS, Chlordiazepoxide, Clonazepam, Flunitrazepam, Flurazepam, Midazolam, Nitrazepam, Temazepam

Benzoic acid

See KERATOLYTICS

Benzoyl peroxide

See KERATOLYTICS

Benzthiazide

See THIAZIDE DIURETICS

Benztropine

TRADE NAME

Cogentin.

DRUG CLASS

Antiparkinsonian

US ES

Parkinsonism.

DOSAGE

 Individualised dose depending on response. Must be closely monitored by doctor.

FORMS

Tablet of 2mg. (white), injection.

PRECAUTIONS

Use with caution in pregnancy (B2) and breast feeding. Not for use in children under 3 years.

Use with caution with enlarged prostate gland, rapid heart rate, psychiatric conditions, glaucoma.

SIDE EFFECTS

Common: Rapid heart rate, constipation, dry mouth, nausea, confusion, blurred vision.

Unusual: Vomiting, hallucinations, difficulty passing urine, rash.

INTERACTIONS

Other drugs:

- Phenothiazines, Tricyclic antidepressants.

PRESCRIPTION

Yes

PERMITTED IN SPORT

Yes

OVERDOSE

Confusion, nervousness, psychiatric disturbances, dizziness, weakness, rapid heart rate, incoordination, palpitations and vomiting may occur. Administer activated charcoal or induce vomiting if medication taken recently. Seek medical assistance.

Benzydamine hydrochloride

TRADE NAME

Difflam, Difflam Oral.

DRUG CLASS

Topical anti-inflammatory.

USES

Reduces inflammation and pain.

DOSAGE

 Cream: Massage into affected area three to six times a day
Oral: Use every 90 minutes as required

FORMS

Cream, gargle, mouth spray.

PRECAUTIONS

Safe in pregnancy, breast feeding and children.

Avoid eyes with all preparations.

Cream should not be used in mouth, nose, anus and vagina.

Use with caution in severe liver disease.

SIDE EFFECTS

Common: Minimal

Unusual: Skin reaction.

INTERACTIONS

None significant

PRESCRIPTION

No

PERMITTED IN SPORT

Yes

OVERDOSE

Unlikely to be a problem.

OTHER INFORMATION

Does not cause addiction or dependence.

Benzyl benzoate

TRADE NAME

Ascabiol.

Anugesic HC (with Hydrocortisone, Paramoxine, Zinc oxide, Bismuth oxide and other ingredients).

Anusol HC (with Hydrocortisone, Zinc oxide, Bismuth oxide and other ingredients).

DRUG CLASS

Antiparasitic

USES

Scabies, head and body lice. Used in combination with other ingredients for piles and anal itch.

DOSAGE

 Lotion: Apply to small area of skin for ten minutes before using to test for sensitivity. Apply to whole body from neck down after a hot bath. Remove by washing after one day. Repeat after five days. More applications may be necessary for lice
Suppositories and anal cream: Insert into and apply around anus twice a day.

FORMS

Lotion, cream, suppository.

PRECAUTIONS

Use with caution in pregnancy (B2). Safe for use in breast feeding. Dilute for use in children.

Avoid use on face, head and around vagina, head of penis and anus.

SIDE EFFECTS

Common: Skin irritation.
Unusual: Skin burning.

INTERACTIONS

None significant.

PRESCRIPTION

No

PERMITTED IN SPORT

Yes

OVERDOSE

If swallowed, administer activated charcoal or induce vomiting if medication taken recently. May cause convulsions. Seek urgent medical advice.

OTHER INFORMATION

Commonly used and effective treatment for parasites. All members of family must be treated at same time. Change and wash all bed linen and clothing in hot water with each treatment.

Benzyl penicillin

See Penicillin G

BETA -2 AGONISTS (ß2 AGONISTS)

(Relieve airway constriction)

TRADE and GENERIC NAMES

Aerocrom (Salbutamol with Sodium cromoglycate).

Aerolin, Airomir, Asmasal, Salamol, Salbulin, Ventmax SR, Ventodisks, Ventolin, Volmax (Salbutamol).

Bambec (Bambuterol).

Berotec (Fenoterol).

Bricanyl (Terbutaline).

Bronchodil (Reproterol).

Combivent (Salbutamol, Ipratropium bromide).

Duovent (Fenoterol, Ipratropium).

Ventide (Salbutamol, Beclomethasone)

DRUG CLASS

Bronchodilators.

USES

Asthma, bronchitis, emphysema, spasm of airways in lung.

DOSAGE

 Inhalers and sprays: Two inhalations every four to six hours.
Tablets: One three times a day.
Elixir: 5mLs to 10mLs three or four times a day.

PRECAUTIONS

Safe to use in pregnancy (A), breast feeding and children.

Not designed for long term constant use.

Use with care in high blood pressure, heart disease, overactive thyroid gland, diabetes, liver and kidney disease.

Lower doses necessary in elderly.

Seek urgent medical assistance if no response to medication.

FORMS

Tablets, elixir, injection, spray, inhaler, nebuliser solution, dischaler, rotacaps.

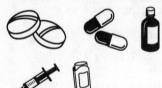

SIDE EFFECTS

Common: Tremor, rapid heart rate, palpitations, headache.

Unusual: Nausea, flush, mouth irritation.

INTERACTIONS

Other drugs:

• Sympathomimetics, Beta-blockers, Theophyllines, Steroids, Diuretics, Digoxin.

Other substances:

• Tablets and capsules may react with alcohol and caffeine.

PRESCRIPTION

Yes

PERMITTED IN SPORT

Tablets, elixir, discs, Isoprenaline: No
Other

OVERDOSE

Exacerbation of side effects likely. May be dangerous in patients with heart disease or high blood pressure.

OTHER INFORMATION

These medications are designed for intermittent occasional use, and are not to be taken regularly. Other medication should be used to prevent asthma if repeated doses of these medications are needed. Do not cause dependence or addiction. First introduced in the 1960s, they have revolutionised life for asthmatics.

See also Eformoterol, Salmeterol.

BETA-BLOCKERS (ß ADRENERGIC BLOCKING AGENTS)

TRADE and GENERIC NAMES

Beta-Adalat, Tenif (Atenolol, Nifedipine).

Beta-Cardone, Sotacor (Sotalol).

Beta-Prograne, Inderal (Propranolol).

Betagan (Levobunolol).

Betaloc, Lopresor (Metoprolol).

Betim, Timoptol (Timolol).

Betoptic, Kerione (Betaxolol).

Brevibloc (Esmolol).

Cardicor, Emcor, Monocor (Bisoprolol).

Celectol (Celiprolol).

Co-Betaloc (Metoprolol, Hydrochlorthiazide).

Corgard (Nadolol).

Corgaretic (Nadolol, Bendrofluazide).

Cosopt (Timolol, Dorzolamide).

Inderetic, Inderex (Propranolol, Bendrofluazide).

Kalten (Atenolol, Hydrochlorthiazide, Amiloride).

Minims Metipranolol (Metipranolol).

Moducren (Timolol, Hydrochlorthiazide).

Monozide (Bisoprolol, Hydrochlorthiazide).

Nebilet (Nebivolol).

Prestim (Timolol, Bendrofluazide).

Secadrex (Acebutalol, Hydrochlorthiazide).

Sectral (Acebutalol).

Slow-Trasicor, Trasicor (Oxprenolol).

Tenben (Atenolol, Bendrofluazide).

Tenoret 50, Tenoretic (<u>Atenolol</u>, Chlorthalidone).

Tenormin (<u>Atenolol</u>).

Teoptic (<u>Carteolol</u>).

Trasidrex (<u>Oxprenolol</u>, Cyclopenthiazine).

Visaldix (<u>Pindolol</u>, Clopamine)

Visken (Pindolol).

USES

All except Bisoprolol , Carteolol, Esmolol, Sotalol, Timolol, Levobunolol & Betaxolol: High blood pressure, angina, over active thyroid gland, rapid heart rate, irregular heart beat, paroxysmal atrial tachycardia, heart attack.

Metoprolol: In addition to above - prevention of migraine.

Propranolol: In addition to above - prevention of migraine, tremors, phaeochromocytoma, prevention of anxiety related symptoms (eg: stage fright, exam nerves)

Esmolol: Short term control of rapid heart rate.

Betaxolol, Carteolol, Levobunolol, Metipranolol , Timolol: Glaucoma.

Bisoprolol: Some types of heart failure and high blood pressure.

Sotalol: Irregular heart rhythm.

DOSAGE

Tablets: Variable dosage depending on form From one tablet a day, to three or four tablets three times a day. Eye drops: One drop twice a day.

FORMS

Tablets, capsules, eye drops, injection.

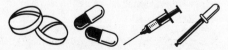

PRECAUTIONS

Should be used in pregnancy (C) only if medically essential. Eye drops unlikely to cause problems in pregnancy.

Safe to use in breast feeding.

May be used with caution in children.

Use with care if suffering from alcoholism, liver or kidney failure or about to have surgery.

 Do not take if:

- suffering from diabetes, asthma, or allergic conditions.

- suffering from heart failure, shock, slow heart rate, or enlarged right heart.

- if undertaking prolonged fast.

SIDE EFFECTS

Common: Low blood pressure, slow heart rate, cold hands and feet, asthma.

Unusual: Loss of appetite, nausea, diarrhoea, impotence, tiredness, sleeplessness, nightmares, rash, loss of libido, hair loss, noises in ears.

Severe but rare (stop medication, consult doctor): Severe asthma.

INTERACTIONS

Other drugs:

- Calcium channel blockers, Disopyramide, Clonidine, Adrenaline, other medications for irregular heart beat, Lignocaine, Ergotamine, Indomethacin, Chlorpromazine.

PRESCRIPTION

Yes

PERMITTED IN SPORT

No

OVERDOSE

Slow heart rate, low blood pressure, asthma and heart failure may result. Administer activated charcoal or induce vomiting if tablets taken recently. Use Salbutamol or other asthma sprays for difficulty in breathing. Seek medical assistance.

OTHER INFORMATION

An amazing group of drugs that can help an extraordinarily wide range of problems. Except for asthmatics, very safe and effective. First developed in 1960's.

See also Carvedilol, Labetalol.

Betahistine

TRADE NAME

Serc.

DRUG CLASS

Vasodilator.

USES

Meniere's syndrome, dizziness, nausea, vomiting, noises in ears (tinnitus), some forms of poor hearing.

DOSAGE

 Two tablets three or four times a day.

FORMS

Tablet of 8 and 16mg. (white).

SIDE EFFECTS

Common: Minimal

Unusual: Rash, diarrhoea, dizziness, headache, nausea, sleeplessness.

PRECAUTIONS

Should not be used in pregnancy, breast feeding or children.

 Do not take if:

- suffering from phaeochromocytoma, asthma, peptic ulcer.

INTERACTIONS

None significant

PRESCRIPTION

Yes

PERMITTED IN SPORT

Yes

OVERDOSE

No serious effects

Betaine

TRADE NAME

Kloref (with Potassium salts).

DRUG CLASS

Detoxifying agent.

USES

Treatment of the rare metabolic condition homocystinuria. In combination with potassium used to treat potassium deficiency.

DOSAGE

 One or two tablets three times a day dissolved in water.

FORMS

Effervescent tablet.

PRECAUTIONS

Not to be used in pregnancy (C) or breast feeding.

SIDE EFFECTS

Common: Nausea, diarrhoea.

INTERACTIONS

Other drugs:

• Affects the absorption of all other medications taken at the same time.

PRESCRIPTION

No

PERMITTED IN SPORT

Yes

OVERDOSE

Significant diarrhoea only likely effect.

Betamethasone

TRADE NAME

Betacap, Betnelan, Betnesol, Betnovate,Bettamousse, Diprosone.

Betnesol N, Betnovate N (with Neomycin).

Betnovate Rectal (with Phenylephrine, Lignocaine).

Betnovate C (with Clioquinol).

Diprosalic (with Salicylic acid).

Fucibet (with Fusidic acid).

Lotriderm (with Clotrimazole).

DRUG CLASS

Corticosteroid.

USES

Skin preparations: Severe inflammation of skin (eczema, dermatitis etc.).

Tablets, injections: Above uses plus severe asthma, rheumatoid and other forms of severe arthritis, auto-immune diseases (eg: Sjøgren's Syndrome), severe allergy reactions, and other severe and chronic inflammatory diseases.

DOSAGE

 Tablets: One to ten tablets a day as directed by doctor
Creams, ointments: Apply two or three times a day.
Lotions, mousse: Apply once or twice a day.

FORMS

Tablets, cream, ointment, gel, lotion, hair mousse, injection.

PRECAUTIONS

Should be used in pregnancy (C), breast feeding and children only on specific medical advice. Skin preparations safe in pregnancy, breast feeding and children over three years.

Use tablets and injections with caution if under stress, and in patients with under active thyroid gland, liver disease, diverticulitis, high blood pressure, myasthenia gravis or kidney disease.

Avoid eyes with all forms.

Use for shortest period of time possible.

 Do not take if:

• suffering from any form of infection, peptic ulcer, or osteoporosis.

• having a vaccination

SIDE EFFECTS

Common: Skin preparations - minimal. Tablets and injections - may cause bloating, weight gain, rashes and intestinal disturbances.

Unusual: Skin preparations - thinning of skin, premature ageing, itching, scarring of skin. Tablets and injections - Biochemical disturbances of blood, muscle weakness, bone weakness, impaired wound healing, skin thinning, tendon weakness, peptic ulcers, gullet ulcers, bruising, increased sweating, loss of fat under skin, premature ageing, excess facial hair growth in women, pigmentation of skin and nails, acne, convulsions, headaches, dizziness, growth suppression in children, aggravation of diabetes, worsening of infections, cataracts, aggravation of glaucoma, blood clots in veins and sleeplessness.

Most significant side effects occur only with prolonged use of tablets or injections.

Medication should not be ceased abruptly, but dosage should be slowly reduced.

Severe but rare (stop medication, consult doctor): Any significant side effect should be reported to a doctor immediately.

INTERACTIONS

Other drugs:

• Tablets and injections may be affected by Oral contraceptives, Barbiturates, Phenytoin, and Rifampicin.

PRESCRIPTION

Yes

PERMITTED IN SPORT

Tablets, injections: No.
Skin preparations: Yes

OVERDOSE

Medical treatment is required. Serious effects and death rare.

OTHER INFORMATION

Extremely effective and useful medication if used correctly. Tablets must be used with extreme care under strict medical supervision. Lowest dose and shortest possible course should be used. Not addictive.

Betaxolol

See BETA BLOCKERS

Bethanechol

TRADE NAME

Myotonine.

USES

Inability to pass urine, reflux of stomach contents in children.

DOSAGE

 10 to 25mg, 3 or 4 times a day.

FORMS

Tablets of 10 and 25mg.

PRECAUTIONS

Use with caution in pregnancy (B2). Use with caution if taking blood pressure medication.

 Do not take if:

• suffering from bowel obstruction.

SIDE EFFECTS

Common: Discomfort in the belly, excess production of saliva, flushing of skin, sweating.

Unusual: Tiredness, headache, diarrhoea, nausea, belching.

Severe but rare (stop medication, consult doctor): Severe belly pain, asthma attack.

INTERACTIONS

None significant.

PRESCRIPTION

Yes

PERMITTED IN SPORT

Yes

OVERDOSE

Atropine is a specific antidote. Seek medical assistance.

Bezafibrate

TRADE NAME

Bezalip.

DRUG CLASS

Hypolipidaemic.

USES

Some types of excess lipids (fats such as cholesterol and triglyceride) in blood.

DOSAGE

 One to three tablets a day with or after food.

PRECAUTIONS

Not to be used in pregnancy, breast feeding and children.

Use with caution with any kidney disease.

 ## Do not take if:

- suffering from severe liver or kidney disease (eg. nephrotic syndrome).

FORMS

Tablets of 200 and 400mg.

SIDE EFFECTS

Common: Diarrhoea, nausea, rash.

Unusual: Vomiting, muscle damage.

Severe but rare (stop medication, consult doctor): Impotence, hair loss.

INTERACTIONS

Other drugs:

- Warfarin, Anticoagulants, MAOI, other Hypolipidaemics, Hypoglycaemics (used in diabetes).

PRESCRIPTION

Yes

PERMITTED IN SPORT

Yes See also HYPOLIPIDAEMICS

Bicalutamide

TRADE NAME

Casodex

DRUG CLASS

Antineoplastic.

USES

Severe cancer of the prostate gland.

DOSAGE

 One tablet a day.

PRECAUTIONS

Not to be used in women or children.

Use with caution in liver disease.

FORMS

Tablets (white) of 50 and 150mg.

SIDE EFFECTS

Common: Hot flushes, itchy skin, breast enlargement and tenderness, nausea, diarrhoea.

Unusual: Liver damage, vomiting.

INTERACTIONS

Other drugs:

• Warfarin.

PRESCRIPTION

Yes

PERMITTED IN SPORT

Yes

OVERDOSE

Serious. seek urgent medical attention.

OTHER INFORMATION

Introduced in 1997 to treat cases of prostate cancer that are not responding to other treatment.

Bicarbonates

See ANTACIDS

Biotin

(Vitamin H)

TRADE NAMES

A large number of preparations include Biotin (Vitamin H) alone or in combination with other vitamins and minerals.

DRUG CLASS

Vitamin.

USES

No specific medical use.

DOSAGE

 Recommended daily allowance: 100 to 200 mcg per day

FORMS

Tablets, capsules, mixture.

PRECAUTIONS

Safe in pregnancy, breast feeding and children.

Do not take in high doses or for prolonged periods of time.

SIDE EFFECTS

Minimal.

INTERACTIONS

None significant.

PRESCRIPTION

No

PERMITTED IN SPORT

Yes

OVERDOSE

Unlikely to have serious adverse effects.

OTHER INFORMATION

Remember, vitamins are merely chemicals that are essential for the functioning of the body, and if taken to excess, act as a drug.

Biperiden

TRADE NAME

Akineton.

DRUG CLASS

Antiparkinsonian.

USES

Parkinson's disease, night time leg cramps, some movement disorders.

DOSAGE

 Night time leg cramps: One or two tablets at night
Other conditions: Half to two tablets three or four times a day.

FORMS

Tablets of 2mg. (white).

PRECAUTIONS

Use with caution in pregnancy (B2) and breast feeding.

Use with caution in prostate gland disease, rapid heart rate.

 Do not take if:
• suffering from glaucoma, megacolon, intestinal obstruction.

SIDE EFFECTS

Common: Dry mouth, drowsiness, blurred vision, dizziness.

Unusual: Rapid heart rate, confusion, constipation.

Severe but rare (stop medication, consult doctor): Severe constipation.

INTERACTIONS

Other drugs:

• Other antiparkinsonian drugs, Quinidine, Tricyclic antidepressants, Tetracyclic antidepressants.

Other substances:

• Reacts with alcohol to cause sedation.

PRESCRIPTION

Yes

PERMITTED IN SPORT

Yes

Bisacodyl

TRADE NAME

Bisacodyl, Dulcolax.

DRUG CLASS

Laxative.

USES

Constipation, preparing bowel for surgery or x-rays.

DOSAGE

 Tablets: Two to four tablets at night
Suppository: One or two at night.

FORMS

Tablets, suppository.

PRECAUTIONS

Safe in pregnancy (A), breast feeding and children.

Designed for short term use only.

 Do not take if:
• suffering from belly pains or bowel obstruction

SIDE EFFECTS

Common: Minimal.

Unusual: Diarrhoea, belly discomfort.

Severe but rare (stop medication, consult doctor): Severe belly pain.

INTERACTIONS

Other drugs:

• Do not take Antacids within 30 minutes of Bisacodyl.

PRESCRIPTION

No

PERMITTED IN SPORT

Yes

OVERDOSE

Diarrhoea and belly pain only effects likely.

OTHER INFORMATION

Widely used and very safe.

Bismuth

TRADE NAME

De-Noltab (Bismuth subcitrate [Tripotassium dicitratobismuthate]).

Pylorid (Bismuth citrate with Ranitidine).

DRUG CLASS

Antiulcerant.

USES

Treatment of stomach and duodenal (upper small intestine) ulcers.

DOSAGE

 Up to four tablets a day, in two to four doses, half hour before meals and last thing at night.

FORMS

Tablets of 120mg. (white).

PRECAUTIONS

Safety in pregnancy and breast feeding not established.

 Do not take if:

• suffering from kidney failure.

SIDE EFFECTS

Common: Black faeces, coated tongue and teeth, nausea, vomiting.

INTERACTIONS

Other drugs:

• Do not take Antacids within one hour of Bismuth subcitrate.

• Tetracycline efficacy may be reduced.

• Efficacy of Cimetidine, Ranitidine, Nizatadine and other Antiulcerants may be reduced.

Other substances:

• Reacts with food and milk to reduce drugs efficiency.

• Avoid carbonated drinks (eg: beer).

PRESCRIPTION

No

PERMITTED IN SPORT

Yes

OVERDOSE

Giving activated charcoal, or induction of vomiting and stomach washout recommended. No reported serious effects.

BISPHOSPHONATES

(Prevent loss of bone density)

See Alendronate, Disodium clodronate, Etidronate, Pamidronate, Risedronate, Sodium clodronate, Tiludronic acid

Botulinum toxin

TRADE NAME

Botox, Dysport.

USES

Spasms of eyelids, facial nerve disorders, facial muscle spasms, foot spasticity and deformity in children with cerebral palsy.

DOSAGE

 Complex. As determined by doctor for each individual patient.

FORMS

Injection.

PRECAUTIONS

Use with caution in pregnancy (B3), breast feeding and children.

Use with caution in myasthenia gravis, Eaton-Lambert syndrome, amyotrophic lateral sclerosis, other nerve-muscle diseases.

Avoid areas of local inflammation when injecting.

SIDE EFFECTS

General: Nerve damage, muscle weakness and pain, rash, irregular heart rhythm.

Eyelid injections: Eye irritation, drooping eyelid, dry eye surface and ulceration.

Facial spasm: Blurred vision, facial muscle weakness.

Severe but rare (stop medication, consult doctor): Heart attack.

INTERACTIONS

Other drugs:

• Aminoglycosides, drugs acting on nerves and muscles.

PRESCRIPTION

Yes

PERMITTED IN SPORT

Yes

OVERDOSE

Potentially fatal.

OTHER INFORMATION

Derived from the bacteria that causes botulism, one of the most severe forms of food poisoning.

Brimonidine tartrate

TRADE NAME

Alphargan.

USES

Glaucoma.

DOSAGE

 One drop in affected eye twice a day.

FORMS

Eye drops (keep refrigerated).

PRECAUTIONS

Use with caution in pregnancy (B1), breast feeding and children.

Use with caution in severe heart disease, poor liver and kidney function, poor blood supply to heart or brain, low blood pressure.

May aggravate Raynaud's phenomenon.

Eye drops are absorbed into the bloodstream and may cause effects in other parts of the body.

 Do not take if:
- using soft contact lenses.

SIDE EFFECTS

Common: Dry mouth, red eyes, irritated eyes, eye stinging, eye itching, headache, tiredness.

Unusual: Eye irritation, eye ulceration, light sensitivity of eye, swelling of eyelid, inflamed eye, intestinal upset.

Severe but rare (stop medication, consult doctor): Rare and serious complications.

INTERACTIONS

Other drugs:
- Must not be used with MAOI (see separate entry).

PRESCRIPTION

Yes

PERMITTED IN SPORT

Yes

OVERDOSE

Unlikely to be serious if swallowed. Wash out eye thoroughly with water if excess drops used.

OTHER INFORMATION

Introduced in 1998 for forms of glaucoma that cannot be controlled by other medications.

Brinzolamide

TRADE NAME

Azopt.

USES

Additional treatment in difficult cases of glaucoma.

DOSAGE

 One drop in affected eye two or three times a day.

FORMS

Eye drops.

PRECAUTIONS

Use with caution in pregnancy. Not for use in breast feeding and children.

Use with caution in some types of glaucoma, dry eyes and with contact lenses (wait 15 minutes after using drops before inserting lenses).

Use with caution in diabetes.

Progress and eye pressure must be monitored closely.

 Do not take if:
- suffering from significant liver or kidney disease.
- allergic to sulpha.

SIDE EFFECTS

Common: Blurred vision, eye discomfort.

Unusual: Headache, abnormal tastes.

INTERACTIONS

Other drugs:
- Some other drops used for glaucoma. Wait 5 minutes before use.

PRESCRIPTION

Yes

PERMITTED IN SPORT

Yes

OVERDOSE

Eye damage possible. Wash out eye thoroughly with water if excess drops used.

OTHER INFORMATION

Introduced in 1999 for otherwise uncontrolled glaucoma.

See also Brimonidine tartrate

Bromazepam

See ANXIOLYTICS

Bromocriptine

TRADE NAME

Parlodel.

DRUG CLASS

Antiparkinsonian.

USES

Parkinson's disease, acromegaly, abnormal production of breast milk, stopping production of breast milk when breast feeding ceased.

DOSAGE

 Depends on purpose. Usually start low, and increase slowly until desired result obtained. Taken three or four times a day.

FORMS

Tablets, capsules.

PRECAUTIONS

Safe in pregnancy (A). Not to be used during breast feeding or in children.

Use with caution in psychiatric conditions, high or low blood pressure, heart disease, diabetes, peptic ulcer, eye disease and liver disease.

Use with caution in women who wish to fall pregnant, as Bromocriptine may reduce fertility.

 Do not take if:

- suffering from high blood pressure in or immediately after pregnancy.

SIDE EFFECTS

Common: Nausea very common. Dizziness, headache, nasal congestion, vomiting, tiredness, reduced blood pressure (fainting).

Unusual: Hallucinations, confusion, behavioural disturbances, unwanted muscle movements, psychiatric disturbances, peptic ulcer.

Severe but rare (stop medication, consult doctor):Vomiting blood, severe psychiatric disturbances.

INTERACTIONS

Other drugs:

- Medications that lower blood pressure, Erythromycin.

Other substances:

- Reacts adversely with alcohol.

PRESCRIPTION

Yes

PERMITTED IN SPORT

Yes

OVERDOSE

May cause vomiting, tiredness, low blood pressure and hallucinations. Not likely to be life threatening. Administer activated charcoal or induce vomiting if taken recently. Seek medical assistance.

OTHER INFORMATION

A very useful drug with an extraordinary range of activities. Tumours of the pituitary gland in the brain cause both acromegaly (excess bone growth) and abnormal breast milk production (in both sexes).

Brompheniramine

See ANTIHISTAMINES, SEDATING

BRONCHODILATORS

(Open airways in lungs)

See BETA-2 AGONISTS, Eformoterol, Ephedrine, Ipratropium bromide, Orciprenaline, Salmeterol, THEOPHYLLINES

Buclizine

TRADE NAME

Only available in combination with other ingredients.

Migraleve Pink (with Paracetamol, Codeine).

USES

Relieves nausea of migraine and causes sedation.

DOSAGE

 Two pink tablets at onset of migraine attack.

PRECAUTIONS

Use with caution in pregnancy, breast feeding and children.

FORMS

Tablets (pink). Yellow Migraleve tablets do not contain Buclizine.

SIDE EFFECTS

Common: Sedation.

INTERACTIONS

Other drugs:

• Other sedatives and pain relievers.

PRESCRIPTION

Yes

PERMITTED IN SPORT

Yes

OVERDOSE

May be very serious due to Paracetamol in contents of tablets (see separate entry). Buclizine alone unlikely to have serious effects.

Budesonide

TRADE NAME

Budenofalk, Entocort, Pulmicort, Rhinocort Aqua.

DRUG CLASS

Corticosteroid.

USES

Prevention of asthma, prevention of hay fever and chronic nasal drip, Crohn's disease.

DOSAGE

 Asthma spray (Pulmicort): One or two inhalations, once a day
Nasal sprays (Rhinocort): One spray, once a day in each nostril
Capsules (Budenofalk, Entocort): One three times a day
Enema (Entocort): One at night.

FORMS

Inhaler, nasal spray, nebuliser solution, capsule, enema.

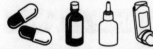

PRECAUTIONS

Use with caution in pregnancy (B3), breast feeding and children.

Sprays and inhalers: Use with caution in lung or throat infection and tuberculosis. Lung function should be checked regularly to ensure adequate dose is received.

Capsules and enema: Use with caution in high blood pressure, diabetes, osteoporosis, peptic ulcer, glaucoma, cataracts and liver disease.

Do not use capsules or enema if

• suffering from bacterial, fungal or viral infections.

SIDE EFFECTS

Common: Fungal (thrush) infections of mouth, sore throat and mouth, dry mouth.

Unusual: Hoarseness, unusual bleeding and bruising, slowed growth, stomach upsets, muscle weakness, high blood pressure.

INTERACTIONS

Inhalers and sprays:

• None significant

Capsules and enema:

• Cholestyramine, Digoxin, Diuretics, live vaccines, some high blood pressure medications.

PRESCRIPTION

Yes

PERMITTED IN SPORT

Yes

OVERDOSE

Unlikely to have any serious effects.

OTHER INFORMATION

The introduction of the turbuhaler for the inhalation of Budesonide was a major advance in asthma prevention as it is far easier to use than pressurised sprays. Budesonide is extremely effective in preventing hay fever and other forms of constantly dripping nose. Inhalers and sprays designed for long term use, but capsules and enemas should not be used for more than a couple of months. Does not cause dependence or addiction.

See also Beclomethasone, Fluticasone

Bumetanide

TRADE NAMES

Burinex.

Burinex A (with Amiloride)

Burinex K (with Potassium).

DRUG CLASS

Diuretic.

USES

Excess fluid in body.

PRECAUTIONS

Should not be used in pregnancy (C) unless medically essential. Should not be used in breast feeding or children.

Use with caution in elderly, diabetes, gout and heart failure.

May require regular blood tests to check on level of salts (electrolytes) in blood.

 ### Do not take if:

• suffering from severe kidney or liver disease.

DOSAGE

 One or more tablets in morning to maximum of 10mg.

FORMS

Tablets, injection.

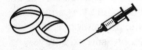

SIDE EFFECTS

Common: Muscle cramps, dizziness, headache, nausea.

Unusual: Deafness, rash, itch, weakness, arthritis, belly pains, vomiting.

Severe but rare (stop medication, consult doctor): Fainting.

INTERACTIONS

Other drugs:

• Digoxin, Lithium, Probenecid, Anticoagulants, Indomethacin.

• Medications that lower blood pressure.

PRESCRIPTION

Yes

PERMITTED IN SPORT

No

OVERDOSE

May lead to severe dehydration and blood clots. Symptoms include weakness, dizziness, confusion, cramps and vomiting. Induce vomiting if tablets taken recently. Give extra fluids. Seek medical assistance.

OTHER INFORMATION

Introduced in 1980's. Similar to Frusemide, but faster and shorter acting.

See also Frusemide.

Bupivacaine

See ANAESTHETICS, LOCAL

Buprenorphine

TRADE NAME

Subutex, Temgesic.

DRUG CLASS

Narcotic, analgesic.

USES

Moderate to severe pain.

DOSAGE

 One or two tablets under tongue every six to eight hours as required.

FORMS

Tablets for use under tongue, injection.

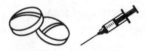

PRECAUTIONS

Should not be used in pregnancy (C) unless medically essential. Not for use in breast feeding or children.

Use with caution in head injury, liver disease and severe lung disease.

 Do not take if:

• operating machinery or driving a vehicle.

SIDE EFFECTS

Common: Drowsiness, nausea.

Unusual: Headache, vomiting, dry mouth, constipation, dizziness, difficulty in passing urine.

Severe but rare (stop medication, consult doctor): Difficulty in breathing.

INTERACTIONS

Other drugs:

• MAOI, Sedatives, other Narcotics.

Other substances:

• Alcohol should be avoided.

PRESCRIPTION

Yes (very restricted).

PERMITTED IN SPORT

No

OVERDOSE

Symptoms may include drowsiness, confusion, difficulty in breathing and coma. Induce vomiting if medication taken recently and patient alert. Seek urgent medical attention.

OTHER INFORMATION

May cause addiction or dependence if used inappropriately. Introduced in the late 1980s for use in more intractable pain conditions.

Bupropion

TRADE NAME

Zyban.

USES

Aids cessation of smoking and counteracts nicotine addiction.

DOSAGE

 One tablet a day for three days, increasing if necessary to one tablet twice a day.

FORMS

Tablet of 150mg. (white).

PRECAUTIONS

Not to be used in pregnancy, breast feeding and children.

Use with caution in any liver or kidney disease, head injury, brain tumour, alcoholism and diabetes.

Blood pressure should be checked regularly.

 Do not take if:

• suffering from epilepsy or other condition causing seizures, bipolar disorder, eating disorder, severe liver disease (eg. cirrhosis).

• under other circumstances

SIDE EFFECTS

Common: Sleeplessness, headache, fever. dry mouth, nausea.

Unusual: Diarrhoea or constipation, brain irritation, skin reaction, taste disorders.

Severe but rare (stop medication, consult doctor): Convulsion.

INTERACTIONS

Other drugs:

• MAOI, Antipsychotics, Antidepressants, Theophylline, Steroid tablets, Benzodiazepines, medications used to treat epilepsy and convulsions, Levodopa.

Other substances:

• Alcohol, stimulants.

PRESCRIPTION

Yes

PERMITTED IN SPORT

No

OVERDOSE

May be very serious. Seek urgent medical attention. Administer activated charcoal or induce vomiting if tablets taken recently and patient alert.

Buserelin

TRADE NAME

Suprecur, Suprefact.

USES

Endometriosis, prostate cancer, control of ovulation during in vitro fertilisation for infertility.

DOSAGE

 Nasal sprays as determined by doctor for each patient, depending on condition.

FORMS

Nasal spray.

PRECAUTIONS

Must not be used in pregnancy, breast feeding or children.

Barrier contraception must be used.

Use with caution if patient at risk of osteoporosis.

 Do not take if:

- suffering from undiagnosed vaginal bleeding.
- testes have been surgically removed.

SIDE EFFECTS

Common: Hot flushes, nasal irritation, loss of libido, dry vagina, emotional upsets, headache, breast tenderness.

Unusual: Change in breast size, ovarian cysts.

INTERACTIONS

Other drugs:

- Contraceptive pill, nasal decongestants, sex hormones.

PRESCRIPTION

Yes

PERMITTED IN SPORT

Yes

OVERDOSE

The effects of an overdose, and the first aid treatment of an overdose. See section on "Overdose" and "Poisoning" in Introduction for further information.

OTHER INFORMATION

Seek medical attention. Exacerbation of side effects likely.

Buspirone

TRADE NAME

Buspar.

DRUG CLASS

Anxiolytic.

USES

Relief of anxiety.

PRECAUTIONS

Should only be used in pregnancy if medically essential. Breast feeding should be ceased before Buspirone taken. Not for use in children.

Should be used with caution in epilepsy, liver and kidney disease.

Lower doses required in elderly.

 Do not take if:

- suffering from severe liver disease.
- operating machinery, driving a vehicle, or undertaking tasks that require concentration, alertness and coordination.

DOSAGE

 5mg. to 20mg. (one to three tablets), three times a day.

FORMS

Tablets of 5mg. and 10mg. (white).

SIDE EFFECTS

Common: Dizziness, sleeplessness, drowsiness, light headedness, nausea, headache.

Unusual: Excitement, chest pain, nightmares.

INTERACTIONS

Other drugs:

• Benzodiazepines and other anxiolytics.

• MAOI.

Other substances:

• No reaction with alcohol.

• Food increases absorption of Buspirone.

PRESCRIPTION

Yes

PERMITTED IN SPORT

No

OVERDOSE

May cause vomiting, drowsiness and stomach pains. Not believed to be serious. Administer activated charcoal or induce vomiting if tablets taken recently and patient alert. Seek medical attention.

OTHER INFORMATION

Introduced in early 1990s as an non-addictive alternative to Benzodiazepines. Does not cause dependence. Very safe, but not as rapid in its effect as other Anxiolytics.

Busulphan

TRADE NAME:

Myleran.

DRUG CLASS:

Alkylater.

USES:

Leukaemia, polycythaemia rubra vera, myelofibrosis, thrombocythaemia.

DOSAGE:

Must be individualised by doctor for each patient depending on disease, severity, age and weight of patient.

FORMS:

Tablets of 2mg. (white)

PRECAUTIONS:

Must not be used in pregnancy (D) unless mother's life is at risk as damage to the foetus may occur. Breast feeding must be ceased before use. May be used in children if medically essential.

Regular blood tests to monitor blood cells and liver function essential.

Adequate contraception must be used by women while medication taken.

Must be used with caution in all patients.

SIDE EFFECTS:

Common: Damage to bone marrow, skin pigmentation.

Unusual: Nausea, vomiting, diarrhoea, lung damage (cough), eye damage, hair loss, rash, itch.

INTERACTIONS:

None significant.

PRESCRIPTION:

Yes

PERMITTED IN SPORT:

Yes

OVERDOSE:

Very serious. Permanent damage to bone marrow with subsequent death likely. Administer activated charcoal or induce vomiting if medication taken recently. Seek urgent medical assistance.

OTHER INFORMATION:

Although Busulfan has serious side effects, it may be life saving in patients with some types of malignancy or blood disorders.

Butobarbitone

See BARBITURATES

Butoxyethyl nicotinate

TRADE NAME

Only available in Britain in combination with other ingredients.

Actinac (with Chloramphenicol, Hydrocortisone, Allantoin, Sulphur compounds).

USES

Acne. When used alone acts as a liniment.

DOSAGE

 Apply twice a day for four days, then once a day.

FORMS

Powder and solvent to make lotion.

PRECAUTIONS

Safe in pregnancy and breast feeding. Do not use on infants.

Avoid eyes, mouth, nose, ears, anus and vagina.

Do not use on broken, diseased, infected or inflamed skin.

SIDE EFFECTS

Common: Skin irritation and redness.

INTERACTIONS

None significant.

PRESCRIPTION

Yes

PERMITTED IN SPORT

Yes

Cabergoline

TRADE NAME

Cabaser, Dostinex.

USES

Parkinson's disease, stopping breast milk production, excess production of the hormone prolactin.

DOSAGE

 Stopping breast feeding: Two 0.5mg tablets taken once. Excess prolactin production: 0.5 to 2mg., once a week.
Parkinson's: 1 to 6mg a day in divided doses. Increase dose very slowly.

FORMS

Tablets.

PRECAUTIONS

Not to be used in pregnancy (C), breast feeding and children.

Use with caution in heart disease, kidney disease, liver disease, peptic ulcer disease.

May aggravate some psychiatric conditions.

High blood pressure after childbirth may be made worse.

SIDE EFFECTS

Common: Low blood pressure, fainting, dizziness, headache, tiredness.

Unusual: Fatigue, depression, stomach upsets, breast pain, hot flushes.

INTERACTIONS

Other drugs:

• Ergot alkaloids, methyl ergotamine, dopamine agonists, drugs that inhibit liver function.

PRESCRIPTION

Yes

PERMITTED IN SPORT

Yes

Caffine

TRADE NAME

Cabaser, Dostinex.

USES

Parkinson's disease, stopping breast milk production, excess production of the hormone prolactin.

DOSAGE

 Stopping breast feeding: Two 0.5mg tablets taken once. Excess prolactin production: 0.5 to 2mg., once a week.
Parkinson's: 1 to 6mg a day in divided doses. Increase dose very slowly.

PRECAUTIONS

Not to be used in pregnancy (C), breast feeding and children.

Use with caution in heart disease, kidney disease, liver disease, peptic ulcer disease.

May aggravate some psychiatric conditions.

High blood pressure after childbirth may be made worse.

FORMS

Tablets.

SIDE EFFECTS

Common: Low blood pressure, fainting, dizziness, headache, tiredness.

Unusual: Fatigue, depression, stomach upsets, breast pain, hot flushes.

INTERACTIONS

Other drugs:

• Ergot alkaloids, methyl ergotamine, dopamine agonists, drugs that inhibit liver function.

PRESCRIPTION

Yes

PERMITTED IN SPORT

Yes

Caffeine

TRADE NAME

Found in multiple over the counter minor stimulants.

Cafergot (with Ergotamine).

Migril (with Ergotamine, Cyclizine).

DRUG CLASS

Stimulant.

USES

Fatigue, additive to assist motion sickness and migraines.

DOSAGE

 One tablet every three hours or as directed by doctor. One suppository up to three times a day.

FORMS

Tablets, suppository.

PRECAUTIONS

Safe in pregnancy and breast feeding. Use with caution in children.

 Do not take if:

• suffering from peptic ulcer, heartburn.

SIDE EFFECTS

Common: Anxiety, nervousness, sleeplessness, passing increased amount of urine.

INTERACTIONS

Other substances:

• Reacts with coffee, tea and cola drinks containing caffeine.

PERMITTED IN SPORT

No

OVERDOSE

Anxiety, restlessness, irritability and sleeplessness are likely.

OTHER INFORMATION

Used for centuries in tea and coffee as a mild stimulant. Also found in cola drinks. 100mL. of brewed coffee contains 60 to 130mg. of caffeine. 100mL. of instant coffee contains 40 to 100mg. caffeine. 100mL. of tea contains 40 to 60mg. caffeine. 100mL. of cola drink contains 10mg. of caffeine. Stimulant sport drinks may contain more.

Calamine

TRADE NAMES

Found in numerous soothing non-prescription preparations.

Calamine lotion.

Vasogen (with Dimethicone, Zinc oxide).

USES

Minor skin irritations, insect bites, sunburn, leg ulcers.

DOSAGE

 Apply several times a day as required.

FORMS

Cream, lotion.

PRECAUTIONS

Safe to use in pregnancy, breast feeding and children. Avoid eyes, mouth and nostrils.

 Do not take if:
- suffering from blistered, raw or oozing skin.

SIDE EFFECTS

Minimal

INTERACTIONS

None

PRESCRIPTION

No

PERMITTED IN SPORT

Yes

OTHER INFORMATION

Widely used, effective old fashioned treatment for everything from bites to chickenpox.

Calciferol

See Cholecalciferol, Calcitriol and Ergocalciferol (Vitamin D)

Calcipotriol

TRADE NAME

Dovonex.

USES

Psoriasis.

DOSAGE

 Apply twice a day. Reduce frequency if possible.

FORMS

Ointment, cream, scalp lotion.

PRECAUTIONS

Use with caution in pregnancy (B1), breast feeding and children.

Avoid contact with eyes.

Use with caution on face, scalp and in skin flexures.

Use with care long term.

Avoid sun exposure during use.

 Do not take if:
- suffering from disorders of calcium metabolism.
- suffering from severe or pustular psoriasis.

SIDE EFFECTS

Common: Skin irritation, sun sensitivity.

INTERACTIONS

Other drugs:

• Calcium, vitamin D supplements.

PRESCRIPTION

Yes

PERMITTED IN SPORT

Yes

OVERDOSE

Skin damage possible if overused.

Calcitonin

TRADE NAME

Forcaltonin.

USES

Paget's disease of bone, excess blood calcium levels (hypercalcaemia).

DOSAGE

 By injection in a dose determined by doctor for each patient.

FORMS

Injection.

PRECAUTIONS

Not to be used in pregnancy, or breast feeding.

Use with great caution in children.

Not for long term use.

SIDE EFFECTS

Common: Nausea, vomiting, injection site inflammation.

INTERACTIONS

Other drugs:

• Digoxin, Biphosphonates, Calcium antagonists.

PRESCRIPTION

Yes

PERMITTED IN SPORT

Yes

OTHER INFORMATION

Derived from a natural hormone found in salmon.

See also Salcatonin

Calcitriol

See Cholecalciferol, Calcitriol and Ergocalciferol (Vitamin D).

Calcium

TRADE NAMES

Calcium in various forms is found in numerous nutritional supplements, dressings and antacids, some of which are listed below.

Adcal-D3, Calceos, Calcichew D3 Forte (Calcium carbonate, Vitamin D).

Cacit, Calcichew, Calcidrink (Calcium carbonate).

Calcium-Sandoz (Calcium lactobionate, Calcium glubionate).

Gaviscon, Peptac (Calcium carbonate with Antacids).

Ostram (Calcium phosphate).

Phosex (Calcium acetate).

Sandocal (Calcium lactate gluconate, Calcium carbonate).

Titralac (Calcium carbonate, Glycine).

DRUG CLASS

Mineral.

USES

Antacid, improves circulation, poor nutrition, osteomalacia, osteoporosis, excess phosphate in body, lack of calcium in body.

DOSAGE

 Recommended daily intake 800mg. per day.

FORMS

Tablets, capsules, mixtures, injections.

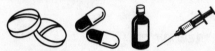

PRECAUTIONS

Safe in pregnancy, breast feeding and children.

Use with caution in kidney stones, kidney disease and diabetes.

 Do not take if:
- suffering from severe kidney disease, high blood calcium.

SIDE EFFECTS

Common: Constipation, hot flushes, sweating.

Unusual: Low blood pressure.

Severe but rare (stop medication, consult doctor): Kidney stones (severe loin pain).

INTERACTIONS

Other drugs:
- Iron, Digoxin, Tetracycline, Fluoride, Calcium channel blockers, Vitamin D.

PRESCRIPTION

No

PERMITTED IN SPORT

Yes

OVERDOSE

Exacerbation of side effects likely.

OTHER INFORMATION

Essential mineral found mainly in dairy products (eg: cheese, milk, yoghurt), bony fish (eg: sardines, salmon); and to a lesser extent in peas, beans, broccoli, almonds and whole grain cereals.

See also ANTACIDS

Calcium acetate

TRADE NAME

Phosex.

USES

Control of excessively high phosphate levels in blood from kidney failure.

DOSAGE

 One to four tablets three times a day with meals.

FORMS

Tablets (yellow) of 1000mg.

PRECAUTIONS

Not to be used in pregnancy or children unless medically essential. Breast feeding should be ceased before use.

Regular blood tests to monitor kidney function, calcium and phosphate levels essential.

 Do not take if:
- suffering from high blood calcium.

SIDE EFFECTS

Common: Nausea, vomiting, constipation, loss of appetite.

INTERACTIONS

Other drugs:

• Calcium supplements, Tetracycline, Digoxin, Ciprofloxacin, Enoxacin, Verapamil.

PRESCRIPTION

Yes

PERMITTED IN SPORT

Yes

OVERDOSE

Serious. May cause extremely high levels of calcium in blood with consequent confusion, delirium and coma. Induce vomiting if tablets taken recently and patient alert. Seek urgent medical assistance.

Calcium alginate

TRADE NAME

Kaltogel, Kaltostat, Sorbalgon, Sorbsan.

USES

Discharging, purulent, contaminated wounds and ulcers.

DOSAGE

 Dressing applied directly to wound. Changed every twelve to 72 hours depending on nature of wound.

FORMS

Dressing.

PRECAUTIONS

Inert agent. Safe to use on all patients.

Not for use on dry wounds or if significant infection present.

Infected wounds may need antibiotics to reduce infection.

SIDE EFFECTS

None

INTERACTIONS

None

PRESCRIPTION

No

PERMITTED IN SPORT

Yes

OTHER INFORMATION

Derived from seaweed. Soaks up exudate from weeping wounds to keep them dry and aid healing. Forms a protective thick gel over healing tissue.

Calcium carbonate

See ANTACIDS; Calcium

CALCIUM CHANNEL BLOCKERS (CALCIUM ANTAGONISTS)

TRADE and GENERIC NAMES

Adalat, Adalat MR, Angiopine MR, Cardilate MR, Coracten, Fortepine LA, Tensipine MR (Nifedipine).

Adizem, Angtil SR, Dilzem, Slozem, Tildiem, Viazem XL, Zemtard XL (Diltiazem).

Beta-Adalat, Tenif (Nifedipine with Atenolol).

Cardene (Nicardipine).

Cordilox, Securon, Univer, Vertab SR (Verapamil).

Istin (Amlodipine).

Motens (Lacidipine).

Nimotop (Nimodipine).

Plendil (Felodipine).

Prescal (Isradipine).

Syscor MR (Nisoldipine).

Tarka (Verapamil with Trandalopril).

Triapin (Felodipine with Ramipril).

Zanidip (Lercanidipine).

USES

All except Nimodipine: High blood pressure, angina, rapid heart rate. Nimodipine: Poor blood supply to brain.

DOSAGE

 Different forms are longer acting than others. Follow doctors instructions. Dosage varies from one capsule or tablet a day, to two capsules or tablets three times a day. Do not vary dosage without medical advice.

FORMS

Tablets, capsules, slow release capsules, injection.

 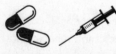

PRECAUTIONS

Should only be used in pregnancy (C) and breast feeding if medically essential. Not designed for use in children.

 Do not take if:

• suffering from severe heart failure, low blood pressure, atrial flutter or fibrillation.

SIDE EFFECTS

Common: Constipation, tiredness, headache, dizziness, indigestion, swelling of feet and ankles.

Unusual: Flushing, palpitations, slow heart rate, scalp irritation, depression, flushes, nightmares, excess wind.

Severe but rare (stop medication, consult doctor): Fainting.

INTERACTIONS

Other drugs:

• Beta blockers (eg: Propranolol), Cyclosporin, Digoxin, Cimetidine, Diazepam, Amiodarone.

• Additive effect with other medications for high blood pressure.

Other substances:

• Smoking may aggravate conditions that these medications are treating.

PRESCRIPTION

Yes

PERMITTED IN SPORT

Yes

OVERDOSE

May continue to be absorbed for up to 48 hours after overdose. Administer activated charcoal or induce vomiting. Purging should be encouraged to eliminate drug from gut. Overdose may cause low blood pressure, irregular heart rhythm, difficulty in breathing, heart attack and death. Obtain urgent medical attention.

OTHER INFORMATION

Commonly used as a first line medication in high blood pressure and to prevent angina. First introduced in early 1970's.

Calcium folinate

(Calcium leucoverin, Folinic acid)

TRADE NAME

Refolinon.

USES

Deficiencies in the body's folic acid level caused by cancer treatment, inadequate intake or anaemia, Methotrexate overdose.

DOSAGE

 Depends on disease, and severity of folic acid deficiency.

FORMS

Tablets (pale yellow) of 15mg., injection.

PRECAUTIONS

May be used safely in pregnancy (A) and children. Use with caution in breast feeding.

 Do not take if:

- suffering from pernicious anaemia.

SIDE EFFECTS

Common: Minimal.

Unusual: Fever.

INTERACTIONS

Other drugs:

- Methotrexate, Droperidol.

PRESCRIPTION

Yes

PERMITTED IN SPORT

Yes

OVERDOSE

No adverse effects expected.

OTHER INFORMATION

Folic acid is essential for formation of red blood cells, but the bacteria that produce it in the gut are destroyed by many anti-cancer drugs.

Calcium Leucoverin

See Calcium folinate

Calcium Salts

See ANTACIDS; Calcium

Camphor

TRADE NAMES

Widely used in many cough mixtures, ointments, creams, liniments, lotions and inhalations.

Balmosa, Salonpas (with Menthol, Methyl salicylate and other ingredients).

Radian B (with Menthol, Methyl salicylate, Aspirin).

DRUG CLASS

Expectorant, rubefacient (liniment).

USES

Soothes muscle and joint pains, and burns.
Eases productive coughs.
Eases nasal congestion.

DOSAGE

 Take every four to six hours. Apply to affected areas or inhale as required.

FORMS

Mixture, ointment, cream, liniment, lotion, inhalation, spray.

PRECAUTIONS

Safe to use in pregnancy, breast feeding and children.

Not to be swallowed.

SIDE EFFECTS

Minimal.

INTERACTIONS

None significant.

PRESCRIPTION

No

PERMITTED IN SPORT

Yes

OVERDOSE

Unlikely to cause any significant adverse effects.

CANCER TREATING DRUGS

(Alkylaters, Antimetabolites, Antineoplastics, Cytotoxics)

See Altretamine, Aminoglutethamide, Amsacrine, Anastrozole, Bicalutamide, Bleomycin sulfate, Busulphan, Carmustine, Chlorambucil, Cyclophosphamide, Daunorubicin, Estramustine, Etoposide, Exemestane, Fluorouracil, Flutamide, Fosfestrol, Goserelin, Hydroxyurea, Idarubicin, Letrozole, Leuprorelin, Medroxyprogesterone, Megestrol, Melphalan, Mercaptopurine, Methotrexate, Paclitaxel, Tamoxifen, Temozolomide, Toremifene, Trilostane,

VINCA ALKALOIDS.

Many other medications are being used experimentally, in trials, or are coming onto the market for brief periods.

Candesartan

See ANGIOTENSIN II RECEPTOR ANTAGONISTS

Cannabis

See Marijuana

Capsaicin

TRADE NAME

Axsain, Zacin.

DRUG CLASS

Rubefacient, analgesic.

USES

Nerve pain in skin after shingles, diabetic nerve pain, arthritic joint pain.

DOSAGE

 Apply to affected area three or four times a day.

FORMS

Cream.

PRECAUTIONS

Safe in pregnancy, breast feeding and children over two years.

Avoid eyes, mouth, nose, anus and vagina.

Avoid broken or infected skin.

SIDE EFFECTS

Common: Minimal

Unusual: Burning, skin irritation.

INTERACTIONS

None significant

PRESCRIPTION

Yes

PERMITTED IN SPORT

Yes

OTHER INFORMATION

Becoming less relevant as more effective treatments for acute shingles (eg: Aciclovir) to prevent nerve pain have become available. Still useful for minor arthritic pain.

Captopril

See ACE INHIBITORS

Carbachol

TRADE NAME

Isopto Carbachol (with Hypromellose).

DRUG CLASS

Miotic

USES

Glaucoma, eye surgery

DOSAGE

 Two drops three times a day.

FORMS

Eye drops.

PRECAUTIONS

May be used in pregnancy, breast feeding and children.

Avoid exceeding recommended dose.

Use with caution in heart failure, asthma, stomach ulcer, over active thyroid gland, Parkinson's disease, gut spasm, difficulty in passing urine.

 Do not use if:
• Eye injured or grazed.

SIDE EFFECTS

Common: Blurred vision, constriction of pupil, headache.

Uncommon: Heart disturbances, gut disturbances.

INTERACTIONS

None significant.

PRESCRIPTION

Yes

PERMITTED IN SPORT

Yes

OVERDOSE

Seek medical attention if swallowed. Antidote available.

See also Acetylcholine chloride

Carbamazepine

TRADE NAME

Tegretol.

DRUG CLASS

Anticonvulsant.

USES

Epilepsy, manic states, mood stabilisation, trigeminal neuralgia (tic douloureux), other forms of neuralgia (nerve pain).

DOSAGE

 Dosage increased slowly under medical supervision until desired effect obtained. Maximum 1200mg. a day. Blood tests help check on dose required.

FORMS

Tablets of 100, 200 and 400mg. (white), controlled release tablet of 200mg. (orange) and 400mg. (brown), suspension, suppositories.

PRECAUTIONS

Not to be used in pregnancy (D) unless medically essential as risk of foetal abnormality is increased by 300%. Breast feeding should be ceased before use. May be used in children over 5 years.

Use with caution in heart disease, glaucoma, psychiatric conditions, prostate disease, kidney and liver disease.

Use with caution in elderly.

Regular blood tests to check liver and kidney function and blood cells recommended.

Do not stop suddenly, but reduce dose slowly.

 Do not take if:

- suffering from heart block, lupus erythematosus, liver failure, porphyria, bone marrow suppression.
- sensitive to Tricyclic antidepressants.
- drinking alcohol.

SIDE EFFECTS

Common: Some side effects are very common for the first few days then get less. Drowsiness, incoordination, reduced alertness, dizziness, double vision, headache, nausea, skin reactions.

Unusual: Vomiting, hallucinations, depression, dry mouth, fluid retention.

Severe but rare (stop medication, consult doctor): Unusual bleeding or bruising.

INTERACTIONS

Other drugs:

- Other anticonvulsants, Oral contraceptives, MAOI within 14 days, Warfarin

Other substances:

- Reacts adversely with alcohol.

PRESCRIPTION

Yes

PERMITTED IN SPORT

Yes

OVERDOSE

Serious. Symptoms very varied but may include vomiting, low blood pressure, rapid heart rate, agitation, hallucinations, blurred vision, coma and death. Administer activated charcoal or induce vomiting if medication recently taken and patient alert. Seek urgent medical assistance.

OTHER INFORMATION

Used for many decades to control epilepsy and neuralgia. Not addictive or dependence forming. Does not cause dependence or addiction.

Carbaryl

TRADE NAME

Carylderm.

USES

Head lice..

DOSAGE

 Apply once to affected hair. Leave for 12 hours before washing out.

FORMS

Lotion, liquid.

PRECAUTIONS

Safe to use in pregnancy, breast feeding and children.

Use with caution under six months of age.

Not for continued or repeated use.

Avoid eyes and areas of broken skin or eczema.

SIDE EFFECTS

Common: Scalp irritation.

INTERACTIONS

Other drugs:

• None significant.

PRESCRIPTION

Yes

PERMITTED IN SPORT

Yes

OVERDOSE

If swallowed seek urgent medical attention. Administer activated charcoal or induce vomiting if medication recently taken and patient alert.

Carbenoxolone

TRADE NAME

Bioplex.

Pyrogastrone (with Antacids).

USES

Heals mouth ulcers.

DOSAGE

 Use mouthwash four times a day after meals, reflux oesophagitis (heartburn).

FORMS

Bioplex: Granules to make mouthwash.
Pyrogastrone: Tablets, liquid.

PRECAUTIONS

Bioplex: Safe in pregnancy, breast feeding and children. Seek medical advice if mouth ulcer not healed in two weeks. Do not swallow mouthwash.

Pyrogastrone: Not for use in pregnancy, breast feeding or children. Use with caution in water and salt retention.

Do not take Pyrogarstone if:

• suffering from heart, liver or kidney failure.

• blood potassium level low

• elderly

SIDE EFFECTS

Bioplex: Minimal Pyrogastrone: Swelling of hands and feet, low blood potassium levels, high blood pressure.

Severe but rare (stop medication, consult doctor): Heart failure.

INTERACTIONS

None significant. Antacids in Pyrogastrone interact with a wide range of medications.

PRESCRIPTION

Yes

PERMITTED IN SPORT

Yes

Carbidopa

See LEVODOPA COMPOUNDS

Carbimazole

TRADE NAME

Neomercazole.

DRUG CLASS

Antithyroid.

USES

Over active thyroid gland.

DOSAGE

 20 to 60mg. a day in divided doses, strictly as directed by doctor.

FORMS

Tablets (pink) of 5mg. and 20mg

PRECAUTIONS

Not to be used in pregnancy (C) or breast feeding. Use in children only if medically essential.

SIDE EFFECTS

Common: Dose related.

Unusual: Nausea, headache, rash.

INTERACTIONS

None significant

PRESCRIPTION

Yes

PERMITTED IN SPORT

Yes

OVERDOSE

Rash likely. Damage to bone marrow possible.

OTHER INFORMATION

Often used to control overactive thyroid gland before surgery to remove gland, or irradiation to destroy gland.

Carbocisteine

TRADE NAME

Mucodyne

DRUG CLASS

Mucolytic

USES

Excessive thick mucus, glue ears, tracheostomy clearance in children.

DOSAGE

 Initially 750mg three times a day, reducing to 500mg. three times a day.

PRECAUTIONS

Use with caution in pregnancy. Safe to use in children.

Use with caution if past history of peptic ulcer.

 Do not take if:
• suffering from active peptic ulcer.

FORMS

Syrup, capsules.

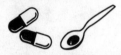

SIDE EFFECTS

Common: Nausea, diarrhoea, rash.

Severe but rare (stop medication, consult doctor): Peptic ulcer.

INTERACTIONS

None significant.

PRESCRIPTION

Yes (very restricted on NHS)

PERMITTED IN SPORT

Yes

OVERDOSE

Significant stomach irritation possible.

Carbomer 940

See EYE LUBRICANTS

Carboxymethylcellulose

TRADE NAME

Glandosane, Luborant.

USES

Artificial saliva for dry mouth.

DOSAGE

 Use spray as required, normally three or four times a day.

FORMS

Mouth spray.

PRECAUTIONS

Safe to use in pregnancy and breast feeding.

Use with caution in children.

SIDE EFFECTS

Minimal.

INTERACTIONS

None significant.

PRESCRIPTION

No

PERMITTED IN SPORT

Yes

OVERDOSE

Unlikely to have serious effects.

OTHER INFORMATION

Normally used after radiotherapy to the mouth and throat, or in the Sicca syndrome, but may also be useful in the elderly to moisturise the mouth.

CARDIAC GLYCOSIDE

(Regulate heart beat)

See Digoxin

Carisoprodol

TRADE NAME

Carisoma

DRUG CLASS

Muscle relaxant.

USES

Muscle spasms.

DOSAGE

 125 to 350mg. three times a day.

FORMS

Tablets of 125 and 350mg. (white).

PRECAUTIONS

Not for use in pregnancy, breast feeding or children.

Reduce dose in elderly.

Use with caution in liver or kidney disease, alcoholism or history of drug dependence.

Avoid long term use. Do not stop suddenly but reduce dose gradually.

 Do not take if:

• suffering from acute intermittent porphyria.

SIDE EFFECTS

Common: Drowsiness, dizziness, nausea. flushes, headache, constipation.

Unusual: Rash.

INTERACTIONS

Other drugs:

• Sedatives, Hypnotics, Anticoagulants, Contraceptive pills, Steroids, Phenytoin, Griseofulvin, Tricyclic antidepressants, Phenothiazines, Rifampicin.

Other substances:

• Alcohol.

PRESCRIPTION

Yes

PERMITTED IN SPORT

Yes

OVERDOSE

Exacerbation of side effects likely. Induce vomiting or administer activated charcoal if swallowed recently. Seek medical attention.

OTHER INFORMATION

May cause dependence if used inappropriately.

Carmellose sodium

TRADE NAME

Orabase, Orahesive (with Pectin and Gelatin).

USES

Mouth ulcers and ulcers on other moist body surfaces (eg. vagina).

DOSAGE

 Cover affected area as necessary.

FORMS

Ointment, powder.

PRECAUTIONS

Safe in pregnancy, breast feeding and children.

No specific precautions.

SIDE EFFECTS

None significant.

INTERACTIONS

None significant.

PRESCRIPTION
No

PERMITTED IN SPORT
Yes

OVERDOSE
Diarrhoea only likely effect if swallowed.

OTHER INFORMATION
Sometimes used in other forms as an eye lubricant.

Carmustine

TRADE NAME
Bicnu.

DRUG CLASS
Antineoplastic.

USES
Hodgkin's disease, multiple myeloma, lymphomas, some types of brain cancer, palliation of other cancers.

DOSAGE
 As determined by doctor for each patient.

PRECAUTIONS
Must not be used in pregnancy (D) or breast feeding. Adequate contraception essential.

Blood tests must be performed regularly to monitor liver function and blood cells.

Use with caution in lung disease.

 Do not take if:
- suffering from bleeding disorders due to low platelet count.

FORMS
Injection.

SIDE EFFECTS
Common: Liver and kidney damage, lung damage.

Unusual: Numerous possibilities that should be discussed with your doctor.

INTERACTIONS
None significant.

PRESCRIPTION
Yes

PERMITTED IN SPORT
Yes

OVERDOSE
Serious organ damage likely. Only given under strict medical supervision.

Carteolol
See BETA BLOCKERS

Carvedilol

TRADE NAME
Eucardic.

DRUG CLASS
Beta-blocker.

USES
Heart failure, prevention of angina, high blood pressure.

DOSAGE

 Start with 12.5mg. twice a day with food. Increase dose slowly to maximum of 25mg. twice a day (may be higher for very heavy patients).

FORMS

Tablets of 12.5 and 25mg.

PRECAUTIONS

Should not be used in pregnancy (C) unless essential for the mother's health. Use with considerable caution in breast feeding and children.

Use with caution in poor circulation to hands and feet, kidney disease, diabetes, overactive thyroid gland.

Do not stop medication suddenly, but reduce dose slowly.

 Do not take if:

- suffering from asthma, slow heart rate, low blood pressure, heart block, poor liver function.

SIDE EFFECTS

Common: Tissue swelling, slow heart rate, low blood pressure, dizziness, diarrhoea, nausea.

Unusual: Vomiting, ankle swelling, joint pain, muscle pain, blurred vision, fainting, chest pain.

Severe but rare (stop medication, consult doctor): Unusual bleeding, wheezing, shortness of breath.

INTERACTIONS

Other drugs:

- Rifampicin, Cimetidine, Clonidine, Calcium Channel Blockers, Hypoglycaemics, Insulin, Quinidine, Paroxetine, Fluoxetine, Digoxin, MAOI, Reserpine, other Beta Blockers.

Other substances:

- Grapefruit.

PRESCRIPTION

Yes

PERMITTED IN SPORT

No

OVERDOSE

Low blood pressure, fainting, slow heart rate, seizures, reduced breathing, collapse, heart failure and death may occur. Lie patient flat on side in coma position. Induce vomiting or administer activated charcoal if swallowed recently. Seek urgent medical attention.

OTHER INFORMATION

Introduced in 1998, mainly to treat more difficult cases of heart failure,

See also BETA BLOCKERS.

Cefaclor, Cefadroxil, Cefamandole, Cefoixime, Cefotaxime, Cefoxitin, Cefpiromine, Cefpodoxime, Cefprozil, Ceftazidime, Ceftriaxone, Cefuroxime.

See CEPHALOSPORINS

Celecoxib

TRADE NAME

Celebrex.

DRUG CLASS

COX-2 Inhibitor.

USES

Rheumatoid arthritis and osteoarthritis.

DOSAGE

 200 to 400mg. a day

FORMS

Capsules (white) of 100 and 200 mg.

PRECAUTIONS

Use with considerable caution in pregnancy (B3).

Use with caution in breast feeding and children.

Use with caution with previous peptic ulcer, high blood pressure, fluid retention, heart failure, asthma, dehydration, liver or kidney disease.

Lower doses may be necessary in the elderly and with long term use.

 Do not take if:

• allergic to sulpha drugs

• asthma occurs with NSAID medications or aspirin

SIDE EFFECTS

Common: Fluid retention (swollen feet).

Unusual: Gut irritation, indigestion.

Severe but rare (stop medication, consult doctor): Liver and kidney damage.

INTERACTIONS

Other drugs:

• Non-steroidal anti-inflammatory drugs (NSAID), steroids, anticoagulants, diuretics, ACE inhibitors, lithium, antacids, fluconazole.

PRESCRIPTION

Yes

PERMITTED IN SPORT

Yes

OVERDOSE

Lethargy, drowsiness, nausea, vomiting and indigestion may occur. Give activated charcoal. Seek medical attention.

OTHER INFORMATION

Revolutionary new class of medications first released in 1999 to treat all forms of arthritis and inflammation with much reduced side effects.

See also NSAID; Rofecoxib

Celiprolol

See BETA BLOCKERS

Cellulose, sodium phosphate

See Sodium cellulose phosphate

Cephalexin

See CEPHALOSPORINS

CEPHALOSPORINS

TRADE and GENERIC NAMES

Baxan (Cefadroxil).

Cefrom (Cefpirome).

Cefzil (Cefprozil).

Ceporex, Keflex (Cephalexin).

Claforan (Cefotaxime).

Distaclor (Cefaclor).

Fortum, Kefadim (Ceftazidime).

Kefadol (Cefamandole).

Kefzol (Cephazolin).

Metoxin (Cefoxitin).

Orelox (Cefpodoxime).

Rocephin (Ceftriaxone).

Suprax (Cefixime).

Velosef (Cephadrine).

Zinacef, Zinnat (Cefuroxime).

DRUG CLASS

Antibiotic, broad spectrum.

USES

Treats infections caused by susceptible bacteria.

DOSAGE

 One or two capsules two to four times a day.

FORMS

Capsules, tablets, suspension, injection.

PRECAUTIONS

Safe to use in pregnancy (Cephalexin - A, other forms - B1), breast feeding and children.

Use with caution in severe kidney disease and colitis (inflammation of large bowel).

Use short term if possible.

SIDE EFFECTS

Common: Diarrhoea,

Unusual: Nausea, vomiting, belly pain, rash.

Severe but rare (stop medication, consult doctor): Bloody diarrhoea, severe itchy rash, yellow skin (jaundice).

INTERACTIONS

Other drugs:

• Diuretics, other Cephalosporins.

Other substances:

• May cause false positive test for sugar in urine.

PRESCRIPTION

Yes

PERMITTED IN SPORT

Yes

OVERDOSE

Exacerbation of side effects only likely effect.

OTHER INFORMATION

Very effective antibiotics, used particularly in skin, lung, sinus, ear, kidney and bladder infections. Does not cause dependence or addiction.

Cephazolin, Cephradine

See CEPHALOSPORINS

Cerivastatin

TRADE NAME

Lipobay

DRUG CLASS

Hypolipidaemic.

USES

Lowers blood fat (cholesterol and triglyceride) levels.

DOSAGE

 100 to 400mcg. in evening.

FORMS

Tablets of 100, 200, 300 and 400mcg.

PRECAUTIONS

Not to be used in pregnancy (C) or breast feeding. Ensure adequate contraception.

Use with caution in children.

Use with caution in alcoholism.

Regular blood tests to check liver function and blood fat levels advisable.

 Do not take if:

- suffering from liver disease or abnormal liver function blood tests.

SIDE EFFECTS

Common: Belly pain, headache, nausea, diarrhoea, tiredness.

Unusual: Liver damage, muscle and joint pain, sleeplessness, pins and needles sensation, dizziness

Severe but rare (stop medication, consult doctor): Muscle and eye damage.

INTERACTIONS

Other drugs:

- Erythromycin, Cholestyramine, Cyclosporin, Nicotinic acid, some antifungals, Rifampicin, Phenytoin.

Other substances:

- Alcohol.

PRESCRIPTION

Yes

PERMITTED IN SPORT

Yes

OVERDOSE

Liver damage possible.

Cetalkonium chloride

TRADE NAME

Only available in combination with other medications.

Bonjela (with Choline salicylate).

DRUG CLASS

Antiseptic.

USES

Mouth and gum irritation, teething.

DOSAGE

 Apply to gums every three hours.

FORMS

Gel.

PRECAUTIONS

Safe in pregnancy, breast feeding, children and infants over four months.

SIDE EFFECTS

Minimal.

INTERACTIONS

Other drugs:

- Aspirin.

PRESCRIPTION

No

PERMITTED IN SPORT

Yes

OTHER INFORMATION

Widely and safely used for infant teething.

Cetirizine

See ANTIHISTAMINES, SEDATING

Cetomacrogol

TRADE NAMES

Found in numerous over the counter skin moisturisers and cosmetics.

DRUG CLASS

Moisturiser

USES

Dry skin, cracked skin, soap substitute.

DOSAGE

 Apply as required.

FORMS

Cream.

PRECAUTIONS

Safe to use in pregnancy, breast feeding and children.

SIDE EFFECTS

None

INTERACTIONS

None

PRESCRIPTION

No

PERMITTED IN SPORT

Yes

OTHER INFORMATION

One of the original moisturising creams that has been available for a century. Cheap and effective.

Cetrimide

TRADE NAMES

Cetavlex, Ceanel (with Undecenoic acid).

Drapolene (with Benzalkonium chloride).

Hibicet, Steripod Yellow, Tisept (with Chlorhexidine).

Siopel (with Dimethicone).

DRUG CLASS

Antiseptic.

USES

Disinfection of skin and medical equipment, acne, minor burns, grazes.

DOSAGE

 Apply or use as required.

FORMS

Cream, wash, lotion, liquid.

PRECAUTIONS

Safe to use in pregnancy, breast feeding and children.

Avoid eye contact.

SIDE EFFECTS

Minimal

INTERACTIONS

None significant

PRESCRIPTION

No

PERMITTED IN SPORT

Yes

OVERDOSE

If swallowed may cause nausea, vomiting, diarrhoea and stomach cramps.

Cetylpyridinium

TRADE NAMES

Merocets Calgel (with Lignocaine).
Merocaine (with Benzocaine).
Also found in numerous locally produced over the counter antiseptic preparations.

DRUG CLASS

Antiseptic.

USES

Prevention of infection, treatment of minor infections, teething in infants.

DOSAGE

 Use up to six times a day as directed by instructions on packaging.

FORMS

Lozenges, gel, gargle.

PRECAUTIONS

Safe to use in pregnancy (A), breast feeding and children.

Use with caution under three years.

SIDE EFFECTS

None significant

INTERACTIONS

None significant

PRESCRIPTION

No

PERMITTED IN SPORT

Yes

OVERDOSE

Swallowing gargle or lozenges may cause belly discomfort, nausea and diarrhoea.

Chamomile

TRADE NAME

Kamillosan
Also used in herbal drinks and other soothing preparations.

USES

Chapped skin, nappy rash, sore nipples.

DOSAGE

 Apply two to four times a day.

FORMS

Ointment.

PRECAUTIONS

Safe in pregnancy, breast feeding and children.

SIDE EFFECTS

None significant.

INTERACTIONS

None significant.

PRESCRIPTION

No

PERMITTED IN SPORT

Yes

OVERDOSE

Swallowing ointment has no serious effects.

Charcoal

TRADE NAME

Actidose-Aqua, Carbomix, Charcodote, Liqui-Char, Medicoal (activated charcoal).

Also available in numerous brands as tablets and capsules.

USES

Excessive amounts of burping, excessive passing of wind, gassy discomfort of stomach, may absorb some forms of poison, drug overdosage.

DOSAGE

 Poisoning: 50 to 100g as a single dose.
Other: 200 to 1200 mg up to four times a day.

FORMS

Suspension, granules, capsules, tablets (store capsules away from heat and moisture).

SIDE EFFECTS

Common: May alter bowel habits.

INTERACTIONS

Other drugs:

• Reduces absorption of many medications.

Other substances:

• Reduces absorption of some foods.

PRECAUTIONS

Safe in pregnancy and breast feeding. Not for use under three years of age.

Do not take from one hour before to two hours after a meal.

 Do not take if:

• taking other medications as charcoal may interfere with absorption of many types of medication.

• suffering from diarrhoea.

PRESCRIPTION

No

PERMITTED IN SPORT

Yes

OVERDOSE

Diarrhoea only likely result. No specific treatment necessary.

OTHER INFORMATION

One of the oldest medications known to mankind, and probably used since prehistoric times for stomach wind and discomfort. Very effective in reducing amount of toxic material absorbed in overdosage of medication or in poisoning. See section on First Aid at front of book.

Chloral betaine

See Chloral hydrate

Chloral hydrate

(Chloral betaine)

TRADE NAME

Welldorm

DRUG CLASS

Sedative, hypnotic.

USES

Insomnia (sleeplessness).

DOSAGE

 One or two tablets at night.

FORMS

Tablet (purple).

PRECAUTIONS

Not to be used in pregnancy and breast feeding.

Use with caution in children.

Should not be used long term.

 Do not take if:

- suffering from porphyria, severe liver or kidney disease, significant heart disease, gastritis (inflamed stomach).

SIDE EFFECTS

Common: Nausea, headache.

Unusual: Vomiting, bloating, passing excess wind, rash.

Severe but rare (stop medication, consult doctor): Allergies, bleeding disorders, blood cell damage.

INTERACTIONS

Other drugs:

- Other sedatives, Anticoagulants, Anticholinergics.

Other substances:

- Alcohol.

PRESCRIPTION

Yes

PERMITTED IN SPORT

Yes

OVERDOSE

Serious. Seek urgent medical attention. Liver and other organ damage possible.

OTHER INFORMATION

Very old fashioned medication that has largely been replaced by more reliable and safer sedatives.

See also **HYPNOTICS** and **SEDATIVES**

Chlorambucil

TRADE NAME

Leukeran.

DRUG CLASS

Alkyllater.

USES

Leukaemia, breast and ovary cancer, Hodgkin's disease, lymphoma, other malignant conditions.

DOSAGE

 Complex. Must be individualised by doctor for each patient.

FORMS

Tablets (brown) of 2mg.

PRECAUTIONS

Must not be used in pregnancy (D) unless the life of the mother is at risk as serious damage to the foetus is likely. Breast feeding must be ceased before use. Use in children only when medically essential.

Regular blood tests to monitor blood cells and liver function essential.

Adequate contraception must be used during treatment.

Must be used with extreme caution in all patients.

SIDE EFFECTS

Common: Bone marrow damage.

Unusual: Nausea, vomiting,diarrhoea, mouth ulcers, lung damage, convulsions in children.

Severe but rare (stop medication, consult doctor): Yellow skin (jaundice).

INTERACTIONS

Other drugs:

• Phenylbutazone, other cancer treatments.

PRESCRIPTION

Yes

PERMITTED IN SPORT

Yes

OVERDOSE

May cause damage to blood and bone marrow cells, convulsions, incoordination and irrational behaviour. Administer activated charcoal or induce vomiting if medication taken recently. Seek medical assistance.

OTHER INFORMATION

Although serious side effects are possible, Chlorambucil may be life saving in some patients.

Chloramphenicol

TRADE NAMES

Chloromycetin, Kemicetine, Minims Chloramphenicol, Sno Phenicol.

Actinac (with Hydrocortisone and other ingredients).

DRUG CLASS

Antibiotic.

USES

Very severe infections, eye and skin infections.

DOSAGE

Eye drops: Two drops every three hours
Eye ointment: Insert three times a day
Cream: Apply once or twice a day.

FORMS

Cream, eye ointment, injection, eye drops.

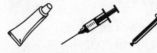

PRECAUTIONS

Eye drops and ointment may be used in pregnancy, breast feeding and children.

Use cream with caution in pregnancy, breast feeding and children.

Injection should not be used in any patient unless no other antibiotic can be successfully used for a severe infection. There are further risks of using injection in pregnancy (C), breast feeding and children.

Never to be used long term.

Use with additional caution in liver and kidney disease.

SIDE EFFECTS

Common: Eye preparations - irritation.

Unusual: Injection - Vomiting, sore mouth, diarrhoea, headache.

Severe but rare: Chloramphenicol can cause (sometimes months after the medication is taken) a severe and usually fatal blood disorder with an incidence between 1:25,000 and 1:100,000 patients using the drug. In children under three months, the "Grey Syndrome" may occur as a result of the undeveloped liver's inability to adequately deal with the drug.

INTERACTIONS

Other drugs:

• Anticonvulsants, Anticoagulants.

PRESCRIPTION

Yes

PERMITTED IN SPORT

Yes

OVERDOSE

Exacerbation of side effects and increased risk of serious reactions possible.

OTHER INFORMATION

Chloramphenicol is a very effective and well tolerated antibiotic, but because if taken by mouth or injection it can rarely cause death by destroying the red blood cells, it is only used when no other antibiotic can control a severe infection. It is widely used in eye and skin preparations quite safely, as the drug is not absorbed in any significant concentration into the blood stream. The use of Chloramphenicol is usually restricted to topical creams and eye preparations. It is used by mouth or injection in certain serious life threatening situations, such as meningitis, when it worth the risk of the rare side effects.

Chlordiazepoxide

TRADE NAME

Librium.

DRUG CLASS

Anxiolytic, benzodiazepine.

USES

Anxiety disorders, acute alcohol withdrawal, relaxation before operations, muscle spasms caused by brain injury.

DOSAGE

 Varies widely from one capsule every few days as required for mild anxiety to 300 mg (30 capsules) a day in several doses for alcohol withdrawal. Most patients would not exceed one 10mg capsule three times a day. Higher dose requires strict medical supervision.

PRECAUTIONS

Should not be used in pregnancy (C) unless essential. Should be used with caution in breast feeding.

Should be used with caution in patients with liver and kidney disease, chronic bronchitis, asthma, emphysema.

Should not be ceased suddenly in epileptics as this may cause a convulsion.

Should only be used for short periods of time if possible.

Should not be used while driving or operating machinery.

Should be used with caution in elderly patients.

 Do not take if:

• Elderly and suffering from heart failure.

• Suffering from myasthenia gravis, glaucoma, some psychiatric conditions.

FORMS

Capsules of 5mg and 10mg.

SIDE EFFECTS

Common: Drowsiness, confusion, poor coordination.

Unusual: Rash, swelling, irregular periods, nausea, constipation, decreased sex drive.

Severe but rare (stop medication, consult doctor):Patient becomes violent and irrational, jaundice (yellow skin) develops.

INTERACTIONS

Other drugs:

• Reacts with Barbiturates, Sedatives, Anti-depressants, Phenothiazines, Antihistamines and muscle relaxants to cause sedation.

• Reacts with Cimetidine and Disulfiram to cause increased effect of Chlordiazepoxide.

• Reacts with Anticonvulsants to change their effectiveness.

Other substances:

• Reacts with alcohol to cause sedation.

PRESCRIPTION

Yes

PERMITTED IN SPORT

Yes

OVERDOSE

May cause drowsiness, coma and very rarely death. First aid involves inducing vomiting and seeking urgent medical attention.

OTHER INFORMATION

May cause dependence if used long term. One of the older and more potent Benzodiazepines.

Chlorhexidine

TRADE NAMES

Bactigras Corsodyl, CX Powder, Hibiscrub, Hibisol, Hibitane'serotulle, Steripod Pink, Unisept, Uriflex C, Uro-Tainer.

Dermol (with Paraffin, Benzalkonium chloride and other ingredients).

Hibicet, Steripod Yellow, Tisept (with Cetrimide).

Instillagel (with Lignocaine and other ingredients).

Naseptin (with Neomycin).

Nystaform (with Nystatin).

Also found in other locally produced antiseptics.

DRUG CLASS

Antiseptic

USES

Prevention of infection, skin cleaning, minor infections of skin and mouth.

DOSAGE

 Depends on form. Normally use several times a day.

PRECAUTIONS

Safe to use in pregnancy (A), breast feeding and children.

Avoid eye contact.

Use with caution on open wounds and in nose, mouth and ears.

FORMS

Cream, solution, wash, oil, powder, tincture, gel, mouth wash, tulle (netting).

SIDE EFFECTS

Minimal

INTERACTIONS

Other drugs:

• None significant

Other substances:

• Detergents

PRESCRIPTION

No

PERMITTED IN SPORT

Yes

OVERDOSE

Diarrhoea, belly discomfort and vomiting only likely effects if swallowed. Seek medical advice, particularly in children.

OTHER INFORMATION

The most widely used antiseptic cleansing agent in hospitals, general practice and operating theatres. Very safe and effective.

Chlormethiazole

TRADE NAME

Heminevrin.

DRUG CLASS

Hypnotic, sedative.

USES

Control of alcohol withdrawal and delirium tremens, short term control of extreme agitation and confusion.

DOSAGE

 One capsule or 5mls. three times a day, then reduce dosage slowly, ceasing within ten days. Higher doses sometimes given initially. Only prescribed in circumstances of strict medical supervision.

FORMS

Capsules, syrup, infusion.

PRECAUTIONS

Safe in pregnancy (A). Breast feeding should be ceased if medication necessary. Not for use in children.

Lower doses required in elderly.

Caution needed in patients with heart disease, and severe liver disease.

 Do not take if:

• suffering from severe lung disease.

• operating machinery, driving vehicles, or undertaking tasks requiring coordination, concentration and alertness.

SIDE EFFECTS

Common: Drowsiness, nasal irritation, eye irritation, facial burning.

Unusual: Rash, red skin, itch, excessive phlegm in throat.

INTERACTIONS

Other drugs:

• Propranolol, Cimetidine.

Other substances:

• Reacts adversely with alcohol.

PRESCRIPTION

Yes

PERMITTED IN SPORT

Yes

OVERDOSE

Low blood pressure, low body temperature, slow heart rate and coma may occur. Symptoms worse if taken with alcohol. Rarely fatal. Administer activated charcoal or induce vomiting if patient alert and tablets taken recently. Seek urgent medical attention.

OTHER INFORMATION

Rarely used outside hospital. Very useful in very disturbed patients or alcohol withdrawal. Addictive.

Chloroquine

TRADE NAME

Avloclor, Nivaquine.

DRUG CLASS

Antimalarial.

USES

Prevention and treatment of malaria, treatment of rheumatoid arthritis, amoebic hepatitis, systemic lupus erythematosus (SLE).

DOSAGE

 Malaria prevention: Two tablets on same day once a week for two weeks before and four weeks after entering malarious area.
Treatment: Start with high daily dose and slowly decrease as directed by doctor.

FORMS

Tablets

PRECAUTIONS

Not to be used in pregnancy (D) unless mother's life threatened by severe malaria. May be used in breast feeding and children over one year.

Use with caution in liver and kidney disease, psoriasis and porphyria.

Regular eye checks required if used daily long term.

 Do not take if:

• suffering from alcoholism.

• trying to become pregnant.

SIDE EFFECTS

Common: Minimal.

Unusual: Nausea, vomiting, diarrhoea, skin pigmentation, hair loss, rash.

Severe but rare (stop medication, consult doctor): Deteriorating vision.

INTERACTIONS

Other drugs:

• Nil significant.

Other substances:

• Reacts with alcohol.

PRESCRIPTION

Yes

PERMITTED IN SPORT

Yes

OVERDOSE

Very serious. Depresses the function of the heart and lungs, and may cause fatal liver damage. Administer activated charcoal or induce vomiting if taken recently. Seek urgent medical assistance.

OTHER INFORMATION

Chloroquine is the traditional mainstay for the prevention of malaria, but malaria in many areas (including most of southeast Asia and New Guinea) is now resistant to Chloroquine. Found serendipitously to assist in the treatment of rheumatoid and other autoimmune diseases. Very dangerous to the foetus in pregnancy, and in overdose.

Chloroxylenol

TRADE NAME

Zeasorb (with other ingredients).

DRUG CLASS

Antiseptic.

USES

Minor skin cuts and grazes, minor skin infections.

DOSAGE

 Apply as required.

FORMS

Powder.

PRECAUTIONS

Safe in pregnancy, breast feeding and children.

Do not use for prolonged period.

Avoid eye contact.

SIDE EFFECTS

Minimal

INTERACTIONS

None significant

PRESCRIPTION

No

PERMITTED IN SPORT

Yes

Chlorpheniramine

See ANTIHISTAMINES, SEDATING

Chlorpromazine

See PHENOTHIAZINES

Chlortetracycline

TRADE NAME

Aureomycin.

Aureocort (with Triamcinolone).

Declo (with Tetracycline, Demeclocycline).

DRUG CLASS

Tetracycline, antibiotic.

USES

Bacterial skin infections, acne.

DOSAGE

 Ointment: Apply once or twice a day.
Tablets: Take one twice a day.

FORMS

Ointment, tablet

PRECAUTIONS

External use during pregnancy (D) is unlikely to cause the serious adverse effects on the foetus that may occur if Tetracyclines are taken internally. May be used in breast feeding, but not on the breast. Use with caution in children.

Seek further medical advice if infection does not settle rapidly.

SIDE EFFECTS

Ointment: None significant Tablets: Nausea, diarrhoea, rash.

Severe but rare (stop medication, consult doctor): Severe headache.

INTERACTIONS

Ointment:

• None significant Tablets:

• Oral contraceptives, Antacids, Penicillins, Anticoagulants.

• Milk, mineral supplements.

PRESCRIPTION

Yes

PERMITTED IN SPORT

Yes

OTHER INFORMATION

Very safe and effective antibiotic for skin use. Widely used. Available for over forty years.

Chlorthalidone
See THIAZIDE DIURETICS

Cholecalciferol, Calcitriol and Ergocalciferol
(Vitamin D)

TRADE NAMES

Vitamin D consists of a number of chemicals including Cholecalciferol, Calcitriol and Ergocalciferol.

It is found in many non-presciption mineral and vitamin supplements, and on prescription as **Calcijex** and **Rocaltrol** (Calcitriol).

DRUG CLASS

Fat soluble essential vitamin.

USES

Nutritional deficiency, osteomalacia, rickets, hypoparathyroidism, osteoporosis.

DOSAGE

 Daily requirement is 5mcg. Much higher doses used to treat diseases listed above.

FORMS

Tablets, capsules, injection.

PRECAUTIONS

Safe for use pregnancy, breast feeding and children. Use with caution in infants.

Use with caution in kidney disease.

SIDE EFFECTS

Common: Drowsiness, constipation.

Unusual: Calcium deposits in tissue, dehydration.

INTERACTIONS

Other drugs:

• Cholestyramine, Thiazide diuretics, Digoxin, Magnesium.

PRESCRIPTION

Calcijex, Rocaltrol: Yes
Other forms: No

PERMITTED IN SPORT

Yes

OVERDOSE

Serious. Symptoms include loss of appetite, tiredness, vomiting, diarrhoea, sweating, excess urine production, extreme thirst and headache. This may progress to high blood pressure and kidney failure. Administer activated charcoal or induce vomiting if taken recently. Seek medical assistance.

OTHER INFORMATION

Remember, vitamins are merely chemicals that are essential in minute doses for the functioning of the body, and if taken to excess, act as a drug. Vitamin D can be found naturally in fatty fish (sardines, tuna, salmon, herrings etc.), margarine and egg yolk. It is also produced in the body by the action of sunlight on the skin.

CHOLESTEROL LOWERING DRUGS (HYPOLIPIDAEMICS)

See Acipimox, Atorvastatin, Cerivastatin, Cholestyramine, Ciprofibrate, Colestipol, Fenofibrate, Fluvastatin, Gemfibrizol, Pravastatin, Simvastatin

Cholestyramine

TRADE NAME

Questran.

DRUG CLASS

Hypolipidaemic.

USES

High blood cholesterol level, relief of itch caused by liver failure, relief of diarrhoea caused by small intestine disease.

DOSAGE

 4g. to 16g. of powder per day with copious fluids in divided doses through the day.

FORMS

Powder

PRECAUTIONS

Should be used with caution in pregnancy (B2). Not to be used in breast feeding. Use with caution in children.

May interfere with vitamin absorption.

Lower doses required in elderly.

 Do not take if:
- suffering from gall bladder obstruction, phenylketonuria.

SIDE EFFECTS

Common: Constipation.

Unusual: Belly discomfort, excess wind, vomiting, heartburn, loss of appetite, rash, osteoporosis.

Severe but rare (stop medication, consult doctor): Unusual bleeding.

INTERACTIONS

Other drugs:

- Other medications should be taken 30 minutes before Cholestyramine or four to six hours after Cholestyramine.

- Warfarin, Digoxin, Phenylbutazone, Chlorthiazide.

PRESCRIPTION

Yes

PERMITTED IN SPORT

Yes

OVERDOSE

No significant problems. Severe constipation probable.

OTHER INFORMATION

One of the earlier forms of treatment for excess blood cholesterol. Effective, but patient compliance often poor due to taste and method of taking.

Choline salicylate

See SALICYLATES

Choline theophyllinate

See THEOPHYLLINES

Chorionic gonadotrophin, human (HCG)

TRADE NAME

Pregnyl, Profasi.

DRUG CLASS

Sex hormone.

USES

Infertility in women, delayed puberty in girls, failure of testicular development, failure of sperm production.

DOSAGE

 As determined for each patient by doctor.

FORMS

Injection.

PRECAUTIONS

Do not use before puberty.

May cause multiple foetus pregnancy.

Use with caution in fluid retention.

Not normally used for more than six months.

 Do not take if:
- suffering from some types of cancer affecting sex organs.

SIDE EFFECTS

Common: Minimal.

Unusual: Multiple foetus pregnancy, fluid retention, rash.

INTERACTIONS

None significant.

PRESCRIPTION

Yes

PERMITTED IN SPORT

No

OVERDOSE

Not likely to be serious. Given under strict medical supervision.

Cilastatin and Imipenem

TRADE NAME

Primaxin (only available as combination of the two medications).

DRUG CLASS

Antibiotic.

USES

Serious bacterial infections of the lungs, belly, pelvis, bones, joints, heart and blood stream.

DOSAGE

 Administered by a slow infusion through a drip into a vein, or deep injection into muscle. Dosage determined by doctor.

FORMS

Injection.

PRECAUTIONS

Use with caution in pregnancy (B3), breast feeding and infants.

Safe to use in children.

Use with caution in kidney disease, colitis, meningitis, brain abscess and other brain diseases.

Not for long term use.

Regular blood tests necessary during use to monitor blood and liver.

SIDE EFFECTS

Common: Rash, itch, other infections, fever, abnormal taste.

Unusual: Seizures, confusion, dizziness, tiredness, nausea, diarrhoea.

Severe but rare (stop medication, consult doctor): Vein inflammation, low blood pressure, pseudomembranous colitis (bowel inflammation), abnormal blood cells, abnormal liver function.

INTERACTIONS

Other drugs:

• Other antibiotics, Ganciclovir, Probenecid.

PRESCRIPTION

Yes

PERMITTED IN SPORT

Yes

OTHER INFORMATION

Introduced in 1999 for the treatment of serious infections that do not respond to other antibiotics.

Ciliazapril

See ACE INHIBITORS

Cimetidine

TRADE NAMES

Dyspamet, Tagamet, Zita.

DRUG CLASS

Antiulcerant, H2 receptor antagonist.

USES

Prevention and treatment of ulcers of the stomach, oesophagus (gullet) and duodenum (upper small intestine). Prevention of acid reflux into the oesophagus (heartburn).

DOSAGE

 Up to 1600mg a day in one, two or three doses.

FORMS

Tablets, soluble tablets, syrup, injection.

PRECAUTIONS

Care should be taken with use in pregnancy (B1) and breast feeding. Children under twelve may be treated at the discretion of the doctor.

 Do not take if:

• suffering from severe kidney disease or phenylketonuria.

SIDE EFFECTS

Common: Headache, diarrhoea, tiredness, dizziness, drowsiness, rash.

Unusual: Constipation, breast enlargement and tenderness (both sexes), confusion in elderly.

Severe but rare (stop medication, consult doctor): Hepatitis (jaundice - yellow skin), pancreatitis (severe stomach pain), rapid or irregular heart beat.

INTERACTIONS

Other drugs:

• Toxicity may result with Warfarin, Phenytoin, Lignocaine, Theophylline, Quinidine, Procainamide, Flecainide, Nifedipine.

• Effectiveness of many medications affecting the heart, blood pressure and diabetes may be altered.

Other substances:

• No reaction with alcohol, caffeine, exercise etc.

PRESCRIPTION

Yes

PERMITTED IN SPORT

Yes

OVERDOSE

No serious effects reported.

OTHER INFORMATION

Introduced in 1978, cimetidine was the first of a group of drugs (H2 antagonists) that radically improved the treatment of peptic ulcers. It is very safe, and available without prescription in some countries.

Cinchocaine
See ANAESTHETICS, LOCAL

Cinnarizine

TRADE NAME

Stugeron.

DRUG CLASS

Sedating antihistamine.

USES

Poor circulation to hands and feet, Raynaud's disease, dizziness, motion sickness.

DOSAGE

 15 to 75 mg., two or three times a day.

FORMS

Tablet of 15mg. (white), capsule of 75mg. (orange/cream).

PRECAUTIONS

Use with caution in pregnancy and breast feeding.

Safe to use in children in low doses.

Not for use in infants.

Use with caution in low blood pressure and Parkinson's disease.

SIDE EFFECTS

Common: Drowsiness.

Unusual: Rash.

INTERACTIONS

Other drugs:

• Sedatives and Antidepressants.

Other substances:

• Alcohol.

PRESCRIPTION

No

PERMITTED IN SPORT

Yes

OVERDOSE

May result in convulsions, hallucinations, delirium, anxiety, muscle spasms, rapid heart rate, flushing, dry skin, dry mouth and coma. First aid involved inducing vomiting and seeking urgent medical attention.

See also ANTIHISTAMINES, SEDATING

Cinoxacin

TRADE NAME

Cinobac.

DRUG CLASS

Quinolone antibiotic.

USES

Urinary infections (eg. cystitis, pyelonephritis).

DOSAGE

 One capsule twice a day.

FORMS

Capsule 500mg. (orange/green).

PRECAUTIONS

Not to be used in pregnancy (C), breast feeding and children.

Use with caution in poor kidney and liver function.

 Do not take if:

• suffering from severe kidney disease.

SIDE EFFECTS

Common: Rash, nausea, diarrhoea.

Unusual: Vomiting, restlessness, tremor, headache, dizziness, itch.

INTERACTIONS

Other drugs:

• NSAID, Warfarin, Theophylline.

PRESCRIPTION

Yes

PERMITTED IN SPORT

Yes

OVERDOSE

Exacerbation of side effects most likely. Administer activated charcoal or induce vomiting if medication taken recently.

See also QUINOLONE ANTIBIOTICS

Ciprofibrate

TRADE NAME

Modalim.

DRUG CLASS

Hypolipidaemic.

USES

High blood fat (eg. cholesterol and triglyceride) levels.

DOSAGE

 One tablet a day.

FORMS

Tablets of 100mg. (white).

PRECAUTIONS

Use in pregnancy (B3) only if medically essential. Not for use in breast feeding and children.

Use with caution in thyroid disease.

Regular blood tests to check blood fat levels, liver enzymes and blood cells are recommended.

 ## Do not take if:

- suffering from liver or kidney disease.

- trying to get pregnant as drug may reduce fertility.

SIDE EFFECTS

Common: Headache, dizziness, rash, nausea, diarrhoea.

Unusual: Muscle pain, impotence, hair loss, dizziness.

Severe but rare (stop medication, consult doctor): Muscle damage.

INTERACTIONS

Other drugs:

- Warfarin, diabetes medications, oral contraceptives, other medications to lower blood fat levels (Hypolipidaemics).

PRESCRIPTION

Yes

PERMITTED IN SPORT

Yes

OVERDOSE

Exacerbation of side effects most likely. Administer activated charcoal or induce vomiting if medication taken recently.

See also HYPOLIPIDAEMICS

Ciprofloxacin

TRADE NAME

Ciproxin, Ciloxan.

DRUG CLASS

Quinolone antibiotic.

USES

Serious bacterial infections.

DOSAGE

 Tablets: One to three tablets twice a day
Eye drops: Two drops every 15 to 60 minutes.

FORMS

Tablets, eye drops, infusion.

PRECAUTIONS

Use in pregnancy (B3) and breast feeding only if medically essential. Not for use in children.

Use with caution in cystic fibrosis and kidney disease.

Designed for short term use.

SIDE EFFECTS

Common: Nausea.

Unusual: Diarrhoea, vomiting, rash, restlessness, tremor, headache, dizziness, itch.

INTERACTIONS

Other drugs:

- Antacids, Theophylline, Probenecid.

PRESCRIPTION

Yes

PERMITTED IN SPORT

Yes

OVERDOSE

Exacerbation of side effects most likely. Administer activated charcoal or induce vomiting if medication taken recently.

OTHER INFORMATION

Very effective and useful medication in dealing with severe bacterial infections that are not controlled by other antibiotics. Introduced in the late 1980s.

Cisapride

TRADE NAME

Prepulsid.

DRUG CLASS

Prokinetic agent. Increases emptying rate of stomach.

USES

Reflux oesophagitis (heartburn), delayed emptying of food from stomach.

DOSAGE

 5 to 10mg three times a day 15 minutes before food, and last thing at night.

PRECAUTIONS

Caution required with use in pregnancy (B1) and breast feeding. Safe in children.

Use with caution in heart disease.

Lower doses may be necessary in elderly.

 Do not take if:

- Suffering from significant liver or kidney disease, irregular heart rhythm.
- Premature infant.

FORMS

Tablets of 10mg and 20mg., mixture.

SIDE EFFECTS

Common: Belly cramps and noises, diarrhoea.

Unusual: Blurred vision, increased cholesterol levels.

Severe but rare (stop medication, consult doctor): Jaundice (yellow skin), convulsions, urinary frequency, severe belly pain, irregular hear rhythm.

INTERACTIONS

Other drugs:

- Digoxin absorption reduced. Many other drugs have their absorption slightly altered due to increased emptying rate of stomach.

Other substances:

- Reacts with alcohol to increase its effect.

PRESCRIPTION

Yes

PERMITTED IN SPORT

Yes

OVERDOSE

Abdominal cramps and diarrhoea only problems. Reversed by giving activated charcoal.

OTHER INFORMATION

Very effective for babies that vomit easily. Safe and effective medication. Often used in combination with other medications to treat stomach and oesophageal (gullet) ulcers.

Citalopram

TRADE NAME

Cipramil.

DRUG CLASS

SSRI antidepressant.

USES

Depression, panic disorders, agoraphobia.

DOSAGE

 20mg. to 60mg. once a day.

FORMS

Tablets of 10, 20 and 40mg. (white), drops.

PRECAUTIONS

Use with caution in pregnancy (B3), breast feeding and children.

Use with caution in heart disease, mania and liver disease.

Reduce dose slowly, do not stop suddenly.

 Do not take if:

• taking other SSRI antidepressants.

SIDE EFFECTS

Common: Nausea, diarrhoea, tiredness, dry mouth, impotence.

Unusual: Sweating, loss of appetite, tremor, agitation, watery nose, low libido.

INTERACTIONS

Other drugs:

• Other SSRI antidepressants, MAOI, Cimetidine, Lithium, Tryptophan.

Other substances:

• Alcohol.

PRESCRIPTION

Yes

PERMITTED IN SPORT

Yes

OVERDOSE

Tiredness, vomiting, rapid heart rate, tremor, sweating, poor circulation (blue tinged colour to skin), coma, convulsions and death can occur. Induce vomiting or administer activated charcoal if tablets taken recently. Seek urgent medical attention.

OTHER INFORMATION

Introduced in 1998 as a further advance within an excellent class of drugs that are very effective in treating depression. Claimed to have a faster effect and fewer side effects than other SSRI antidepressants.

See also SSRI.

Citric acid

See URINARY ALKALINISERS

Clarithromycin

TRADE NAME

Klaricid.
Heliclear (with Lansoprazole, Amoxycillin).

DRUG CLASS

Macrolide antibiotic.

USES

Treatment of infections caused by susceptible bacteria.

DOSAGE

 250 to 500mg. twice a day.

FORMS

Tablets of 250 and 500mg., suspension, powder in sachet.

PRECAUTIONS

Use with caution in pregnancy (B3), breast feeding and children.

Not designed for prolonged or repeated use.

Use with caution in kidney disease.

Do not take if:

- suffering from severe liver disease, jaundice (yellow skin).
- using Terfenadine or Astemizole.

SIDE EFFECTS

Common: Nausea, vomiting, diarrhoea, rash, headache.

Unusual: Belly pain, loss of appetite, excess wind, dizziness, ear noises, temporary deafness.

Severe but rare (stop medication, consult doctor): Yellow skin (jaundice), irregular heart beat.

INTERACTIONS

Other drugs:

- Terfenadine, Astemizole, Theophylline, Carbamazepine, Oral contraceptives.

PRESCRIPTION

Yes

PERMITTED IN SPORT

Yes

OVERDOSE

Severe diarrhoea, stomach pains and deafness may occur.

Clavulanic acid (Potassium clavulanate)

TRADE NAMES

Augmentin (with Amoxycillin).

Timentin (with Ticarcillin).

USES

Only available as an additive to Penicillin antibiotics to decrease bacterial resistance.

DOSAGE

 One or two capsules, two or three times a day.

FORMS

Capsules, tablets, suspension, injection.

PRECAUTIONS

Safe to use in pregnancy (B1), breast feeding and children.

SIDE EFFECTS

Related to the form of Penicillin with which it is combined. Diarrhoea very common.

INTERACTIONS

None significant.

PRESCRIPTION

Yes

PERMITTED IN SPORT

Yes

OVERDOSE

Diarrhoea and vomiting only likely effects.

OTHER INFORMATION

The combination of Amoxycillin and Potassium clavulanate is becoming very widely prescribed as very few bacteria are resistant to this potent combination.

Clemastine

See ANTIHISTAMINES, SEDATING

Clindamycin

TRADE NAMES

Dalacin C, Dalacin Cream, Dalacin T.

DRUG CLASS

Antibiotic.

USES

Solution: Acne.

Cream: Vaginal infections.

Capsules and injection:

Serious bacterial infections (eg: lung, belly and skin abscesses).

DOSAGE

Solution: Apply to acne twice a day.
Vaginal cream: Once a day at night.
Capsules: One or two capsules, three or four times a day.

FORMS

Capsules of 75 and 150mg., injection, lotion, solution, vaginal cream.

  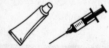

PRECAUTIONS

Safe to use in pregnancy (A). May be used with caution in breast feeding and infants. Safe in children.

Capsules and syrup not to be used long term.

Capsules and syrup to be used with caution in kidney and liver disease.

Cream not to be used on skin or in eyes.

SIDE EFFECTS

Common: Solution - dry skin. Capsules - nausea, rash.

Unusual: Capsules - vomiting, diarrhoea, belly pains, itch.

Severe but rare (stop medication, consult doctor): Severe or bloody diarrhoea, severe belly pain, yellow skin (jaundice).

INTERACTIONS

Other drugs:

• Erythromycin.

Other substances:

• Capsules and syrup react with alcohol.

PRESCRIPTION

Yes

PERMITTED IN SPORT

Yes

OVERDOSE

Exacerbation of side effects likely.

OTHER INFORMATION

Effective medication that is reserved for more severe internal infections, but commonly used as a topical preparation to control acne.

Clioquinol

TRADE NAMES

Only available in combination with other medications.

Betnovate C (with Betamethasone).

Locacorten Vioform (with Flumethasone).

Synalar C (with Fluocinolone).

Vioform-Hydrocortisone (with Hydrocortisone).

DRUG CLASS

Antiseptic

USES

Minor bacterial and fungal infections of skin.

DOSAGE

 Apply three or four times a day.

FORMS

Cream, ear drops

PRECAUTIONS

Safe to use in pregnancy, breast feeding (avoid application to breasts) and children over two years.

Avoid eye contact.

Not designed for long term use.

May interfere with blood tests for thyroid function.

SIDE EFFECTS

Common: Staining, skin irritation.

Severe but rare (stop medication, consult doctor): Brain irritation in children.

INTERACTIONS

None significant.

PRESCRIPTION

Yes

PERMITTED IN SPORT

Yes

OTHER INFORMATION

Dangerous brain inflammation may rarely occur if used in children under two years.

Clobazam

See ANXIOLYTICS

Clobetasol

TRADE NAMES

Dermovate
Dermovate NN (with Neomycin, Nystatin).

DRUG CLASS

Corticosteroid.

USES

Psoriasis, severe eczema and dermatitis, lichen planus, discoid lupus.

DOSAGE

 Apply very sparingly once or twice a day.

FORMS

Cream, ointment, scalp lotion.

PRECAUTIONS

Use with caution in pregnancy, breast feeding and children. Not for use in infants.

Do not use around mouth, nose, nipple, vagina or anus.

Not for long term use.

Do not take if:

- suffering from acne, scabies, broken or ulcerated skin, tuberculosis, fungal or bacterial skin infection.

SIDE EFFECTS

Common: Exacerbation of infections, skin reaction.

Unusual: Skin thinning and damage, bleeding under skin, hair growth in skin.

Severe but rare (stop medication, consult doctor): Swelling of tissues, weight gain.

INTERACTIONS

None significant.

PRESCRIPTION

Yes

PERMITTED IN SPORT

Yes

OVERDOSE

Skin damage if overused.

OTHER INFORMATION

Very potent medication that is only used when others have failed.

Clobetasone

TRADE NAMES

Cloburate, Eumovate
Trimovate (with Oxytetracycline, Nystatin).

DRUG CLASS

Corticosteroid.

USES

Eye inflammation, eczema, dermatitis.

DOSAGE

 Eye drops: One or two drops every three to six hours
Skin preparations: Apply three or four times a day.

FORMS

Eye drops, cream, ointment

PRECAUTIONS

Do not use excessively in pregnancy, breast feeding and children. Not for use in infants.

Do not use eye drops if:

- suffering from viral, fungal or bacterial eye infection, glaucoma, contact lenses.

Do not take if:

- suffering from tuberculosis, broken or ulcerated skin

- under other circumstances

SIDE EFFECTS

Eye drops: Damage to eye surface, eye irritation, worsening of eye infections, glaucoma. Skin preparations: Exacerbation of infections, skin reaction.

INTERACTIONS

None significant.

PRESCRIPTION

Yes

PERMITTED IN SPORT

Yes

OVERDOSE

Unlikely to be harmful.

OTHER INFORMATION

Medium strength steroid.

Clofazime

TRADE NAME

Lamprene.

USES

Leprosy in combination with other drugs.

DOSAGE

 Complex. As directed by doctor.

FORMS

Capsules (red/brown) of 100mg.

PRECAUTIONS

Not to be used in pregnancy (C) or breast feeding. May be used in children.

Use with caution in liver or kidney disease.

SIDE EFFECTS

Common: Reversible discolouration of skin and hair, nausea, dry skin, diarrhoea.

Unusual: Itch, light sensitive skin, acne, vomiting, belly pain, weight loss.

Severe but rare (stop medication, consult doctor): Blood in faeces or urine, severe belly pain.

INTERACTIONS

Nil significant.

PRESCRIPTION

Yes

PERMITTED IN SPORT

Yes

OVERDOSE

Serious exacerbation of side effects possible. Seek medical assistance.

Clofibrate

TRADE NAME

Atromid S.

DRUG CLASS

Hypolipidaemic.

USES

Lowers excessively high blood cholesterol and triglyceride levels.

DOSAGE

 One or two tablets, two or three times a day after meals.

FORMS

Gel capsules of 500mg.

PRECAUTIONS

Should be used with caution in pregnancy (B1). Should not be used during breast feeding. Use only if medically essential in children.

Regular blood tests to measure blood fat levels and check on liver function recommended.

 Do not take if:

- suffering from kidney or liver failure

SIDE EFFECTS

Common: Nausea.

Unusual: Vomiting, diarrhoea, burping, excess wind, belly discomfort, headache, dizziness, muscle aches and cramps, rash, itch, allergy reaction, dry hair, hair loss.

Severe but rare (stop medication, consult doctor): Yellow skin (jaundice).

INTERACTIONS

Other drugs:

• Anticoagulants, Phenytoin, Diuretics.

• Drugs that lower blood sugar in diabetes.

PERMITTED IN SPORT

Yes

OVERDOSE

No specific problems.

OTHER INFORMATION

One of the earlier drugs used to control excess cholesterol and triglycerides. No longer widely used.

Clomiphene

TRADE NAME

Clomid.

USES

Female infertility.

DOSAGE

 One tablet a day for five days. Repeat monthly for a maximum of six cycles.

FORMS

Tablets (beige) of 50mg.

PRECAUTIONS

Not to be used in pregnancy (B3), breast feeding or children.

Use with caution with ovarian cysts.

Multiple pregnancies (ie: twins, triplets, quads etc.) possible.

Must only be used in carefully selected patients.

 Do not take if:

• suffering from liver disease, abnormal bleeding from uterus.

SIDE EFFECTS

Common: Hot flushes, belly discomfort and bloating.

Unusual: One in 200 chance of birth defect (similar to normal risk).

Severe but rare (stop medication, consult doctor): Blurred vision, yellow skin (jaundice).

INTERACTIONS

None significant

PRESCRIPTION

Yes

PERMITTED IN SPORT

Yes

OVERDOSE

May increase risk of foetal abnormality if taken during pregnancy. Otherwise no serious effects likely.

OTHER INFORMATION

Stimulates ovulation in infertile women, but several eggs may be released, resulting in multiple pregnancies. Has revolutionised the lives of many infertile couples since first introduced in the 1970s.

Clomipramine

See TRICYCLICS

Clonazepam

TRADE NAME

Rivotril.

DRUG CLASSES

Anticonvulsant, Benzodiazepine.

USES

Epilepsy

DOSAGE

 Given twice a day in individually determined dosage. Follow doctors instructions carefully.

FORMS

Tablets of 0.5 and 2mg., injection.

PRECAUTIONS

Not to be used in pregnancy (D) unless medically essential. Use with caution in breast feeding and infants. Safe for use in children.

Use with caution in glaucoma, myasthenia gravis, low blood pressure, heart disease, kidney and liver disease, depression and psychiatric conditions (eg: schizophrenia).

Use with caution if operating machinery or driving a vehicle.

 Do not take if:
• suffering from severe lung disease.

SIDE EFFECTS

Common: Drowsiness (worse in first few days), incoordination, behaviour changes, tiredness, fatigue, muscle weakness, excess salivation, dizziness.

Unusual: Low blood pressure, itch, skin pigmentation, changes in hair distribution, nausea, loss of appetite, weight changes, impotence, low libido, confusion, aggression, depression, irritability, cough.

Severe but rare (stop medication, consult doctor): Unusual bruising or bleeding.

INTERACTIONS

Other drugs:

• Sedatives, Stimulants, other Anticonvulsants, Disulfiram, Cimetidine.

Other substances:

• Reacts adversely with alcohol.

PRESCRIPTION

Yes

PERMITTED IN SPORT

Depends on sport. Check with governing body.

OVERDOSE

May cause drowsiness, confusion, incoordination, slow breathing, coma and rarely death. Administer activated charcoal or induce vomiting if taken recently and patient alert. Seek urgent medical attention.

OTHER INFORMATION

May cause dependence if used inappropriately.

Clonidine

TRADE NAME

Catapres, Dixarit.

DRUG CLASS

Antihypertensive, Antimigraine.

USES

High blood pressure, prevention of migraine and vascular headaches, treatment of menopausal flushing.

DOSAGE

 One or two tablets, three times a day to a maximum of 900mcg. per day.

FORMS

Tablets, capsules, injection.

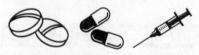

PRECAUTIONS

Should be used only if medically indicated in pregnancy (B3) and breast feeding. Not for use in children.

Medication must not be stopped suddenly, but dosage must be slowly decreased over several days or weeks.

 Do not take if:

- suffering from liver or kidney failure, severe heart disease, diabetes.

SIDE EFFECTS

Common: Drowsiness, dry mouth, stomach upsets.

Unusual: Hair thinning, blurred vision, constipation, delusions, depression, impotence, irritability, low blood pressure on standing.

INTERACTIONS

Other drugs:

- Sedatives, hypnotics, other medications for treatment of high blood pressure, antidepressants.

Other substances:

- Reacts with alcohol.

PRESCRIPTION

Yes

PERMITTED IN SPORT

Yes

OVERDOSE

Slow heart rate, low blood pressure and coma result. First aid involves administering activated charcoal or inducing vomiting if awake and alert, and seeking very urgent medical assistance.

OTHER INFORMATION

Old fashioned, but often effective treatment for migraines. Only used for most severe forms of high blood pressure. Occasionally used to stop symptoms of narcotic withdrawal.

Clopamide

See **THIAZIDE DIURETICS**

Clopidogrel

TRADE NAME

Plavix

DRUG CLASS

Anticoagulant.

USES

Prevention of blood clots (eg. strokes, heart attack).

DOSAGE

One tablet a day.

FORMS

Tablets of 75mg. (pink).

PRECAUTIONS

Not for use in pregnancy (B1). Use with caution in breast feeding and children.

Use with caution in peptic ulcers, other intestinal ulcers, recent heart attack or stroke.

Cease before any elective surgery.

 Do not take if:

- suffering from liver disease or bleeding disorders.

SIDE EFFECTS

Common: Abnormal bleeding, diarrhoea, rash, agitation.

Unusual: Low level of white blood cells.

Severe but rare (stop medication, consult doctor): Jaundice, heavy bleeding.

INTERACTIONS

Other drugs:

- NSAID, Aspirin, Anticoagulants (eg. Warfarin), Phenytoin, Tamoxifen, Tolbutamide.

PRESCRIPTION

Yes

PERMITTED IN SPORT

Yes

OVERDOSE

May be very serious with excessive internal and external bleeding. Administer activated charcoal or inducing vomiting if awake and alert, and seek urgent medical assistance.

OTHER INFORMATION

Introduced 1999 as an additional treatment for patients who have recurrent episodes of abnormal blood clotting.

See also ANTICOAGULANTS

Clorazepate
See ANXIOLYTICS

Clotrimazole
See IMIDAZOLES

Clozapine
See PHENOTHIAZINES

Co-trimoxazole
See Sulphamethoxazole, Trimethoprim

Coal tar
See Tar

Cocaine

OTHER NAMES

Crack, coke.

DRUG CLASS

Local anaesthetic, stimulant.

USES

No recognised medical uses. Used illegally as a psychoactive drug to cause euphoria

DOSAGE

 (artificial happiness).

FORMS

Used illegally in many forms including smoked, injected and sniffed.

PRECAUTIONS

Should never be used in pregnancy (increased risk of malformation and heart disease), breast feeding or children.

 ### Do not take if:

- suffering from psychiatric disturbances.
- driving a car, operating machinery, swimming or undertaking any activity that requires concentration.

SIDE EFFECTS

Common: Damage to nostrils, fever, headache, irregular heart rate, dilation of pupils, loss of libido, infertility, impotence, breast enlargement and tenderness in both sexes, menstrual period irregularities, psychiatric disturbances, abnormal breast milk production, may lead to desire for more frequent use or stronger drugs of addiction.

Unusual: High blood pressure, perforation of nasal septum, difficulty in breathing, convulsions, stroke, dementia, heart attack, death.

INTERACTIONS

Other drugs:

- Stimulants, MAOI, Tricyclics, Sedatives, other medications acting on the brain.

Other substances:

- Reacts with alcohol, Heroin and Marijuana.

PRESCRIPTION

Illegal except in hospitals

PERMITTED IN SPORT

No

OVERDOSE

Convulsions, difficulty in breathing, irregular heart rate, coma and death may occur.

OTHER INFORMATION

The more refined version of Cocaine known as 'crack' is the only form that can be smoked, and is ten times more potent than Cocaine base, and is therefore more dangerous. Highly addictive. When smoked, sniffed or injected, Cocaine works within seconds to cause euphoria (artificial happiness) and stimulates the brain to increase all sensations. After use many people feel worse than before, hence they want to repeat the artificial high. The more frequently it is used, the higher the dose necessary to achieve the same sensations, and the greater the risk of serious side effects.

Codeine Phosphate

TRADE NAMES

Galcodine.

Codaphen Continus (with Ibuprofen).

Kapake, Solpadol, Tylex (with Paracetamol).

Migraleve (with Buclizine, Paracetamol).

Also found in other locally produced cough and cold remedies, and pain relievers.

DRUG CLASS

Narcotic.

USES

Pain, diarrhoea, coughing.

DOSAGE

5mg. to 60mg. every 4 to 6 hours.

FORMS

Mixture as Codeine Phosphate alone.

Tablets, powders and mixtures in combination with other medications.

PRECAUTIONS

Safe in pregnancy (A). Should be used with caution in breast feeding and children.

Should be used with caution in people with an underactive thyroid gland, liver disease, an enlarged prostate gland or lung disease.

Elderly patients should take a reduced dose.

 Do not take if:-

- addicted to Narcotics.
- operating machinery, driving a vehicle or undertaking other activity requiring concentration.

SIDE EFFECTS

Common: Constipation, nausea, drowsiness.

Unusual: Dizziness, vomiting.

INTERACTIONS

Other drugs:

- Increases the effects of Sedatives and Hypnotics.

Other substances:

- Do not drink alcohol while taking Codeine

PRESCRIPTION

Depends on strength and formulation.

PERMITTED IN SPORT

Yes.

OVERDOSE

Moderately serious. May cause initial stimulation, followed by vomiting, drowsiness, convulsions, reduced breathing, coma and very rarely death. Seek urgent medical attention.

OTHER INFORMATION

May cause dependency or addiction if used unnecessarily for long periods. The mildest of the narcotic drugs. Very effective and except for slight risk of dependency, very safe. Widely used in many cough and cold mixtures, pain relievers and preparations for diarrhoea.

Cod liver oil

TRADE NAME

Found in a large range of over the counter and health shop medications.

USES

Tonic, moisturiser.

DOSAGE

 Apply to skin as required, or take one dose a day.

FORMS

Cream, capsule, mixture etc.

PRECAUTIONS

Safe in breast feeding and children.

Small amounts safe, but excess may cause birth defects in pregnancy (D).

SIDE EFFECTS

Common: Foul taste.

Unusual: Nausea, diarrhoea.

INTERACTIONS

None significant.

PRESCRIPTION

No

PERMITTED IN SPORT

Yes

OVERDOSE

Vomiting and diarrhoea only likely effects.

OTHER INFORMATION

Very old form of multivitamin (particularly A and D) and fatty acid supplementation.

See also Retinol

Colchicine

TRADE NAME

Colgout.

USES

Treatment of acute gout, prevention of gout.

DOSAGE

 Two tablets at once, then one tablet every two hours until relief obtained, diarrhoea starts or six tablets taken.

FORMS

Tablets (white) of 500mcg.

PRECAUTIONS

Use with caution in pregnancy (B2) and breast feeding. Not for use in children.

Use with caution in heart disease, kidney disease and bowel disease.

Lower doses necessary in elderly and debilitated.

SIDE EFFECTS

Common: Diarrhoea.

Unusual: Reduced body temperature, reduced urge to breathe, muscle weakness, cold extremities, high blood pressure, rash.

INTERACTIONS

Other drugs:

• Sedatives.

Other substances:

• Alcohol may aggravate gout.

PRESCRIPTION

Yes

PERMITTED IN SPORT

Yes

OVERDOSE

Very serious. Symptoms may be delayed in onset and may include burning mouth, vomiting, diarrhoea, gut pain and spasms, delirium, convulsions and death. Administer activated charcoal or induce vomiting if medication taken recently. Give copious fluids. Seek urgent medical attention.

OTHER INFORMATION

Does not cause addiction or dependence. Effective, but diarrhoea limits its usefulness.

Colestipol

TRADE NAME

Colestid.

DRUG CLASS

Hypolipidaemic.

USES

Lowering high levels of cholesterol in blood.

DOSAGE

 15g. to 30g. two to four times a day with water.

FORMS

Granules (sachets of 5g.).

PRECAUTIONS

Should be used with caution in pregnancy (B2). Should not be used in breast feeding. Use only if medically essential in children.

Regular blood tests to check blood fat levels are recommended.

 Do not take if:

- suffering from underactive thyroid gland, diabetes, severe kidney or liver disease.

SIDE EFFECTS

Common: Constipation.

Unusual: Vitamin deficiency.

Severe but rare (stop medication, consult doctor): Rare and serious complications.

INTERACTIONS

Other drugs:

- Numerous other drugs - check with doctor.
- Do not take at same time as any other medication.

PRESCRIPTION

Yes

PERMITTED IN SPORT

Yes

OVERDOSE

Constipation only likely problem.

Colloidal bismuth

See Bismuth subcitrate

CONTRACEPTIVES

See Etonogestrel, Medroxyprogesterone acetate, ORAL CONTRACEPTIVES, SPERMICIDES

Copper

TRADE NAME

Cuplex (with Salicylic and Lactic acid).

Also found in other non-prescription skin and cosmetic preparations and as part of intrauterine devices.

DRUG CLASS

Mineral.

USES

Mild antiseptic.

DOSAGE

 Massage into skin twice a day.

FORMS

Gel.

PRECAUTIONS

May be used in pregnancy and breast feeding.

Not for use under two years of age.

Do not swallow mouthwash tablets.

Use with caution in kidney and liver failure.

Do not take if:

• suffering from Wilson's disease.

• under other circumstances

SIDE EFFECTS

Common: Dry skin, skin irritation.

INTERACTIONS

None significant.

PRESCRIPTION

No

PERMITTED IN SPORT

Yes

CORTICOSTEROIDS

(Powerful reducers of inflammation)

See Beclomethasone, Betamethasone, Budesonide, Clobetasol, Clobetasone, Cortisone, Deflazacort, Desoxymethasone, Dexamethasone, Diflucortolone, Fludrocortisone, Flucinolone, Fluocinonide, Fluocortolone, Fluorometholone, Flurandrelone, Fluticasone, Halcinonide, Hydrocortisone, Mometasone, Prednisolone, Rimexolone, Triamcinolone.

Cortisol

See Hydrocortisone

Cortisone

TRADE NAME

Cortisyl.

DRUG CLASS

Corticosteroid.

USES

Addison's disease, severe asthma, rheumatoid and other forms of severe arthritis, auto-immune diseases (eg: Sjøgren's syndrome), severe allergy reactions, and other severe and chronic inflammatory diseases.

DOSAGE

One to five tablets a day as directed by doctor.

FORMS

Tablets of 25mg. (white).

PRECAUTIONS

Should be used in pregnancy (C), breast feeding and children only on specific medical advice.

Use with caution if under stress, and in patients with under active thyroid gland, liver disease, diverticulitis, high blood pressure, myasthenia gravis, or kidney disease.

Use for shortest period of time possible.

Do not take if:

• suffering from any form of infection, peptic ulcer, or osteoporosis.

• having a vaccination

SIDE EFFECTS

Common: May cause bloating, weight gain, rashes and intestinal disturbances.

Unusual: Biochemical disturbances of blood, muscle weakness, bone weakness, impaired wound healing, skin thinning, tendon weakness, peptic ulcers, gullet ulcers, bruising, increased sweating, loss of fat under skin, premature ageing, excess facial hair growth in women, pigmentation of skin and nails, acne, convulsions, headaches, dizziness, growth suppression in children, aggravation of diabetes, worsening of infections, cataracts, aggravation of glaucoma, blood clots in veins and sleeplessness. Most significant side effects occur only with prolonged use. Medication should not be ceased abruptly, but dosage should be slowly reduced.

Severe but rare (stop medication, consult doctor): Any significant side effect should be reported to a doctor immediately.

INTERACTIONS

Other drugs:

• Oral contraceptives, Barbiturates, Phenytoin, and Rifampicin.

PRESCRIPTION

Yes

PERMITTED IN SPORT

No

OVERDOSE

Medical treatment is required. Serious effects and death rare.

OTHER INFORMATION

Extremely effective and useful medication if used correctly. Must be used with extreme care under strict medical supervision. Lowest dose and shortest possible course should be used. Not addictive.

COUGH SUPPRESSANTS

(Relieve hard dry cough)

See Codeine, Dihydrocodeine

COX -2 INHIBITORS

(Anti-inflammatory medication for the treatment of arthritis with minimal effects on the stomach compared to other non-steroidal anti-inflammatory drugs - NSAID)

See Celecoxib, Rofecoxib

Cromoglycate, sodium

See Sodium cromoglycate

Crotamiton

TRADE NAME

Eurax.
Eurax-HC (with Hydrocortisone).

DRUG CLASS

Antiseptic

USES

Itchy skin, scabies.

DOSAGE

Itch: Apply to affected area two or three times a day
Scabies: Rub over entire body surface except scalp and face after bathing for three to five consecutive days.

FORMS

Cream, lotion.

PRECAUTIONS

Use with caution in first three months of pregnancy and small children. May be used safely in breast feeding (not on breasts) and older children.

Avoid eye contact.

Do not use if:-

• suffering from weeping or broken skin.

SIDE EFFECTS

Common: Slight stinging.

INTERACTIONS

None significant.

PRESCRIPTION

No

PERMITTED IN SPORT

Yes

Cyanocobalamin

(Vitamin B12)

TRADE NAME

Cytacon, Cytamen.

A large number of other preparations include various forms of Vitamin B12 alone or in combination with other medications.

DRUG CLASS

Vitamin

USES

Pernicious anaemia, pins and needles sensation of feet.

DOSAGE

 Injection: Once every three months, or as determined by doctor. Recommended daily allowance: 2ug a day.

FORMS

Tablets, injection.

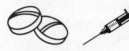

PRECAUTIONS

Safe in pregnancy, breast feeding and children.

Do not take in high doses or for prolonged periods of time.

SIDE EFFECTS

Minimal.

INTERACTIONS

Other drugs:

• Methyldopa, Colchicine, Neomycin, Cholestyramine, some medications for diabetes, Cimetidine, Potassium chloride, Chloramphenicol, Oral contraceptives.

PRESCRIPTION

Injection: Yes

Other forms: No

PERMITTED IN SPORT

Yes

OVERDOSE

Unlikely to cause any serious effects.

OTHER INFORMATION

Several chemical variations of Vitamin B12 exist including Cyanocobalamin and Hydroxocobalamin. They are identical in their actions and use. Cyanocobalamin was the original form of Vitamin B12 used medically. Vitamin B12 is a water soluble vitamin found in animal products. It is essential for the formation of red blood cells, normal growth, and normal fat and sugar metabolism. In pernicious anaemia, the body loses the ability to absorb vitamin B12 from the stomach. Remember, vitamins are merely chemicals that are essential for the functioning of the body, and if taken to excess, act as a drug.

See also Hydroxocobalamin.

Cyclizine

TRADE NAME

Valoid Cyclimorph (with Morphine).

Diconal (with Dipipanone).

Migril (with Ergotamine, Caffeine).

DRUG CLASS

Antiemetic, Antihistamine.

USES

Vomiting caused by migraine or cancer drugs, motion sickness, dizziness.

PRECAUTIONS

Not for use in pregnancy.

Use with caution in breast feeding and children.

 Do not take if:
- suffering from severe heart failure.

FORMS

Tablets, injection.

SIDE EFFECTS

Common: Drowsiness, dry mouth, constipation, restlessness in children, incoordination, blurred vision.

Unusual: Upper belly discomfort, loss of appetite, diarrhoea, irritability.

INTERACTIONS

Other drugs:

- May interfere with Anticoagulants, MAOI (monoamine oxidase inhibitors), Sedatives and relaxants.

PRESCRIPTION

Tablets: No

Injection: Yes

Combined with other medications: Yes

PERMITTED IN SPORT

Alone: Yes.

Combined with narcotics: No.

OVERDOSE

May result in convulsions, hallucinations, delirium, anxiety, muscle spasms, rapid heart rate, flushing, dry skin, dry mouth and coma. First aid involved inducing vomiting and seeking urgent medical attention.

Cyclopenthiazide
See THIAZIDE DIURETICS

Cyclopentolate
See MYDRIATICS

Cyclophosphamide

TRADE NAME

Endoxana.

DRUG CLASS

Alkylater.

USES

Leukaemia, lymphomas, multiple myeloma, Hodgkin's disease, cancer of the ovary and retina (eye). Prevents rejection of transplanted organs.

DOSAGE

Must be individualised by doctor for each patient depending on disease, severity, response, weight and age of patient.

FORMS

Tablets, injection.

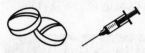

PRECAUTIONS

Use in pregnancy (D) will cause damage or death to the foetus, and therefore Cyclophosphamide must not be used unless life of mother is threatened. Breast feeding must be ceased before use. Use in children only if child's life at risk.

Regular blood tests to follow course of disease and the effect of medication on blood cells, bone marrow and liver function essential.

Adequate contraception must be used during use of Cyclophosphamide.

Must be used with caution in all patients.

Ensure adequate fluid intake.

 Do not take if:-
- suffering from recent surgery.

SIDE EFFECTS

Common: Nausea, vomiting, mouth ulcers, hair loss, dermatitis, nail damage, delayed wound healing, infertility.

Unusual: Yellow skin (jaundice), blood in urine, fluid retention.

INTERACTIONS

Other drugs:
- Barbiturates.

PRESCRIPTION

Yes

PERMITTED IN SPORT

Yes

OVERDOSE

Extremely serious. May cause severe damage to kidney, bone marrow and blood cells leading to destruction of immune system and subsequent fatal infections. Administer activated charcoal or induce vomiting if medication taken recently. Seek urgent medical assistance.

OTHER INFORMATION

Although Cyclophosphamide has multiple serious side effects, it may be life saving in patients with severe or widespread cancer or leukaemia.

Cyclosporin

TRADE NAME

Neoral, Sandimmun, SangCya.

DRUG CLASS

Immunomodifier

USES

Prevents rejection of transplanted organs (eg: kidney, liver, heart), severe rheumatoid arthritis, severe psoriasis.

DOSAGE

 Taken twice a day with milk or food.

FORMS

Capsules, solution, infusion.

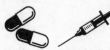

PRECAUTIONS

Not to be used in pregnancy (C) unless mother's life at risk. Breast feeding must be ceased before use. Must be used with caution in children.

Careful monitoring of all patients by clinical examination and blood tests essential.

 Do not take if:

- suffering from high blood pressure, significant infection, immune deficiency, poor kidney function.

SIDE EFFECTS

Common: Excess hair growth, tremor, sore gums, nausea, vomiting, high blood pressure, increased risk of infection.

Unusual: Fluid retention, convulsions, diarrhoea, peptic ulcer formation, acne, rash, itch, muscle cramps, headache, hearing loss, ringing in ears, confusion, tiredness, anaemia, pins and needles, flushing, sinusitis, weight loss.

INTERACTIONS

Other drugs:

- Reacts with a wide range of medications. Check all with a doctor.

PRESCRIPTION

Yes

PERMITTED IN SPORT

Yes

OVERDOSE

Serious. Administer activated charcoal or induce vomiting if medication taken recently. Seek urgent medical assistance.

OTHER INFORMATION

Potent medication which can be of great benefit if used appropriately and carefully.

Cyproheptadine

See ANTIHISTAMINES, SEDATING

Cyproterone Acetate

TRADE NAME

Androcur, Cyprostat.

Dianette (with Ethinyloestradiol - see Oral Contraceptives).

DRUG CLASS

Sex hormone

USES

Excessive body hair in women, loss of scalp hair in women, severe acne in women. Reduction of sexual drive in men, premature puberty, cancer of the prostate gland. Dianette: Oral contraception.

DOSAGE

 Androcur, Cyprostat: Usually one morning and evening Depends on use and response to medication

Follow doctors instructions
Dianette: Take one daily, including 7 days of sugar drug free pills.

FORMS

Tablets.

PRECAUTIONS

Not to be used in pregnancy or breast feeding. Adequate contraception must be used in sexually active women. Not to be used in girls. For use in boys only if medically indicated.

Use Androcur and Cyprone with caution if operating machinery or undertaking tasks that require concentration.

Use with caution in diabetes, liver tumours.

Do not take if:

- suffering from severe liver disease, blood clots, sickle cell anaemia.

SIDE EFFECTS

Common: Male infertility, reduced libido, tiredness, increased weight, nausea, headache, irregular menstrual periods (Androcur and Cyprostat only).

Unusual: Breast enlargement in men, depression, breast milk production, sleeplessness, hot flushes.

Severe but rare (stop medication, consult doctor): Calf or chest pain.

INTERACTIONS

None significant

PERMITTED IN SPORT

Yes

OVERDOSE

Aggravation of side effects likely.

OTHER INFORMATION

Does not cause addiction or dependence. Must be used strictly according to doctor's instructions.

Cysteamine

TRADE NAME

Cystagon.

DRUG CLASS

Detoxifying agent.

USES

Cystinosis affecting the kidneys.

DOSAGE

 Depends on body weight. Gradually increased over six weeks to maintenance dose level.

FORMS

Capsules of 50mg and 150mg.

PRECAUTIONS

Use with caution in pregnancy (B2), breast feeding and children.

Use with caution if brain symptoms or rash present due to cystinosis.

Liver function and blood condition must be monitored regularly by blood tests.

Do not take if:

- hypersensitive to Penicillamine.

SIDE EFFECTS

Common: Rash, drowsiness, depression, stomach ulcers,nausea.

Unusual: Bleeding from bowel, vomiting blood, abnormal liver function, fever, low white blood cell count.

Severe but rare (stop medication, consult doctor): Seizures, brain inflammation.

INTERACTIONS

None significant.

PRESCRIPTION

Yes

PERMITTED IN SPORT

Yes

OTHER INFORMATION

Introduced in 1997 for treatment of the rare condition, cystinosis.

Cytarabine

TRADE NAME

Cytosar.

DRUG CLASS

Antimetabolite.

USES

Treatment of leukaemia and lymphomas.

DOSAGE

 As determined for each patient by doctor.

FORMS

Injection.

PRECAUTIONS

Never to be used in pregnancy (D).

Use with caution in breast feeding.

Regular blood tests necessary to monitor function of kidney, liver and blood cells.

SIDE EFFECTS

Common: Ulcers of mouth and anus, nausea, vomiting, fever, muscle pain, bone pain, chest pain, rash, tiredness, red irritated eyes, diarrhoea, loss of appetite.

Unusual: Liver dysfunction, infections, skin ulcers, nerve inflammation, sore throat, pain on swallowing, retention of urine, dizziness, hair loss, itchy skin, headache.

Severe but rare (stop medication, consult doctor): Pneumonia, blood clots, severe belly pain.

INTERACTIONS

Other drugs:

• Methotrexate.

PRESCRIPTION

Yes

PERMITTED IN SPORT

Yes

OVERDOSE

Very serious. Only given under strict medical supervision.

CYTOTOXIC

See CANCER TREATING DRUGS

Dactinomycin

See **Actinomycin D**

Dalteparin

TRADE NAME

Fragmin.

DRUG CLASS

Anticoagulant.

USES

Prevention and treatment of blood clots.

DOSAGE

 Injection under skin into fat tissue once a day.

FORMS

Injection.

SIDE EFFECTS

Common: Abnormal bruising and bleeding.

Severe but rare (stop medication, consult doctor): Excessive bleeding or bruising, loss of blood from anus, vagina or mouth, coughing blood..

INTERACTIONS

Other drugs:

• Aspirin, NSAIDs, Vitamin K antagonists, dipyridamole, dextran, sulfinpyrazone, probenecid, ethacrynic acid, antihistamines, digoxin, tetracycline antibiotics, ascorbic acid.

Other substances:

• Vitamin C.

PRESCRIPTION

Yes.

PERMITTED IN SPORT

Yes.

OVERDOSE

Very serious. May cause catastrophic excessive bleeding. Seek emergency medical treatment.

PRECAUTIONS

Use only if essential in pregnancy (C) as damage to foetus may occur. Use with caution in breast feeding and children.

Bleeding times must be checked regularly by blood test.

Liver and kidney function must be checked regularly by blood tests if used for prolonged period.

Use with caution in osteoporosis and elderly.

 Do not take if:

• suffering from bleeding disorder, active bleeding, severe coagulation disorders, heart infection, uncontrolled high blood pressure.

• having eye, ear, brain or spinal cord surgery.

• Using aspirin or NSAIDs (anti-inflammatory drugs used for joint pain).

OTHER INFORMATION

Used instead of Heparin in some patients as it is less likely to have serious side effects.

See also Heparin

Danazol

TRADE NAME

Danol.

DRUG CLASS

Sex hormone.

USES

Endometriosis, severe intractable period pain, severe abnormal menstrual bleeding, severe breast pain, rare form of severe tissue swelling.

DOSAGE

 One capsule two to four times a day for three to nine months.

PRECAUTIONS

Not to be used during pregnancy (D) or breast feeding. Adequate non-hormonal contraception must be used by women taking Danazol. Not to be used in children.

Regular blood tests to check liver function recommended. Use with caution in liver disease, high blood pressure, heart disease, diabetes.

 Do not take if:

• suffering from undiagnosed genital disease, severe liver disease, pelvic infection, cancer of sex organs, heart failure, recent blood clot, porphyria.

FORMS

Capsules of 100mg. and 200mg.

SIDE EFFECTS

Common: Acne, weight gain, fluid retention, excess body hair growth, voice deepening, flushing, sweating, dry vagina, menstrual period irregularities.

Unusual: Oily skin, hoarseness, reduced breast size, enlargement of clitoris, nervousness.

Severe but rare (stop medication, consult doctor): Yellow skin (jaundice).

INTERACTIONS

Other drugs:

• Warfarin, Carbamazepine, Cyclosporin, Oral contraceptives.

PRESCRIPTION

Yes.

PERMITTED IN SPORT

No.

OVERDOSE

May cause vomiting, tissue swelling and indigestion.

OTHER INFORMATION

Very effective medication, but significant side effects a problem for some patients. Used for six to nine months only. Does not cause addiction or dependence.

Dantrolene

TRADE NAME

Dantrium.

USES

Muscle spasm caused by cerebral palsy, stroke, multiple sclerosis or spinal cord injury.

DOSAGE

 25mg. once a day initially, then slowly increase as directed by doctor to a maximum of 100mg. four times a day.

FORMS

Capsules of 25 and 100mg.

PRECAUTIONS

Use with caution in pregnancy (B2), breast feeding and children.

Use with caution in liver disease.

Regular blood tests to check on liver function recommended.

 Do not take if:

- suffering from severe liver disease.
- operating machinery or driving a vehicle.

SIDE EFFECTS

Common: Drowsiness, weakness, dizziness, diarrhoea.

Unusual: Constipation, bleeding from bowel, slurred speech, headache, rapid heart rate, depression, urinary frequency, skin sensitised to sunlight.

Severe but rare (stop medication, consult doctor): Yellow skin (jaundice).

INTERACTIONS

Other drugs:

- Tranquillisers, Verapamil, Oral contraceptives.

Other substances:

- Reacts adversely with alcohol.

PRESCRIPTION

Yes.

PERMITTED IN SPORT

Yes.

OVERDOSE

May cause drowsiness, irregular heart rate, convulsions and coma. Induce vomiting if medication taken recently and patient alert. Seek urgent medical assistance.

OTHER INFORMATION

Does not cause addiction or dependence.

Dapsone

TRADE NAMES

Dapsone.

Maloprim (with Pyrimethamine).

USES

Dapsone: Leprosy, some rare forms of dermatitis.
Maloprim: Prevention of malaria.

DOSAGE

 Dapsone: One tablet a day
Maloprim: One tablet a week.

FORMS

Dapsone: Tablet (white) of 50 and 100mg.
Maloprim: Tablet (white).

PRECAUTIONS

May be used in pregnancy (B2) if medically essential. May be used in breast feeding and children.

Use with caution in heart disease, lung disease, liver and kidney disease.

SIDE EFFECTS

Common: Loss of appetite, nausea, diarrhoea, headache, dizziness.

Unusual: Rapid heart rate, sleeplessness, rash, vomiting.

INTERACTIONS

Other drugs:

• Rifampicin, Chloroquine, Primaquine.

PRESCRIPTION

Yes.

PERMITTED IN SPORT

Yes.

OVERDOSE

May seriously damage red blood cells. Administer activated charcoal or induce vomiting if medication taken recently. Seek urgent medical assistance.

OTHER INFORMATION

Very effective, but long term use necessary.

Daunorubicin

TRADE NAME

Cerubidin, Daunoxome.

DRUG CLASS

Cytotoxic.

USES

Leukaemia, neuroblastoma, other cancers.

DOSAGE

 As determined by doctor for each patient. Given by drip into vein.

FORMS

Injection.

PRECAUTIONS

Must not be used in pregnancy (D). Use with caution in breast feeding.

Second full course must not be used unless clinically essential.

Use with caution in heart, kidney and liver disease.

Regular blood tests to monitor kidney, liver and bone marrow function essential.

Ensure medication does not leak out of drip into surrounding tissues outside vein.

 Do not take if:

• suffering from suppressed bone marrow from radiotherapy or chemotherapy.

• under other circumstances

SIDE EFFECTS

Common: Nausea, vomiting, hair loss, ulceration of mouth, anus and vagina, inflammation around drip site.

Unusual: Anaemia, diarrhoea, belly pain, fever, chills.

Severe but rare (stop medication, consult doctor): Heart and kidney damage..

INTERACTIONS

Other drugs:

• Doxorubicin, cyclophosphamide, allopurinol, colchicine, heparin, fluorouracil, dexamethasone.

PRESCRIPTION

Yes.

PERMITTED IN SPORT

Yes.

OVERDOSE

Very serious. Given under strict medical supervision.

DECONGESTANTS SYMPATHOMIMETICS

(Clear blocked nose and sinuses)

See Phenylephrine, Pseudoephedrine

Deflazacort

TRADE NAME

Calcort.

DRUG CLASS

Corticosteroid.

USES

Severe asthma, rheumatoid and other forms of severe arthritis, auto-immune diseases (eg: Sjøgren's syndrome), severe allergy reactions, and other severe and chronic inflammatory diseases.

DOSAGE

 Strictly as directed by doctor.

FORMS

Tablets.

PRECAUTIONS

Should be used in pregnancy (C), breast feeding and children only on specific medical advice.

Use with caution if under stress, and in patients with under active thyroid gland, liver disease, diverticulitis, high blood pressure, myasthenia gravis or kidney disease.

Use for shortest period of time possible.

Medication should not be ceased abruptly, but dosage should be slowly reduced.

 Do not take if:

- suffering from any form of infection, peptic ulcer or osteoporosis.

- having a vaccination.

SIDE EFFECTS

Most significant side effects occur only with prolonged use of tablets or rectal preparations.

Common: May cause bloating, weight gain, rashes and intestinal disturbances.

Unusual: Biochemical disturbances of blood, muscle weakness, bone weakness, impaired wound healing, skin thinning, tendon weakness, peptic ulcers, gullet ulcers, bruising, increased sweating, loss of fat under skin, premature ageing, excess facial hair growth in women, pigmentation of skin and nails, acne, convulsions, headaches, dizziness, growth suppression in children, aggravation of diabetes, worsening of infections, cataracts, aggravation of glaucoma, blood clots in veins and sleeplessness.

Severe but rare (stop medication, consult doctor): Any significant side effect should be reported to a doctor immediately.

INTERACTIONS

Other drugs:

• Oral contraceptives, Barbiturates, Phenytoin and Rifampicin.

PRESCRIPTION

Yes.

PERMITTED IN SPORT

No.

OVERDOSE

Medical treatment is required. Serious effects and death rare.

OTHER INFORMATION

Extremely effective and useful medication if used correctly. Must be used with extreme care under strict medical supervision. Lowest dose and shortest possible course should be used. Not addictive.

Demeclocycline

TRADE NAMES

Ledermycin.

Deteclo (with Tetracycline hydrochloride, Chlortetracycline).

DRUG CLASS

Tetracycline antibiotic.

USES

Infections caused by susceptible bacteria.

DOSAGE

 One capsule four times a day.

FORMS

Capsules, tablets

PRECAUTIONS

Not to be used in pregnancy (D) or children under twelve as it may cause permanent staining of teeth of foetus or child. Use with caution in breast feeding.

Use with caution in kidney and liver disease.

 Do not take if:

• suffering from severe kidney disease, systemic lupus erythematosus (SLE), Staphylococcal infection.

SIDE EFFECTS

Common: Loss of appetite, nausea, sore mouth, diarrhoea, difficulty in swallowing, inflamed colon.

Unusual: Vomiting, inflamed pancreas, rash, secondary fungal infection (thrush).

Severe but rare (stop medication, consult doctor): Severe belly pain, severe diarrhoea, tooth discolouration.

INTERACTIONS

Other drugs:

• Anticoagulants, Penicillin, Antacids, Iron, Oral contraceptives.

Other substances:

• Milk may reduce absorption from gut.

PRESCRIPTION

Yes.

PERMITTED IN SPORT

Yes.

OVERDOSE

Exacerbation of side effects only likely effect. See also Doxycycline, Methacycline, Minocycline, Tetracycline

Dequalinium chloride

TRADE NAME

Labosept.

DRUG CLASS

Antiseptic.

USES

Mouth and throat infections, mouth ulcers, denture irritation.

DOSAGE

 One every two or three hours.

FORMS

Lozenges

PRECAUTIONS

Safe in pregnancy (A), breast feeding and children.

SIDE EFFECTS

Minimal

INTERACTIONS

None significant

PRESCRIPTION

No.

PERMITTED IN SPORT

Yes.

Desferrioxamine

TRADE NAME

Desferal.

DRUG CLASS

Detoxifying agent.

USES

Iron poisoning.

DOSAGE

 By drip into vein as determined by doctor for each patient.

FORMS

Injection.

PRECAUTIONS

Use with caution in pregnancy (B3), breast feeding and children.

Not for long term use.

Not to be given rapidly.

Test eye and ear function regularly.

Use with caution in kidney disease.

 Do not take if:
• iron stores in body are normal.

SIDE EFFECTS

Common: Reaction at injection site, nausea, vomiting, diarrhoea.

Unusual: Disturbances to lung, heart, blood, kidney and nerve function. Increased risk of infection.

Severe but rare (stop medication, consult doctor): Growth disturbance in children.

INTERACTIONS

Other drugs:

• Phenothiazines, methyldopa, ascorbic acid.

Other substances:

• Vitamin C.

PRESCRIPTION

Yes.

PERMITTED IN SPORT

Yes.

OVERDOSE

Excessively low iron levels and organ damage may occur.

Desmopressin acetate

TRADE NAME

DDAVP, Desmospray, Desmotabs.

DRUG CLASS

Antidiuretic.

USES

Diabetes insipidus, bed wetting, abnormally frequent passing of urine.

DOSAGE

 Nasal spray: 10mcg to 40mcg a day
Tablets: One or two at night.

FORMS

Nasal spray, tablets, injection.

PRECAUTIONS

Use with caution in pregnancy (B2), breast feeding and children.

Use nasal spray with caution in nasal infection and hay fever.

Use all forms with caution in heart disease and after operations.

Lower doses necessary in elderly.

 Do not take if:

- suffering from some types of von Willebrand's disease.

SIDE EFFECTS

Common: Headache, stomach pain, nausea.

Unusual: Fluid retention, rapid heart rate, low blood pressure, headache, nausea, gut cramps, nasal congestion.

Severe but rare (stop medication, consult doctor): Convulsions.

INTERACTIONS

Other drugs:

- Glibenclamide, Clofibrate, Chlorpropamide.

PRESCRIPTION

Yes.

PERMITTED IN SPORT

Yes.

OVERDOSE

No serious effects expected.

OTHER INFORMATION

One of the few effective treatments for the rare condition of diabetes insipidus which is a totally separate condition to sugar diabetes (diabetes mellitus). Last resort treatment for bed wetting.

Desogestrel

See ORAL CONTRACEPTIVES

Desoxymethasone

TRADE NAME

Stiedex LP

Stiedex Lotion (with Salicylic acid).

DRUG CLASS

Corticosteroid.

USES

Inflammation of skin (eczema, dermatitis etc.).

DOSAGE

 Apply two or three times a day.

FORMS

Cream, lotion.

PRECAUTIONS

Skin preparations safe in pregnancy, breast feeding and children.

Avoid eyes.

Use for shortest period of time possible.

SIDE EFFECTS

Most significant side effects occur only with prolonged use. *Common:* Rarely cause adverse reactions.

Unusual: Thinning of skin, scarring of skin, premature ageing of skin.

INTERACTIONS

None significant.

PRESCRIPTION

Yes.

PERMITTED IN SPORT

Yes.

OVERDOSE

Exacerbation of side effects likely.

OTHER INFORMATION

Extremely effective and useful medication if used correctly. Lowest dose and shortest possible course should be used. Not addictive.

Dexamethasone

TRADE NAMES

Decadron, Dexsol, Minims Dexamethasone.

Dexa-Rhinaspray Duo (Dexamethasone isonicotinate with Tramazoline).

Maxidex (with Hypromellose).

Maxitrol (with Hypromellose, Neomycin, Polymyxin B).

Otomize (with Acetic acid, neomycin).

Sofradex (with Framycetin, Gramicidin).

DRUG CLASS

Corticosteroid.

PRECAUTIONS

Should be used in pregnancy (C), breast feeding and children only on specific medical advice.

Eye, nose and ear preparations safe in pregnancy, breast feeding and children.

Use tablets with caution if under stress, and in patients with under active thyroid gland, liver disease, diverticulitis, high blood pressure, myasthenia gravis, or kidney disease.

Avoid eyes with all forms except eye drops.

Use for shortest period of time possible.

 Do not take if:

- suffering from any form of infection, peptic ulcer, or osteoporosis.
- having a vaccination

USES

Severe inflammation of eyes, ears and nose.

Severe asthma, rheumatoid and other forms of severe arthritis, auto-immune diseases (eg: Sjøgren's syndrome), severe allergy reactions, other severe and chronic inflammatory diseases.

DOSAGE

 Eye drops: Insert every two to four hours
Ear drops: Two drops three times a day
Nose spray: One spray in each nostril two to four times a day
Tablets: O.5mg to 4mg a day strictly as directed by doctor.

FORMS

Injection, tablets, eye drops, ear drops, nose spray.

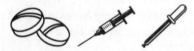

SIDE EFFECTS

Common: Tablets and injection - May cause bloating, weight gain, rashes and intestinal disturbances. Eye, ear and nose drops rarely cause adverse reactions.

Unusual: Tablets and injections - Biochemical disturbances of blood, muscle weakness, bone weakness, impaired wound healing, skin thinning, tendon weakness, peptic ulcers, gullet ulcers, bruising, increased sweating, loss of fat under skin, premature ageing, excess facial hair growth in women, pigmentation of skin and nails, acne, convulsions, headaches, dizziness, growth suppression in children, aggravation of diabetes, worsening of infections, cataracts, aggravation of glaucoma, blood clots in veins and sleeplessness.

Most significant side effects occur only with prolonged use of tablets.

Medication should not be ceased abruptly, but dosage should be slowly reduced.

Severe but rare (stop medication, consult doctor): Any significant side effect should be reported to a doctor immediately.

INTERACTIONS

Other drugs:

• Tablets - Oral contraceptives, Barbiturates, Phenytoin, Rifampicin.

PRESCRIPTION

Yes

PERMITTED IN SPORT

Tablets and injections: No.
Eye, nose and ear drops: Yes

OVERDOSE

Medical treatment is required. Serious effects and death rare.

OTHER INFORMATION

Extremely effective and useful medication if used correctly. Tablets must be used with extreme care under strict medical supervision. Lowest dose and shortest possible course should be used. Not addictive.

Dexamphetamine

TRADE NAME

Dexedrine.

DRUG CLASS

Stimulant, Amphetamine.

USES

Hyperactivity disorders in children, narcolepsy.

DOSAGE

 2.5mg to 60mg. a day in several doses depending upon age, condition and response.

FORMS

Tablets of 5mg. (white).

PRECAUTIONS

Should be used in pregnancy only if medically essential. Not for use in breast feeding. May be used in children over three years.

Use with caution in kidney disease.

 Do not take if:

- suffering from heart disease, high blood pressure, overactive thyroid gland, anxiety, excitability, Tourette syndrome,or twitching.

- MAOI taken within two weeks.

SIDE EFFECTS

Common: Dry mouth, restlessness, difficulty passing urine, sleeplessness, tremor, loss of appetite, twitching.

Unusual: Rapid heart rate, high blood pressure, irregular heart beat, angina.

INTERACTIONS

Other drugs:

- Urinary alkalinisers, MAOI.

PRESCRIPTION

Yes (restricted).

PERMITTED IN SPORT

No.

OVERDOSE

Very serious. May cause vomiting, agitation, tremors, twitching, confusion, hallucinations, convulsions, coma and death. Administer activated charcoal or induce vomiting if tablets taken recently. Seek urgent medical attention.

OTHER INFORMATION

May be addictive if used inappropriately. Very effective in improving the lives of some children with hyperactivity.

Dexketoprofen
See NSAID

Dextran
See EYE LUBRICANTS

Dextranomer

TRADE NAME

Debrisan.

USES

Ulcers and infected or weeping wounds.

DOSAGE

 Apply every one to three days.

FORMS

Micro beads, paste.

PRECAUTIONS

Safe in pregnancy, breast feeding and children.

No other precautions.

SIDE EFFECTS

Minimal.

INTERACTIONS

None significant.

PRESCRIPTION

No.

PERMITTED IN SPORT

Yes.

OVERDOSE

Unlikely to have serious effects if swallowed.

Dextromoramide

TRADE NAME

Palfium.

DRUG CLASS

Narcotic, Analgesic.

USES

Severe pain.

DOSAGE

 One to four tablets as required for pain before meals. Patient should lie down for 30 minutes after first dose.

FORMS

Tablets of 5mg. (white) and 10mg. (peach).

SIDE EFFECTS

Common: Lightheadedness, dizziness, drowsiness, fainting, nausea.

Unusual: Vomiting, difficulty in breathing.

PRECAUTIONS

Should not be used in the last few weeks of pregnancy (C) as medication may cause difficulty in breathing in newborn infant. Use with caution in breast feeding and children.

Not designed for prolonged use except in patients with terminal disease.

 Do not take if:

- suffering from severe lung disease, low blood pressure.

- operating machinery, driving a vehicle or undertaking tasks that require concentration.

INTERACTIONS

Other drugs:

- MAOI, Barbiturates, Tranquillisers, Anaesthetics.

Other substances:

- Do not use alcohol with Dextromoramide.

PRESCRIPTION

Yes (very restricted)

PERMITTED IN SPORT

No

OVERDOSE

Serious. Administer activated charcoal or induce vomiting if medication taken recently and patient alert. May cause drowsiness, difficulty in breathing, convulsions, coma and death. Especially dangerous when taken with other sedatives including alcohol. Seek urgent medical assistance. Antidote available.

OTHER INFORMATION

May cause dependence or addiction if used inappropriately.

Dextropropoxyphene

TRADE NAME

Doloxene.

Distalgesic (with Paracetamol).

DRUG CLASS

Narcotic, Analgesic.

USES

Pain relief.

DOSAGE

 One or two capsules or tablets, three or four times a day.

FORMS

Tablets, capsules.

PRECAUTIONS

Should only be used in pregnancy (C) if medically essential. May cause difficulty in breathing of newborn if used during labour.

Use with caution in breast feeding. Not for use in children. Use with caution in severe lung disease.

Designed for short term use.

 Do not take if:

- suffering from alcoholism.

- operating machinery or driving a vehicle.

SIDE EFFECTS

Common: Sleeplessness, mood changes, rash, dizziness, sedation, nausea.

Unusual: Constipation, belly pains, headache, lightheadedness, weakness, blurred vision.

Severe but rare (stop medication, consult doctor): Yellow skin (jaundice).

INTERACTIONS

Other drugs:

- Sedatives, Anticoagulants, Orphenadrine, Beta blockers, Diazepam, Phenytoin, Carbamazepine.

Other substances:

- Do not use with alcohol.

PRESCRIPTION

Yes.

PERMITTED IN SPORT

No.

OVERDOSE

Serious. Induce vomiting if medication taken recently and patient alert. Symptoms include drowsiness, convulsions, reduced breathing, low blood pressure, coma and possibly death. Seek emergency medical assistance.

OTHER INFORMATION

Widely used for many decades to treat moderate severity pain. May cause dependence if used long term and inappropriately.

Diabetes medications

See **HYPOGLYCAEMICS, Insulin**

Diazepam

See **ANXIOLYTICS**

Diazoxide

TRADE NAME

Eudemine.

DRUG CLASS

Vasodilator, Antihypertensive, Thiazide diuretic.

USES

Severe high blood pressure.

DOSAGE

 Injection into vein every four hours as necessary.

FORMS

Injection.

PRECAUTIONS

Use only if essential in pregnancy (C). Use with caution in breast feeding and children.

Use with caution in kidney disease, brain damage, severe heart disease, diabetes and gout.

Patient must be monitored very carefully during use.

 Do not take if:

- suffering from arteriovenous shunt, sensitive to thiazides.

SIDE EFFECTS

Common: High blood sugar, fluid retention, low blood pressure, headache, sensation of warmth, rapid heart rate.

Unusual: High blood salt levels, vomiting, diarrhoea.

Severe but rare (stop medication, consult doctor): Heart attack, stroke, coma.

INTERACTIONS

Other drugs:

- Thiazide diuretics, Anticoagulants, other medications that lower blood pressure.

PRESCRIPTION

Yes.

PERMITTED IN SPORT

Yes.

OVERDOSE

Extremely serious. Only given under close medical supervision.

OTHER INFORMATION

Only used in cases of extremely high, life threatening high blood pressure.

Dibromopropamidine isethionate

See Propamidine isethionate

Diclofenac

See NSAID

Dicyclomine

TRADE NAME

Merbentyl.

Kolanticon (with Dimethicone and Antacids).

DRUG CLASS

Anticholinergic, Spasmolytic.

USES

Spasm of the intestine, irritable bowel syndrome, colic.

DOSAGE

 Tablets: One to four tablets, three or four times a day. Mixture: 5 to 20mls three or four times a day.

FORMS

Merbentyl: Tablets, mixture. Infacol-C: Mixture.

PRECAUTIONS

Should only be used in pregnancy if medically indicated.

Should not be used while breast feeding.

Should not be used in children under six months of age.

Use with caution in glaucoma, enlarged prostate, reflux oesophagitis and hiatus hernia.

 Do not take if:

- suffering from difficulty in passing urine

- suffering from ulcerative colitis , intestinal obstruction or intestinal underactivity.

- suffering from myasthenia gravis.

SIDE EFFECTS

Common: Dry mouth, difficulty in passing urine, blurred vision.

Unusual: Rapid heart rate, loss of taste, headache, nervousness, weakness, dizziness, constipation, sleeplessness, bloating, rashes.

Severe but rare (stop medication, consult doctor): Cessation of breathing in infants.

INTERACTIONS

None significant

PRESCRIPTION

Merbentyl: Yes
Kolanticon: No

PERMITTED IN SPORT

Yes.

OVERDOSE

Causes headache, dizziness, vomiting, hot dry skin and difficulty in swallowing.

Didanosine

TRADE NAME

Videx.

DRUG CLASS

Antiviral.

USES

Treatment of advanced AIDS (Acquired Immune Deficiency Syndrome).

DOSAGE

 100 to 200mg. twice a day on an empty stomach.

FORMS

Tablets of 25, 100, 150 and 200mg..

PRECAUTIONS

Should not be used in pregnancy (B2) and children unless medically essential. Breast feeding should be ceased before use.

Use with caution in kidney and liver disease, pancreatitis.

SIDE EFFECTS

Common: Diarrhoea, nausea, vomiting.

Unusual: Pins and needles, chills, fever, headache, pancreatitis, muscle pain, tiredness, convulsions, confusion, sleeplessness, rash, itch, arthritis.

INTERACTIONS

Other drugs:

• Ketoconazole, Dapsone, Pentamidine, Tetracycline.

PRESCRIPTION

Yes.

PERMITTED IN SPORT

Yes.

OVERDOSE

Liver damage likely. Seek medical assistance.

OTHER INFORMATION

Introduced in 1993 to help slow the progress (but not cure) of HIV/AIDS.

Dienoestrol

TRADE NAME

Ortho Dienoestrol.

DRUG CLASS

Sex hormone.

USES

Inflammation and dryness of vagina due to lack of oestrogen.

DOSAGE

 Insert cream once or twice a day initially, reducing to one to three times a week long term.

FORMS

Vaginal cream.

PRECAUTIONS

Not designed for use in pregnancy (B1), breast feeding or children.

Use with caution in a history of blood clots.

Use with caution in heart failure, liver or kidney disease, high blood pressure, epilepsy, diabetes, migraine, endometriosis, breast pain, porphyria and high blood fats (cholesterol).

 Do not take if:

• suffering from otosclerosis, blood clots, stroke, breast or genital cancer.

SIDE EFFECTS

Common: Breast tenderness.

INTERACTIONS

None significant.

PRESCRIPTION

Yes.

PERMITTED IN SPORT

Yes.

OTHER INFORMATION

Often used as a mild form of hormone replacement in menopause.

Diethylamine salicylate

See SALICYLATES

Diflucortolone

TRADE NAME

Nerisone.

DRUG CLASS

Corticosteroid.

USES

Inflammation of skin (eczema, dermatitis etc.).

DOSAGE

 Apply two or three times a day.

FORMS

Cream, ointment.

PRECAUTIONS

Safe on skin in pregnancy (C), breast feeding and children over three years.

Avoid eyes.

Use for shortest period of time possible.

 Do not take if:

- suffering from any form of skin infection.

- having a vaccination

SIDE EFFECTS

Common: Minimal.

Unusual: Thinning of skin, premature ageing, itching, scarring of skin

Most significant side effects occur only with prolonged use of tablets or injections.

INTERACTIONS

None significant.

PRESCRIPTION

Yes.

PERMITTED IN SPORT

Yes.

Diflunisal

See NSAID

Digitalis

See Digoxin

Digoxin

TRADE NAME

Lanoxin.

DRUG CLASS

Cardiac glycoside.

USES

Heart failure, irregular heart beat originating in heart atrium (atrial fibrillation).

PRECAUTIONS

Safe in pregnancy (A), breast feeding and children.

Should be used with care in thyroid disease, malabsorption, poor kidney function and elderly.

Regular blood tests recommended to check blood level of medication.

 Do not take if:

- suffering from heart block.

DOSAGE

 Must be carefully individualised by regular blood tests. Usually one or two tablets once a day.

FORMS

Tablets of 62.5, 125 and 250mg., elixir, injection.

SIDE EFFECTS

Common: Usually associated with overdosage. Loss of appetite, nausea.

Unusual: Vomiting, weakness, breast enlargement (both sexes), depression, headache.

Severe but rare (stop medication, consult doctor): Unusual bleeding, slow heart rate.

INTERACTIONS

Other drugs:

- Blood levels of Digoxin increased by Diuretics, Lithium, Steroids, Carbenoxolone, Amiodarone, Captopril, Flecainide, Prazosin, Quinidine, Spironolactone, Tetracyclines, Erythromycin, Propantheline and other drugs.

- Blood levels of Digoxin decreased by Antacids, Kaolin, Pectin, bulking agents, Laxatives, Cholestyramine, Sulfasalazine, Neomycin, Rifampicin, Phenytoin, Metoclopramide, Penicillamine and other drugs. • Variable effects from Calcium channel blockers.

PRESCRIPTION

Yes.

PERMITTED IN SPORT

Yes.

OVERDOSE

May result in life threatening heart beat irregularities. Early symptom of overdosage is a slow heart rate. Administer activated charcoal or induce vomiting if tablets taken recently. Seek urgent medical assistance.

OTHER INFORMATION

In 1785, William Withering identified the active ingredient of an English folk remedy for dropsy (heart failure)distilled from the purple foxglove as digitalis. This has been further refined into Digoxin, which has been the most important medication for the treatment of heart disease for over two centuries.

Dihydrocodeine

TRADE NAMES

DF118, DHC Contiuous.

Remedeine (with Paracetamol).

DRUG CLASS

Cough suppressant, analgesic.

USES

Severe pain.

DOSAGE

 One or two tablets two or three times a day.

FORMS

Tablets.

PRECAUTIONS

Safe to use in pregnancy (A), breast feeding and children over two years.

Use with caution in severe lung disease.

SIDE EFFECTS

Common: Constipation, nausea, dizziness, headache when medication wears off.

INTERACTIONS

Other drugs:

• Sedatives, MAOI.

Other substances:

• Alcohol

PRESCRIPTION

Yes.

PERMITTED IN SPORT

Yes.

OVERDOSE

Sedation and constipation only likely effects.

OTHER INFORMATION

Safe and effective. Risk of dependence if used long term in high doses.

Dihydroergotamine

TRADE NAME

Migranal.

USES

Migraine, cluster headaches, vascular headaches, low blood pressure.

DOSAGE

 Nasal spray, repeated after 15 minutes if necessary. Maximum of four sprays a day.

FORMS

Nasal spray.

PRECAUTIONS

Not for use in pregnancy (C), breast feeding or children.

Use with caution in high blood pressure, nasal disorders,

 Do not take if:

• suffering from kidney or liver disease, heart disease, major infections, poor circulation to legs and arms, high blood pressure, history of stroke, head injury.

SIDE EFFECTS

Common: Nose irritation, nausea, vomiting, pins and needles sensation, muscle cramps, chest pain.

INTERACTIONS

Other drugs:

• Macrolide antibiotics, Glyceryl trinitrate, Beta-blockers, Ritonavir.

PRESCRIPTION

Yes.

PERMITTED IN SPORT

Yes.

OVERDOSE

Very serious. May cause arterial spasm, cessation of breathing, heart attack and death. Administer activated charcoal or induce vomiting if tablets taken recently. Seek emergency medical assistance.

OTHER INFORMATION

The ergot alkaloids are naturally occurring substances from a fungus that grows on rye. In the Middle Ages, accidental overdose of ergotamine and similar substances could follow the use of contaminated rye.

Dihydrotachysterol

TRADE NAME

AT-10.

USES

Conditions associated with low levels of calcium in the body (eg: hypoparathyroidism, rickets, osteomalacia, some forms of kidney and bowel failure).

DOSAGE

 Must be determined by doctor for each patient.

FORMS

Solution.

PRECAUTIONS

Use with caution in pregnancy, breast feeding and children.

Use with caution in kidney stones.

Regular blood tests to check level of calcium necessary.

SIDE EFFECTS

Common: Minimal at correct dose.

INTERACTIONS

Other drugs:

• Thiazide diuretics, Digoxin.

PRESCRIPTION

Yes.

PERMITTED IN SPORT

Yes.

OVERDOSE

May cause effects for many weeks including weakness, fatigue, nausea, vomiting, diarrhoea, headache, and increased frequency of passing urine. Long term overdosage may cause calcium deposits in kidneys, heart, lungs, skin and blood vessels. Give copious fluids and seek medical attention.

OTHER INFORMATION

Does not cause addiction or dependence. Increases absorption of calcium from intestine.

Diltiazem

See CALCIUM CHANNEL BLOCKERS

Dimethicone

(Simethicone)

TRADE NAMES

Infacol.

Altacite Plus (with Hydrotalcite).

Asilone, Maalox Plus (with Antacids).

Conotrane (with Benzalkonium chloride).

Kolanticon (with Dicyclomine and Antacids).

Siopel (with Cetrimide).

Spirilon, Vasogen (with Zinc oxide).

Also found in numerous other preparations.

USES

Skin protection, burping, indigestion, heartburn, dyspepsia, peptic ulcer.

DOSAGE

 Skin preparations: Apply freely as required
Mixtures: Use three or four times a day.

FORMS

Cream, mixture, gel, solution, skin spray.

PRECAUTIONS

Safe to use in pregnancy, breast feeding and children.

SIDE EFFECTS

Nil

INTERACTIONS

Other drugs:

• Tetracycline antibiotics.

PRESCRIPTION

No

PERMITTED IN SPORT

Yes.

Dinoprostone

TRADE NAME

Propess, Prostin.

USES

Inducing labour in late pregnancy.

DOSAGE

 As determined by doctor for each patient.

FORMS

Vaginal gel, tablets, pessary.

PRECAUTIONS

Not to be used until late in pregnancy (C).

Use with caution in liver, heart and kidney disease.

Use with caution in asthma, epilepsy and glaucoma.

Contractions of uterus and health of baby must be monitored regularly.

 Do not take if:

• suffering from ruptured membranes around the baby, head of baby is high, previous pregnancies delivered by Caesarean section, patient has had surgery to uterus, breech or other inappropriate presentation, abnormal vaginal bleeding, more than five previous childbirths.

SIDE EFFECTS

Common: Excessive contractions of uterus, altered heart rate in baby, nausea, diarrhoea, excess bleeding after delivery.

Unusual: Infection after delivery.

Severe but rare: Lung embolism.

INTERACTIONS

Other drugs:

• Oxytocin.

PRESCRIPTION

Yes.

OVERDOSE

Excessive contractions of uterus may lead to rupture of the uterus, a condition which is potentially fatal to mother and child.

OTHER INFORMATION

Normally used when a woman is overdue for delivery and the health of the baby is being affected by a prolonged pregnancy.

Diphenoxylate hydrochloride

TRADE NAME

Lomotil, Tropergen (with Atropine Sulfate).

DRUG CLASS

Antidiarrhoeal.

USES

Diarrhoea.

DOSAGE

 Two tablets, three or four times a day as required for diarrhoea.

FORMS

Tablets.

PRECAUTIONS

Should not be used in the last part of pregnancy (C). Should be used with caution in breast feeding.

Should not be used in children under 12 years.

 Do not take if:

- suffering from diarrhoea caused by use of antibiotics.
- suffering from jaundice, ulcerative colitis, Crohn's disease, bacterial colitis or amoebic colitis.

SIDE EFFECTS

Common: Tiredness, dizziness, confusion, rapid heart rate.

Unusual: Restlessness, mood changes, headache, tissue swelling, rash, vomiting, belly discomfort.

INTERACTIONS

Other drugs:

- Interacts with Barbiturates, Tranquillisers and Monoamine oxidase inhibitors (MAOI).

Other substances:

- Should not be taken with alcohol.

PRESCRIPTION

Yes.

PERMITTED IN SPORT

Yes.

OVERDOSE

Serious. May cause dry skin and mouth, restlessness, rapid heart rate, coma and reduced breathing. Seek urgent medical attention.

OTHER INFORMATION

Possibility of addiction with prolonged use. Very effective medication.

Diphtheria vaccine

TRADE NAME

Diftavax, Diphtheria Vaccine.

ACT-HiB DTP, Infanrix-HiB (with Haemophilus influenzae B, Tetanus and Whooping Cough vaccines).

Dip/Tet (with Tetanus Vaccine).

Infanrix, DTP (with Tetanus and Whooping Cough vaccines).

DRUG CLASS

Vaccine.

USES

Prevention of diphtheria (life threatening throat infection).

DOSAGE

Three doses two months apart at two, four and six months of age; repeat at 18 months, five years and then every ten years.

FORMS

Injection.

PRECAUTIONS

May be used safely in pregnancy (A), breast feeding and children.

SIDE EFFECTS

Common: Local redness, soreness and lump at injection site; fever.

Unusual: Tiredness, irritability.

INTERACTIONS

None significant

PRESCRIPTION

Yes.

PERMITTED IN SPORT

Yes.

OVERDOSE

No serious effect expected if unintentional additional dose given.

OTHER INFORMATION

Normally given in combination with Tetanus and Whooping Cough vaccines as Triple Antigen. Should be given to all infants starting at two months of age. Diphtheria is a very serious infectious disease causing severe and often fatal throat infection. It can be prevented by vaccination.

Dipipanone

TRADE NAME

Diconal (with Cyclizine).

DRUG CLASS

Narcotic.

USES

Moderate to severe pain.

DOSAGE

One tablet, two or three times a day.

FORMS

Tablet (pink).

PRECAUTIONS

Not for use in children.

Use with caution in pregnancy and breast feeding.

Use with caution in patients with history of narcotic dependency. Use with caution in under active thyroid gland, low blood pressure, diabetes and enlarged prostate gland.

 Do not take if:

- suffering from severe lung disease, alcoholism, head injury, ulcerative colitis, liver or kidney disease.

SIDE EFFECTS

Common: Tolerance to drug requiring higher doses, drowsiness, dry mouth.

Unusual: Blurred vision.

INTERACTIONS

Other drugs:

• MAOI, Sedatives.

Other substances:

• Alcohol.

PRESCRIPTION

Yes (restricted).

PERMITTED IN SPORT

No.

OVERDOSE

Moderately serious. May cause initial stimulation, followed by vomiting, drowsiness, convulsions, reduced breathing, coma and very rarely death. Seek urgent medical attention.

OTHER INFORMATION

May cause dependency or addiction if used unnecessarily for long periods. Relatively mild narcotic drugs. Risk of dependency.

Dipivefrine hydrochloride

TRADE NAME

Propine.

USES

Some types of glaucoma.

DOSAGE

 One drop twice a day.

FORMS

Eye drops.

PRECAUTIONS

May be used in pregnancy, breast feeding and children.

 Do not take if:

• suffering from narrow angle glaucoma.

SIDE EFFECTS

Common: Red eyes, eye burning and stinging.

Unusual: Rapid heart rate.

INTERACTIONS

None significant.

PRESCRIPTION

Yes.

PERMITTED IN SPORT

Yes.

Dipyridamole

TRADE NAME

Persantin, Persantin Retard.

Asasartin Retard (with Aspirin)

DRUG CLASS

Anticoagulant.

USES

Prevention and treatment of blood clots and strokes, particularly in patients with previous strokes, transient ischaemic attacks (mini-strokes), kidney disease and after transplantation of heart valves.

DOSAGE

 Persantin - One tablet four times a day one hour before meals.

Asasartin Retard, Persantin Retard - One tablet twice a day.

FORMS

Tablet, capsule.

PRECAUTIONS

Should be used with caution in pregnancy (B1). Not for use in breast feeding. Use with caution in children.

SIDE EFFECTS

Common: Headache.

Unusual: Diarrhoea, nausea, flushing.

PRESCRIPTION

Yes.

PERMITTED IN SPORT

Yes.

OVERDOSE

Unlikely to be serious, but medical assistance should be sought.

OTHER INFORMATION

Often used in combination with other Anticoagulants. Very safe and can be taken long term to prevent heart attacks and strokes.

Disodium clodronate

TRADE NAME

Loron.

USES

High blood calcium blood levels, bone cancer pain.

DOSAGE

 2 to 4 capsules a day in divided doses, one hour before or after food.

FORMS

Capsules, tablets, injection.

PRECAUTIONS

Not to be used in pregnancy, breast feeding and children.

Use with caution in kidney disease.

Blood levels of calcium and phosphate must be checked regularly during use.

 Do not take if:
- suffering severe kidney disease, mouth ulcers.

SIDE EFFECTS

Common: Nausea, diarrhoea.

Unusual: Blood chemistry changes, reduced kidney function, skin reactions.

Severe but rare (stop medication, consult doctor): Damage to kidney or parathyroid glands.

INTERACTIONS

Other drugs:

- Other drugs that alter calcium levels, Antacids.

Other substances:

- Mineral supplements.

PRESCRIPTION

Yes.

PERMITTED IN SPORT

Yes.

OVERDOSE

Potentially very serious. Seek urgent medical attention.

Disodium cromoglycate

See Sodium cromoglycate

Disodium etidronate

See Etidronate

Disodium pamidronate

See Pamidronate

Disopyramide

TRADE NAME

Dirythmin SA, Rythmodan, Rythmodan Retard.

DRUG CLASS

Antiarrythmic.

USES

Control of heart beat irregularities.

DOSAGE

 Rythmodan: One or two tablets, three to four times a day
Dirythmin SA, Rythmodan Retard: One or two, twice a day

FORMS

Capsules, tablets, injection.

 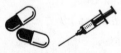

PRECAUTIONS

Should be used with caution in pregnancy (B2) and breast feeding. Not designed for use in children.

Use with caution in heart failure, diabetes, glaucoma, prostate disease, kidney and liver failure.

 Do not take if:

• suffering from heart failure

SIDE EFFECTS

Common: Dose related effects may cause dry mouth, nausea, indigestion, belly pains, bloating, constipation, blurred vision, difficulty in passing urine, dry eyes, dry nose.

Unusual: Dizziness, angina, itch, rash, loss of appetite, bad taste, diarrhoea, frequent urination, burning on urination, impotence, tiredness, pins and needles sensation, headache.

Severe but rare (stop medication, consult doctor): Unable to pass urine, yellow skin.

INTERACTIONS

Other drugs:

• Other drugs for treatment of irregular heart rhythm.

• Phenothiazines, Tricyclic Antidepressants, Phenytoin.

PRESCRIPTION

Yes.

PERMITTED IN SPORT

Yes.

OVERDOSE

Extremely serious. Administer activated charcoal or induce vomiting if conscious. Seek emergency medical assistance. Symptoms include shortness of breath, cessation of breathing, coma and death.

Distigmine

TRADE NAME

Ubretid.

DRUG CLASS

Anticholinesterase.

USES

Myasthenia gravis, inability to pass urine, maintenance of bowel movement after surgery, premedication before general anaesthetic.

DOSAGE

 One to three tablets once or twice a day

FORMS

Tablets.

PRECAUTIONS

Should be used in pregnancy (C) only when medically essential. Safe for use in breast feeding. Use with caution in children.

Dosage must be carefully monitored by doctor.

Use with caution in epilepsy, slow heart rate, asthma, recent heart attack, irregular heart beat, overactive thyroid gland, and peptic ulcer.

 Do not take if:
• suffering from gut obstruction.

SIDE EFFECTS

Common: Slow heart rate, headache, nausea, diarrhoea, excess salivation, cough, wheeze, bowel noises.

Unusual: Confusion, slurred speech, vomiting, belly cramps, desire to pass urine, muscle cramps, contracted pupils.

Severe but rare (stop medication, consult doctor): Difficulty breathing, chest pain.

INTERACTIONS

Other drugs:

• Muscle relaxants, Atropine, Aminoglycosides, drugs used to treat irregular heart beat, some anaesthetics.

PRESCRIPTION

Yes.

OVERDOSE

Serious. May cause diarrhoea, vomiting, difficulty in breathing, weakness, low blood pressure, slow heart rate and heart attack. Seek urgent medical attention.

OTHER INFORMATION

Very useful for the few patients with the distressing muscle disease of myasthenia gravis.

Disulfiram

TRADE NAME

Antabuse.

USES

Alcoholism. Causes violent vomiting if alcohol taken within 24 hours.

DOSAGE

 Half to two tablets once a day.

FORMS

Tablets (white) of 200mg.

SIDE EFFECTS

Common: Numbness, tingling, pain or weakness in hands and feet.

Unusual: Eye pain, blurred vision, psychiatric disturbances, impotence, headache, tiredness, bad taste.

INTERACTIONS

Other drugs:

- Metronidazole and Paraldehyde must not be used.
- Phenytoin, Isoniazid, Chlordiazepoxide, Diazepam, Anticoagulants.

Other substances:

- Reacts severely with alcohol.

PRESCRIPTION

Yes.

PERMITTED IN SPORT

Yes.

OVERDOSE

Severe adverse effects unlikely provided alcohol avoided. Induce vomiting if medication taken recently. Seek medical attention.

PRECAUTIONS

Use in pregnancy (B2) and breast feeding only if medically essential. Not designed for use in children.

Patient and close relatives must be made completely aware of effects of medication before use.

Use with caution in diabetes, thyroid disease, epilepsy, allergic dermatitis, eczema and asthma.

Not designed for prolonged use.

 Do not take if:

- suffering from significant heart disease, severe liver or kidney disease, psychiatric disturbances.
- using cough mixtures or other medicines containing alcohol.
- alcohol taken within previous 24 hours.

OTHER INFORMATION

A very useful incentive in encouraging alcoholics to completely abstain from alcohol. Must be accompanied by appropriate counselling and support. In use for many decades. Does not cause addiction or dependence.

Dithranol

(Anthralin)

TRADE NAMES

Dithrocream, Micanol.

Psorin (with Salicylic acid and Tar).

USES

Psoriasis, fungal skin infections.

DOSAGE

 Apply sparingly twice a day. Wash off if redness occurs.

FORMS

Cream, ointment.

PRECAUTIONS

Safe in pregnancy and breast feeding. Use with caution on children.

Avoid eyes, nostrils, mouth, vagina, penis head and anus.

Use with care in skin folds and thin skin.

Wash hands after use.

 Do not take if:

- suffering from severe or pustular psoriasis.
- suffering from broken skin.

SIDE EFFECTS

Common: Skin irritation.

INTERACTIONS

None significant

PRESCRIPTION

No.

PERMITTED IN SPORT

Yes.

OTHER INFORMATION

Very effective medication for psoriasis, but must be used carefully, starting with lowest concentration cream then slowly increasing strength depending on response.

DIURETICS

(Increase output of urine)

See Amiloride, Bumetanide, Frusemide, Spironolactone, THIAZIDE DIURETICS, Torasemide, Triamterene

Docosahexaenoic acid

See Fatty acids

Docusate sodium

TRADE NAME

Dioctyl, Docusol, Fletcher's Enemette, Norgalax, Waxsol.

Normax (with Danthron).

DRUG CLASS

Laxative, softener.

USES

Constipation, softening faeces, softening ear wax.

DOSAGE

 Tablets: Two tablets, once a day after evening meal
Suppositories: One a day in evening
Ear drops: Ten drops nightly for two or three nights.

FORMS

Tablets, suspension, suppository, liquid enema, ear drops.

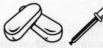

PRECAUTIONS

Safe in pregnancy (A), breast feeding and after medical advice in children.

Designed for short term use only, unless advised otherwise by a doctor.

 Do not take if:
• suffering from belly pains or bowel obstruction.

SIDE EFFECTS

Common: Ear drops - None. Other forms - Belly discomfort.

Unusual: Diarrhoea. Blood chemistry imbalances with prolonged use.

Severe but rare (stop medication, consult doctor): Severe belly pains.

INTERACTIONS

Other drugs:

• Do not use within two hours of any other Laxative.

PRESCRIPTION

Normax: Yes
Others: No

PERMITTED IN SPORT

Yes.

OVERDOSE

Diarrhoea and loss of vital body chemicals may occur.

OTHER INFORMATION

Safe and frequently used medication. Use of ear drops before ear syringing makes wax removal far easier.

Domperidone

TRADE NAME

Motilium.

Domperamol (with Paracetamol).

DRUG CLASS

Antiemetic.

USES

Nausea, vomiting, delayed stomach emptying, migraine.

DOSAGE

 Motilium: One tablet, three or four times a day, 30 minutes before meals
Domperamol: Two every four hours as necessary
maximum eight a day.

PRECAUTIONS

Should be used with caution in pregnancy (B2) and breast feeding and children.

Use with caution in breast cancer, liver and kidney disease.

 Do not take if:
• suffering from some forms of pituitary gland tumour.

FORMS

Motilium: Tablets (white) of 10mg.
Domperamol: Tablet (white).

SIDE EFFECTS

Common: Minimal.

Unusual: Dry mouth, stomach cramps, breast enlargement, breast milk production, reduced libido, rash. Rare: Dizziness.

INTERACTIONS

Other drugs:

• Antacids, Anticholinergics, Narcotics.

PRESCRIPTION

Yes.

PERMITTED IN SPORT

Yes.

OVERDOSE

No serious effects likely. Seek medical advice.

OTHER INFORMATION

A remarkably safe and effective medication introduced in the mid-1980s. Marvellous for motion sickness. Does not cause dependence or addiction, but is designed for short term use.

Donepezil

TRADE NAME

Aricept.

DRUG CLASS

Anticholinesterase.

USES

Mild Alzheimer's disease.

DOSAGE

 5 to 10mg. a day before bed.

FORMS

Tablets of 5mg. (white) and 10mg. (yellow).

PRECAUTIONS

Not for use in breast feeding (B3), breast feeding or children.

Use with caution in irregular heart rhythm, peptic ulcers, asthma, emphysema, seizures, difficulty in passing urine.

SIDE EFFECTS

Common: Nausea, diarrhoea, tiredness, sleeplessness.

Unusual: Muscle cramps, difficulty in passing urine, seizures, dizziness, headache, loss of appetite.

Severe but rare (stop medication, consult doctor): Liver damage (jaundice), psychiatric disturbances, irregular heart rhythm, peptic ulcer.

INTERACTIONS

Other drugs:

• Some anaesthetics, Beta-blockers, other Anticholinergics, NSAID, Ketoconazole, Phenytoin, Quinidine, Carbamazepine, Dexamethasone, Rifampicin, Phenobarbitone.

PRESCRIPTION

Yes.

PERMITTED IN SPORT

Yes.

OVERDOSE

Serious. May cause diarrhoea, vomiting, difficulty in breathing, weakness, low blood pressure, slow heart rate and heart attack. Seek urgent medical attention.

OTHER INFORMATION

Introduced in 1999 as a form of treatment for the otherwise untreatable early stages of Alzheimer's disease.

See also PYRIDOSTIGMINE

Dorzolamide hydrochloride

TRADE NAME

Trusopt.

Cosopt (with Timolol).

USES

Glaucoma.

DOSAGE

 One drop two or three times a day in affected eye.

PRECAUTIONS

Use with caution in pregnancy (B3), breast feeding and children.

Only suitable for certain types of glaucoma (open angle glaucoma).

Use with caution in severe liver and kidney disease.

Use with caution if eye painful from ulcers on surface or other eye disease present.

 Do not useif:

• wearing contact lenses.

FORMS

Eye drops.

SIDE EFFECTS

Common: Eye irritation, bitter taste.

INTERACTIONS

Other drugs:

• Oral carbonic anhydrase inhibitors (eg: Acetazolamide, Dichlorphenamide, Methazolamide).

PRESCRIPTION

Yes.

PERMITTED IN SPORT

Yes.

OVERDOSE

May cause heart and blood pressure irregularities.

OTHER INFORMATION

Introduced in 1996.

Dothiepin

See TRICYCLICS

Doxazosin

TRADE NAME

Cardura.

DRUG CLASS

Alpha blocker.

USES

Control of mild to moderate high blood pressure.

DOSAGE

 Start at low dose and increase very slowly. Maximum 8mg. a day in divided doses.

FORMS

Tablets of 1, 2 and 4mg.

PRECAUTIONS

Use with considerable caution in pregnancy (B3). Use with caution in breast feeding. Not for use in children.

Use lower doses in elderly.

Use with caution in heart disease, blood vessel disease, severe liver and kidney disease.

SIDE EFFECTS

Common: Sudden drop in blood pressure to cause fainting, swelling of ankles, headache, tiredness.

Unusual: Fatigue, change in heart rate.

Severe but rare (stop medication, consult doctor): Low white blood cell count, severe infections.

INTERACTIONS

None significant.

PRESCRIPTION

Yes.

PERMITTED IN SPORT

Yes.

OVERDOSE

Low blood pressure, drowsiness and depressed reflexes only effects.

OTHER INFORMATION

Introduced in 1996.

See also Prazosin.

Doxepin

See ANTIHISTAMINES, SEDATING;
TRICYCLIC ANTIDEPRESSANTS

Doxycycline

TRADE NAME

Vibramycin.

DRUG CLASS

Tetracycline antibiotic, Antimalarial.

USES

Treatment or prevention of infections
caused by susceptible bacteria.
Prevention of malaria.

DOSAGE

 Treatment of infection: Two
tablets or capsules at once, then
one tablet or capsule a day
Prevention of malaria and acne:
One tablet or capsule a day.

FORMS

Capsules, tablets.

SIDE EFFECTS

Common: Loss of appetite, nausea, sore
mouth, diarrhoea, difficulty in
swallowing, inflamed colon.

Unusual: Vomiting, inflamed pancreas,
rash, sun sensitive skin, secondary fungal
infection (thrush).

Severe but rare (stop medication, consult
doctor): Severe belly pain, severe
diarrhoea, tooth discolouration.

PRECAUTIONS

Not to be used in pregnancy (D) or
children under twelve as it may
cause permanent staining of teeth of
foetus or child. Use with caution in
breast feeding.

Use with caution in kidney disease.

 Do not take if:

- suffering from severe
  kidney disease, systemic
  lupus erythematosus
  (SLE), Staphylococcal
  infection.

- Taking Vitamin A or
  Retinoids.

INTERACTIONS

Other drugs:

- Vitamin A, Retinoids, Anticoagulants,
  Penicillin, Antacids, Iron, Oral
  contraceptives, Methoxyflurane.

Other substances:

- Milk and food may reduce absorption
  from gut.

PRESCRIPTION

Yes.

PERMITTED IN SPORT

Yes.

OVERDOSE

Exacerbation of side effects only likely
effect.

OTHER INFORMATION

Used to prevent acne and malaria. Used
to treat a wide variety of bacterial
infections. Does not cause dependence or
addiction.

**See also Demeclocycline, Methacycline,
Minocycline, Tetracycline**

Droperidol

TRADE NAME

Droleptan

DRUG CLASS

Antipsychotic.

USES

Calming manic and agitated patients, severe nausea, some types of anaesthesia.

DOSAGE

 5 to 20mg., every four to eight hours.

FORMS

Tablets, liquid, injection.

PRECAUTIONS

Not to be used in pregnancy (C)

Use with caution in breast feeding.

May be used in children.

Use with caution in liver and kidney disease, and epilepsy.

 Do not take if:

- suffering from head injury, coma, Parkinson's disease, epilepsy.

SIDE EFFECTS

Common: Drowsiness, low blood pressure.

Unusual: Confusion, tremor.

Severe but rare (stop medication, consult doctor): Abnormal heart rhythm, abnormal muscle movements.

INTERACTIONS

Other drugs:

- Narcotics, Sedatives, medications that lower blood pressure.

Other substances:

- Alcohol.

PRESCRIPTION

Yes.

PERMITTED IN SPORT

Yes.

OVERDOSE

Very serious. Seek urgent medical attention. Rapid death possible. Sedation and low blood pressure leading to coma with muscle rigidity.

OTHER INFORMATION

Often used during gastroscopy and colonoscopy procedures to relax patient.

Dydrogesterone

TRADE NAME

Duphaston.

DRUG CLASS

Sex hormone

USES

Abnormal bleeding from uterus, failure of menstrual periods, endometriosis, painful menstrual periods. Used with Oestrogens in post-menopausal hormone replacement.

DOSAGE

 Must be individualised by doctor.

FORMS

Tablets (white) of 10mg.

PRECAUTIONS

Not to be used in pregnancy (D), breast feeding or children.

Use with caution in high blood pressure, heart failure, and depression.

 Do not take if:

• suffering from blood clots, inflamed veins, stroke, angina, heart attack, breast or genital cancer, liver disease, sickle cell anaemia.

SIDE EFFECTS

Common: Dizziness, breast pain.

Severe but rare (stop medication, consult doctor): Blood clot, yellow skin (jaundice).

INTERACTIONS

Other drugs:

• Other Sex Hormones.

PRESCRIPTION

Yes.

PERMITTED IN SPORT

Yes.

OVERDOSE

Vomiting and abnormal vaginal bleeding only likely effects.

OTHER INFORMATION

Does not cause addiction or dependence.

Econazole

See IMIDAZOLES

Efavirenz

TRADE NAME

Sustiva.

DRUG CLASS

Antiviral.

USES

Treatment of HIV/AIDS in combination with other medications.

DOSAGE

 Up to 600mg. once a day.

PRECAUTIONS

Never to be used in pregnancy (D). Use with caution in breast feeding and children.

Use with caution in liver and kidney disease, psychiatric disturbances.

Use lower doses in elderly.

Monitor blood cholesterol and liver enzyme levels by regular blood tests.

 Do not take if:

- suffering from severe liver disease.
- unless using other medications to control HIV/AIDS.

FORMS

Capsules of 50, 100 and 200mg.

SIDE EFFECTS

Common: Rash, dizziness, sleeplessness, nausea, diarrhoea, tiredness.

Unusual: Poor concentration, psychotic reactions, headache.

Severe but rare (stop medication, consult doctor): Liver damage.

INTERACTIONS

Other drugs:

- Terfenadine, Cisapride, Astemizole, Midazolam, Triazolam, Oral contraceptives, Phenobarbitone, Phenytoin.

Other substances:

- Grapefruit,

PRESCRIPTION

Yes

PERMITTED IN SPORT

Yes

OVERDOSE

Serious liver and brain damage may occur. Seek urgent medical attention. Induce vomiting or give activated charcoal if alert and medication taken recently.

OTHER INFORMATION

One of numerous antivirals that are used in combination to control HIV/AIDS.

Eformoterol

TRADE NAME

Foradil, Oxis.

DRUG CLASS

Bronchodilator.

USES

Long term treatment of asthma.

DOSAGE

 Inhale once or twice, two times a day.

FORMS

Capsules containing powder for inhalation, inhaler.

PRECAUTIONS

Use with caution in pregnancy (B3). Safe in breast feeding and children over five years.

Not for use in unstable or deteriorating asthma.

Do not exceed recommended dose.

Do not swallow capsules.

Use with caution in diabetes, heart and thyroid disease.

Lung function should be monitored regularly by use of spirometer.

SIDE EFFECTS

Common: Tremor, palpitations, headache, throat irritation, dizziness.

Unusual: Lung irritation, low blood potassium levels.

INTERACTIONS

Other drugs:

• Other bronchodilators used for treatment of asthma (check with doctor).

PRESCRIPTION

Yes

PERMITTED IN SPORT

No

OVERDOSE

Palpitations, tremor and exacerbation of side effects likely.

OTHER INFORMATION

Introduced in 1996. Enables patients who would otherwise use large quantities of inhaled bronchodilators (eg: Ventolin) to reduce their usage of these medications dramatically.

Eicosapentaenoic acid

TRADE NAME

Used as an ingredient in many skin preparations and nutritional supplements.

Maxepa (with Docosahexaenoic acid).

DRUG CLASS

Nutritional (triglyceride) supplement, moisturiser.

USES

Fatty acid supplement, dry skin.

DOSAGE

 One to five capsules twice a day. Apply to skin three times a day.

PRECAUTIONS

Safe in pregnancy (A), breast feeding and children.

Do not exceed recommended dose.

FORMS

Capsules, liquid, creams, gels.

SIDE EFFECTS

Common: Nausea.

INTERACTIONS

None significant.

PRESCRIPTION

No

PERMITTED IN SPORT

Yes

OVERDOSE

Vomiting and diarrhoea only likely effects.

OTHER INFORMATION

Derived from fish oil.

See also Fatty acids

ELECTROLYTES

TRADE and GENERIC NAMES

Electrolytes such as Sodium chloride (common salt), Potassium bicarbonate, Potassium chloride, Sodium bicarbonate and Sodium acid citrate are found in numerous preparations, sometimes in combination with Antacids, Laxatives and Analgesics.

Algicon (Potassium bicarbonate with Aluminium hydroxide, Calcium carbonate, Magnesium salts, and other ingredients). See ANTACIDS for further details.

Aqsia, Askina, Irriclens, Minims Sodium Chloride, Normasol, Optiflo S, Steripod Blue, Uriflex S, Uriflex SP, Uro-Tainer (Sodium chloride).

Burinex K (Potassium chloride with Bumetanide).

Diumide K, Lasikal (Potassium chloride with Frusemide).

Glandosane, Luborant (Potassium chloride and Sodium chloride with Carboxymethylcellulose).

Iocare (Sodium chloride, Potassium chloride, Sodium acetate and Sodium citrate with Calcium chloride, Magnesium chloride, Sodium citrate).

Kay-Cee-L, Slow-K (Potassium chloride).

Klean-Prep, Movicol (Potassium chloride, Sodium chloride and Sodium bicarbonate with Polyethylene glycol, and other ingredients).

Kloref (Potassium bicarbonate and Potassium chloride with Betaine and Potassium benzoate).

Micralax (Sodium citrate with Sorbic acid, Sodium alkylsulphoacetate).

Microlette (Sodium citrate with Glycerol, Sodium lauryl sulphoacetate)

Mictral (Sodium citrate and Sodium Bicarbonate with Nalidixic acid).

Minims Artificial Tears (Sodium chloride with Hydroxymethycellulose)

Neo-Naclex-K (Potassium chloride with Bendrofluazide).

Pyrogastrone Liquid (Potassium bicarbonate with Carbenoxolone and Antacids).

Relaxit (Sodium citrate with Glycerol, Sodium lauryl sulphoacetate, Sorbitol and other ingredients).

Sando-K (Potassium bicarbonate and Potassium chloride).

Electrolytes are underlined

Electrolytes are also found in many ANTACIDS(see separate entry).

USES

Replacement of essential electrolytes lost because of diarrhoea, vomiting, excess passing of urine, heart disease and other diseases.

DOSAGE

 Tablets: One to four tablets a day in one or more doses **Powder:** Dissolve in water and use as often as necessary to prevent dehydration.

FORMS

Tablets, powder, mixture, enema, injection.

PRECAUTIONS

Safe in pregnancy, breast feeding and children.

Be careful not to exceed necessary dose.

Blood tests to measure severity of electrolyte depletion and response to treatment may be necessary.

Use with caution in kidney and liver disease, stomach ulcers.

Dilute powders with water only, not milk, juice etc.

Use with caution in dehydration as adequate fluid replacement also necessary.

 ## Do not take if:

• suffering from Addison's disease, severe kidney disease, severe injuries or burns.

SIDE EFFECTS

Common: Minimal.

Unusual: Fluid retention.

INTERACTIONS

Other drugs:

• Triamterene, Amiloride.

PRESCRIPTION

No

PERMITTED IN SPORT

Yes

OVERDOSE

Most forms: No serious effects expected.

Potassium salts: Serious. May cause low blood pressure, irregular heart beat, pins and needles sensation, convulsions, paralysis, heart attack, inability to breathe and death. Administer activated charcoal or induce vomiting if medication taken recently. Seek urgent medical assistance.

OTHER INFORMATION

Electrolytes are elements such as Potassium, Sodium, Chlorine and Magnesium that are essential for the biochemical functioning of the body. Diuretics cause increased loss of potassium and specific replacement and regular checks of blood potassium level is advisable.

Emedastine

TRADE NAME

Emadine.

DRUG CLASS

Antihistamine.

USES

Allergic conjunctivitis (eye allergy).

DOSAGE

 One drop into affected eye(s) twice a day.

FORMS

Eye drops.

PRECAUTIONS

Must not be used in pregnancy (D).

Use with caution in breast feeding and kidney disease.

May be used in children over three years.

Use with caution if wearing contact lenses. Do not use long term.

 Do not take if:

- suffering from kidney or liver disease.

SIDE EFFECTS

Common: Eye irritation, blurred vision.

Unusual: Eye surface swelling, headache, eye pain, runny nose.

INTERACTIONS

None significant.

PRESCRIPTION

Yes

PERMITTED IN SPORT

Yes

OVERDOSE

Unlikely to be serious.

OTHER INFORMATION

Introduced in 1999.

See also Levocabastine

Enalapril

See ACE INHIBITORS

Enoxaparin

TRADE NAME

Clexane.

DRUG CLASS

Anticoagulant.

USES

Prevention and treatment of blood clots in veins. Often used after major surgery.

DOSAGE

 As determined by doctor for each patient.

FORMS

Injection.

PRECAUTIONS

Not to be used in pregnancy (C) unless essential. Use with caution in breast feeding.

Must not be injected into muscle.

Use with caution in severe kidney and liver disease, history of peptic ulcer and uncontrolled high blood pressure.

Not for use in association with a spinal or epidural anaesthetic.

 Do not use if:

- suffering from heart infections, bleeding disorders, active peptic ulcer, stroke caused by bleeding in brain.

- Taking aspirin or NSAIDs (anti-inflammatory drugs used for arthritis).

SIDE EFFECTS

Common: Abnormal bruising and bleeding, bruising at injection site.

Unusual: Liver damage.

Severe but rare (stop medication, consult doctor): Bleeding from anus, coughing blood.

INTERACTIONS

Other drugs:

• Warfarin, other anticoagulants, NSAIDs, aspirin, dextran.

Other substances:

• Celery tablets.

PRESCRIPTION

Yes

PERMITTED IN SPORT

Yes

OVERDOSE

Very serious. Excessive bleeding may occur. Antidote available. Given under strict medical supervision.

OTHER INFORMATION

Introduced in 1996. Has fewer side effects than Heparin.

See also Heparin.

Entacapone

TRADE NAME

Comtess.

DRUG CLASS

Antiparkinsonian.

USES

Severe Parkinson's disease, unmanageable by other medications.

DOSAGE

 One tablet, four to seven times a day.

FORMS

Tablets of 200mg. (orange).

PRECAUTIONS

Use with caution in pregnancy (B3), breast feeding and children.

Use with caution in low blood pressure.

Avoid taking with fatty meal.

Do not cease suddenly, but reduce dose slowly.

 Do not take if:

• suffering from phaeochromocytoma, liver disease.

SIDE EFFECTS

Common: Incoordination, dry mouth, nausea, diarrhoea, belly pains, discoloured urine.

Unusual: Sleep disturbances, psychiatric disturbances, chest pain, confusion, shortness of breath.

Severe but rare (stop medication, consult doctor): Pneumonia, anaemia.

INTERACTIONS

Other drugs:

• MAOI, Isoprenaline, Adrenaline, Methyldopa, Apomorphine, Iron, Diazepam, Venlafaxine, Antidepressants, Ibuprofen, Benserazide.

Other substances:

• Fatty foods.

PRESCRIPTION

Yes

PERMITTED IN SPORT

Yes

OVERDOSE

Likely to be serious. Seek urgent medical attention.

OTHER INFORMATION

Introduced in 1999 to assist the most severely affected cases of Parkinson's disease.

See also ANTIPARKINSONIANS

ENZYMES

See PANCREATIC ENZYMES

Ephedrine

TRADE NAME

CAM.

Franol (with Theophylline).

Haymine (with Chlorpheniramine).

DRUG CLASS

Sympathomimetic, Bronchodilator.

USES

Asthma, spasm of bronchi in lungs, severe allergy, bed wetting.

DOSAGE

 One or two tablets, three or four times a day.

FORMS

Tablets, injection

PRECAUTIONS

May be used in pregnancy (A), breast feeding and children.

Use with caution in heart disease, angina and prostate gland enlargement.

Do not exceed recommended dose.

 Do not take if:

- suffering from narrowing of heart arteries, heart attack, glaucoma, high blood pressure, overactive thyroid gland.

SIDE EFFECTS

Common: Alertness, sleeplessness, dizziness, headache, nausea, sweating, palpitations.

Unusual: Vomiting, diarrhoea, rapid heart rate, difficulty in passing urine, weakness.

INTERACTIONS

Other drugs:

- MAOI, Digoxin.

Other substances:

- Reacts with caffeine.

PRESCRIPTION

Yes

PERMITTED IN SPORT

No

OVERDOSE

Exacerbation of side effects leading to convulsions and possible heart attack possible. Seek urgent medical assistance.

Epoetin

See Erythropoietin

Eprosartan

See ANGIOTENSIN II RECEPTOR ANTAGONISTS

Ergocalciferol

See Cholecalciferol, Calcitriol and Ergocalciferol

TRADE NAME

(Vitamin D).

Ergometrine

TRADE NAME

Ergometrine.

Syntometrine (with Oxytocin).

USES

Stopping abnormal bleeding after delivery or abortion.

DOSAGE

 One injection immediately after delivery of baby.

FORMS

Injection.

PRECAUTIONS

Safe to use after delivery in pregnancy (A), but should not otherwise be used in pregnancy. Safe for use in breast feeding. Not for use in children.

Use with caution in heart disease.

Do not take injection if:

• previous Caesarean section.

SIDE EFFECTS

Common: Rapid heart rate, retention of fluid.

PRESCRIPTION

Yes

PERMITTED IN SPORT

Yes

OVERDOSE

Unlikely to have serious effects.

OTHER INFORMATION

Injection commonly used to increase intensity of labour and immediately after delivery to reduce bleeding.

Ergotamine

TRADE NAME

Lingraine.

Migril (with Caffeine, Cyclizine).

Cafergot (with Caffeine).

DRUG CLASS

Antimigraine.

USES

Migraine, vascular headaches.

DOSAGE

 Tablets and capsules: One or two tablets or capsules immediately symptoms detected. Repeat every half hour. Maximum six a day
Suppository: One immediately symptoms detected. Maximum three a day.

FORMS

Tablets, capsules, suppositories.

SIDE EFFECTS

Common: Nausea, vomiting, diarrhoea, leg weakness, pins and needles sensation, chest pain.

Unusual: Swelling of feet, itch, slow heart rate.

Severe but rare (stop medication, consult doctor): Severe chest pain, irregular heart beat.

INTERACTIONS

Other drugs:

•Vasoconstrictors.

Other substances:

• Alcohol, caffeine, smoking and exercise may be migraine triggers.

PRESCRIPTION

Yes

PERMITTED IN SPORT

Yes

PRECAUTIONS

Should not be used in pregnancy (C) as it may cause premature labour. Not for use in breast feeding or children.

Should not be used for prolonged period.

Not designed for prevention of migraine.

 ### Do not take if:

• suffering from poor circulation to arms or legs, angina, high blood pressure, hardening of arteries, severe infection, severe liver or kidney disease.

OVERDOSE

May be serious. Symptoms include vomiting, diarrhoea, thirst, tingling, itching, cold skin, rapid weak pulse, confusion and coma. If tablets or capsules taken recently, induce vomiting. Seek urgent medical assistance.

OTHER INFORMATION

May become ineffective if used too frequently.

See also Dihydroergotamine.

Erythromycin

TRADE NAME

Aprimycin, Eryacne, Erymax, Erythrocin, Erythroped, Ilosone, Stiemycin, Tiloryth.

Benzamycin (with Benzoyl peroxide).

Isotrexin (with Isotretinoin).

Zineryt (with Zinc acetate and other ingredients).

DRUG CLASS

Macrolide antibiotic.

USES

Treatment of infections caused by susceptible bacteria, acne.

DOSAGE

 One tablet or capsule, two to four times a day
Gel: Apply twice a day.

FORMS

Tablets, capsules, injection, syrup, suspension, gel.

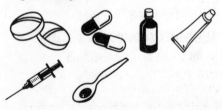

PRECAUTIONS

Safe to use in pregnancy (A), breast feeding and children.

Not designed for prolonged or repeated use.

Use with caution in liver disease.

 Do not take if:

- suffering from severe liver disease, jaundice (yellow skin).
- using Terfenadine or Astemizole.

SIDE EFFECTS

Common: Nausea, vomiting, diarrhoea, rash, headache.

Unusual: Belly pain, loss of appetite, excess wind, dizziness, ear noises, temporary deafness.

Severe but rare (stop medication, consult doctor): Yellow skin (jaundice), irregular heart beat.

INTERACTIONS

Other drugs:

- Terfenadine, Astemizole, Theophylline, Carbamazepine, Warfarin, Cyclosporin, Triazolam, Phenytoin, Digoxin, Oral contraceptives, Dihydroergotamine.

PRESCRIPTION

Yes

PERMITTED IN SPORT

Yes

OVERDOSE

Severe diarrhoea, stomach pains and deafness may occur.

OTHER INFORMATION

Used for a wide range of infections in general practice. Does not cause addiction or dependence. Some forms may cause fewer side effects than others.

Erythropoietin

(Epoetin)

TRADE NAME

Eprex, Neorecormon.

USES

Stimulates red blood cell production in anaemia associated with kidney failure.

DOSAGE

 One to three injections a week as determined by doctor.

FORMS

Injection.

PRECAUTIONS

Use in pregnancy (B3) only if medically essential. Not for use in breast feeding or children.

Use with caution in heart disease, epilepsy, porphyria and gout.

 Do not take if:

- suffering from uncontrolled high blood pressure.

SIDE EFFECTS

Common: Chills, bone pains, headache, fluid retention.

Unusual: Rash, high blood pressure.

INTERACTIONS

Other drugs:

- Iron

PRESCRIPTION

Yes

PERMITTED IN SPORT

No. Occasionally used illegally in endurance sports, when it may cause blood clots and sudden death.

OTHER INFORMATION

Has dramatically improved life expectancy and quality of life for patients on dialysis for kidney failure, but expense limits its use. Has been used illegally by athletes to improve the oxygen uptake of their body and increase endurance.

Esmolol

See BETA BLOCKERS

Estradiol

See Oestradiol

Estramustine

TRADE NAME

Estracyt.

USES

Cancer of prostate gland.

DOSAGE

 One to three capsules, two to three times a day depending on body weight.

FORMS

Capsules of 140mg. (off white).

SIDE EFFECTS

Common: Nausea, diarrhoea, fluid retention, breast enlargement and tenderness, reduced libido.

Unusual: Blood clots, heart damage.

INTERACTIONS

Other drugs:

• None significant.

Other substances:

• Reacts with milk and milk products.

PRECAUTIONS

Must not be used in women or children.

Use with caution with history of blood clots, heart disease, diabetes, bone marrow damage.

 Do not take if:

• suffering from liver disease, peptic ulcer, severe heart disease or blood clots.

PRESCRIPTION

Yes

PERMITTED IN SPORT

Yes

OVERDOSE

Serious exacerbation of side effects possible. Seek medical assistance.

OTHER INFORMATION

Although significant side effects occur, this medication may prolong life.

Estropipate

TRADE NAME

Harmogen.

DRUG CLASS

Sex hormone.

USES

Female hormone replacement in menopause.

DOSAGE

 One or two tablets a day, combined with Progestogen for 10 to 14 days if uterus intact.

FORMS

Tablets of 1.5mg. (peach).

PRECAUTIONS

Not to be used in pregnancy (B1), breast feeding or children. Accidental usage in these situations unlikely to be harmful.

Use with caution in epilepsy, migraine, heart failure, high blood pressure, kidney disease, diabetes, porphyria or uterine disease.

 Do not take if:

- suffering from liver disease, breast or genital cancer, blood clots.

SIDE EFFECTS

Common: Abnormal uterine bleeding, vaginal thrush, nausea, fluid retention, weight gain, breast tenderness.

Unusual: Rash, blurred vision, vomiting, bloating, intestinal cramps, pigmentation of skin on face.

Severe but rare (stop medication, consult doctor): Blood clots, calf or chest pain, yellow skin (jaundice).

INTERACTIONS

Other drugs:

- Other Sex hormones.

Other substances:

- Smoking increases risk of serious side effects.

PRESCRIPTION

Yes

PERMITTED IN SPORT

Yes

OVERDOSE

Vomiting and abnormal vaginal bleeding only likely effects.

OTHER INFORMATION

Does not cause addiction or dependence. Very useful in managing the effects of menopause, and reduces the risk of osteoporosis and heart disease after the menopause.

See also Oestrogen

Ethanol

TRADE NAME

Ethanol is common alcohol (ethyl alcohol), and is used in a large number of medications, particularly as a solvent in mixtures, gels and lotions.

Ethanol is the alcohol that is present in all alcoholic drinks (beer, wine, spirits etc.).

DRUG CLASS

Alcohol.

PRECAUTIONS

Use in pregnancy should be avoided. May be used in small quantities in breast feeding. Not to be given to children except when used in approved medications.

 Do not take if:

- suffering from liver damage, alcoholism, depression, other psychiatric conditions, pancreatitis, any abnormal bleeding.

- operating machinery, driving a vehicle or undertaking tasks that require concentration.

USES

In medication: Dissolves other medications, acts as a preservative, mild sedative, mild cough suppressant. In drinks: Relaxes, reduces inhibitions.

DOSAGE

 As directed or desired.

FORMS

Mixture, liquid, gel, lotion.

SIDE EFFECTS

Common: Drowsiness, flush, rapid heart rate.

Unusual: Nausea, vomiting, headache.

INTERACTIONS

Other drugs:

• Interacts with a wide range of medications. Should not be taken while using any other medication without consulting a pharmacist or doctor.

Other substances:

• Reacts adversely with exercise, Cocaine, Marijuana and Narcotics.

PRESCRIPTION

No

PERMITTED IN SPORT

Yes. Impairs sport performance.

OVERDOSE

Vomiting, poor coordination, loss of inhibitions, headache, blurred vision, loss of control of bodily functions, convulsions, coma and rarely death may occur. Seek medical assistance if massive rapid overdose consumed.

OTHER INFORMATION

Ethanol has been produced by fermenting various fruits, vegetables and cereals for thousands of years and is mankind's most widely used drug. May cause dependence and addiction. Long term use at moderate to high dosage can cause damage to liver, brain and other organs.

Ethinyloestradiol

See **MORNING AFTER PILL, ORAL CONTRACEPTIVES**

Ethoheptazine

TRADE NAME

Equagesic (with Meprobamate, Aspirin).

DRUG CLASS

Narcotic.

USES

Moderate to severe muscle and bone pain.

DOSAGE

 One or two tablets, two or three times a day.

FORMS

Tablets (pink, white, yellow).

SIDE EFFECTS

Common: Tolerance to drug requiring higher doses, drowsiness, dizziness, nausea, dry mouth.

Unusual: Blurred vision, poor coordination, pins and needles sensation, excitation.

Severe but rare (stop medication, consult doctor): Damage to blood cells, intestinal bleeding.

INTERACTIONS

Other drugs:

• MAOI, Sedatives, Anticoagulants.

Other substances:

• Alcohol.

PRECAUTIONS

Not for use in pregnancy, breast feeding and children.

Use with caution in patients with history of narcotic dependency.

Use lower dose in elderly.

Use with caution in under active thyroid gland, epilepsy, depression'suicide tendency, low blood pressure, diabetes and enlarged prostate gland.

 ### Do not take if:

• suffering from severe lung disease, alcoholism, head injury, ulcerative colitis, peptic ulcer, liver or kidney disease, haemophilia, porphyria.

PRESCRIPTION

Yes (restricted).

PERMITTED IN SPORT

No

OVERDOSE

Moderately serious. May cause initial stimulation, followed by vomiting, drowsiness, convulsions, reduced breathing, coma and very rarely death. Seek urgent medical attention.

OTHER INFORMATION

May cause dependency or addiction if used unnecessarily for long periods. Relatively mild narcotic drugs.

Ethosuximide

TRADE NAME

Emeside, Zarontin.

DRUG CLASS

Anticonvulsant.

USES

Petit mal epilepsy (absences).

DOSAGE

 One to four capsules twice a day.

FORMS

Capsule of 250mg., syrup.

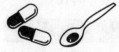

PRECAUTIONS

Not to be used in pregnancy (D) unless medically essential. Breast feeding should be ceased before use. May be used in children.

Regular blood tests to check on liver function and blood cells recommended.

Do not stop medication suddenly, but reduce dosage slowly.

Use with caution if operating machinery or driving a vehicle.

SIDE EFFECTS

Common: Loss of appetite, nausea, belly cramps, drowsiness, headache.

Unusual: Belly pain, weight loss, diarrhoea, hiccups, irritability, rash, abnormal liver function.

INTERACTIONS

Other substances:

• Reacts adversely with alcohol.

PRESCRIPTION

Yes

PERMITTED IN SPORT

Yes

OVERDOSE

Administer activated charcoal or induce vomiting if medication taken recently and patient alert. Seek medical attention.

OTHER INFORMATION

Widely and successfully used in treatment of petit mal absences. Does not cause dependence or addiction.

Ethynodiol diacetate

See ORAL CONTRACEPTIVES

Etidronate

(Disodium etidronate)

TRADE NAME

Didronel.

DRUG CLASS

Bisphosphonate.

USES

Paget's disease, osteoporosis.

DOSAGE

 Once a day at bedtime on an empty stomach. Usually combined with calcium supplement.

FORMS

Tablets, effervescent tablet.

PRECAUTIONS

Use in pregnancy only if medically essential. Not for use in breast feeding or children.

Use with caution in peptic ulcer, inflamed bowel, kidney stones.

Diet must contain adequate calcium and vitamin D.

 Do not take if:

• suffering from osteomalacia, severe kidney disease.

SIDE EFFECTS

Common: Diarrhoea, nausea.

Unusual: Bone pain.

Severe but rare (stop medication, consult doctor): Bleeding from bowel.

INTERACTIONS

Other drugs:

• Antacids, vitamin and mineral supplements.

Other substances:

• High calcium foods (eg: cheese, sardines).

PRESCRIPTION

Yes

PERMITTED IN SPORT

Yes

OVERDOSE

Unlikely to be serious unless taken long term in excessive doses.

OTHER INFORMATION

Does not cause dependence or addiction.

Etodolac

See NSAID

Etonogestrel

TRADE NAME

Implanon

DRUG CLASS

Sex hormone.

USES

Long term contraception. One implant gives three years protection.

DOSAGE

 One implant inserted under skin at inside of upper arm every three years. Implant initially during a menstrual period.

FORMS

Implant.

PRECAUTIONS

Not for use in pregnancy (B3), breast feeding or children.

Implantation must be preceded by a thorough medical history and examination.

 Do not take if:

- suffering from blood clots (thromboses), liver disease or tumours, breast cancer.
- cause of any abnormal vaginal bleeding has not been diagnosed.

SIDE EFFECTS

Common: Breast discomfort, heavy periods, acne, headaches, belly pain, emotional upsets, weight increase, pain at implant site.

Unusual: Chloasma (skin pigmentation), hair loss, dizziness, nausea, depression, increased libido.

Severe but rare (stop medication, consult doctor): Blood clot in vein or artery, lumps in breast, constant vaginal bleeding.

INTERACTIONS

Other drugs:

- Barbiturates, primidone, carbamazepine, rifampicin, other sex hormones.

PRESCRIPTION

Yes

PERMITTED IN SPORT

Yes

OTHER INFORMATION

Introduced in 1999 as an improved long term contraceptive that requires no regular dosing schedule or planning.

Etoposide

TRADE NAME

Vepesid.

Etopophos (Etoposide phosphate).

USES

Leukaemia, lung cancer, Hodgkin's disease, lymphoma.

PRECAUTIONS

Not to be used in pregnancy (D) unless mother's life is threatened. Breast feeding must be ceased before use. Use in children only if medically essential.

Adequate contraception must be used by women while taking Etoposide.

Regular blood tests to check blood cells, kidney and liver function essential.

Use with caution in infections.

Do not allow infusion to come in contact with skin.

 Do not take if:

- suffering from severe liver or bone marrow disease.

DOSAGE

 Complex. Must be determined individually for each patient by doctor depending on diseases, severity, response and size of patient.

FORMS

Capsules (pink) of 50mg. and 100mg., drip infusion.

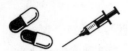

SIDE EFFECTS

Common: Reduced blood white cells and increased risk of infection, unusual bleeding and bruising, total hair loss, nausea, vomiting, loss of appetite, sore mouth, diarrhoea.

Unusual: Low blood pressure, fever, rapid heart rate, shortness of breath, pins and needles.

INTERACTIONS

Other drugs:

• Other medications used to treat cancer.

PRESCRIPTION

Yes

PERMITTED IN SPORT

Yes

OVERDOSE

Worsening of side effects likely. Seek medical attention.

OTHER INFORMATION

Despite serious side effects, Etoposide may be life saving for patients with some severe forms of cancer.

Evening primrose oil (Linoleic acid)

See FATTY ACIDS

Exemestane

TRADE NAME

Aromasin.

USES

Advanced breast cancer.

DOSAGE

 One tablet a day.

FORMS

Tablet of 25mg. (white).

SIDE EFFECTS

Common: Hot flushes, nausea, fatigue, sweating, headache, dizziness, sleeplessness, muscle pain.

Unusual: Rash, loss of appetite, weight loss, belly pains, depression, swelling of feet, hair loss, constipation, indigestion.

Severe but rare (stop medication, consult doctor): Blood cell damage, liver damage.

PRECAUTIONS

Not to be used in pregnancy (D), breast feeding or children.

Use with caution in liver and kidney disease.

Blood tests to check liver function required regularly.

 Do not take if:

• still menstruating regularly.

INTERACTIONS

Other drugs:

• Oestrogen.

PRESCRIPTION

Yes

PERMITTED IN SPORT

Yes

OVERDOSE

Very serious. Seek urgent medical attention.

OTHER INFORMATION

Introduced in 1999 to treat breast cancer patients in whom no other treatment is helping.

EYE LUBRICANTS

TRADE and GENERIC NAMES

Geltears (Carbomer 940).

Hypotears, LiquifilmTears, Sno Tears (Polyvinyl alcohol).

Ilube (Hypromellose with Acetylcysteine).

Isopto Alkaline, Isopto Plain (Hypromellose).

Isopto Atropine (Hypromellose with Atropine).

Isopto Carbachol (Hypromellose with Carbachol).

Isopto Carpine (Hypromellose with Pilocarpine).

Isopto Frin (Hypromellose with Phenylephrine).

Lacri Lube, Lubri-Tears (Paraffin, wool fat).

Maxidex (Hypromellose with Dexamethasone).

Maxitrol (Hypromellose with Dexamethasone, Neomycin, Polymixin).

Minims Artificial Tears (Hydroxymethylcellulose).

Oculotect (Povidone)

Tears Naturale (Hypromellose with Dextran).

Viscotears (Polyacrylic acid).

NB: Eye lubricants are underlined.

USES

Dry, itchy, irritated eyes

DOSAGE

 Use drops as required several times a day.

FORMS

Eye drops, eye ointment, eye gel.

PRECAUTIONS

May be used safely in pregnancy (use Carbomer 940 with caution), breast feeding and children.

Use with caution if wearing contact lenses.

SIDE EFFECTS

Common: Mild stinging, blurred vision.

INTERACTIONS

None significant.

PRESCRIPTION

No

PERMITTED IN SPORT

Yes

OVERDOSE

No adverse effects likely if swallowed.

OTHER INFORMATION

Widely and commonly used for dry itchy eyes.

Famciclovir

TRADE NAME

Famvir.

DRUG CLASS

Antiviral

USES

Treatment of herpes zoster infections (genital herpes, shingles).

DOSAGE

 One tablet two or three times a day.

FORMS

Tablets (white) of 250, 500 and 750mg.

PRECAUTIONS

Use with caution in pregnancy (B1), breast feeding and children.

Use with caution in serious kidney disease.

SIDE EFFECTS

Common: Headache.

Unusual: Nausea, fatigue.

INTERACTIONS

Other drugs:

• Probenecid, Diuretics (fluid tablets).

PRESCRIPTION

Yes

PERMITTED IN SPORT

Yes

OVERDOSE

Exacerbation of side effects likely.

OTHER INFORMATION

Introduced in 1996. Very safe and effective medication that has a very high success rate in treating Herpes infections. Chickenpox and shingles are caused by Herpes zoster, and cold sores and genital herpes by Herpes simplex. It is vital that any patient who suspects they have shingles must see their doctor immediately as medication only works if started within 72 hours of onset of rash.

Famotidine

TRADE NAME

Pepcid.

DRUG CLASS

Anti-ulcerant.

USES

Ulceration of the stomach, duodenum (upper small intestine) and oesophagus (gullet). Zollinger-Ellison syndrome (a rare cause of severe stomach ulceration).

DOSAGE

 20 to 40mg. once a day at night. Higher doses with Zollinger-Ellison syndrome and severe ulceration.

FORMS

Tablets of 20mg. and 40mg.

PRECAUTIONS

Caution required in pregnancy (B1), and with children.

Do not take if:

- suffering from stomach cancer, significant kidney disease, breast feeding.

SIDE EFFECTS

Common: Headache, dizziness, irregular bowel habits.

Unusual: Dry mouth, nausea, loss of appetite, bloating, tiredness, itchy skin, arthritis.

INTERACTIONS

None significant.

PRESCRIPTION

Yes

PERMITTED IN SPORT

Yes

OVERDOSE

No serious adverse effects expected.

OTHER INFORMATION

An effective and safe medication for rapidly easing the pain of peptic ulcers, and curing them. May be used safely long term.

FATTY ACIDS

TRADE and GENERIC NAMES

Evening Primrose Oil (Linoleic acid).

Maxepa (Eicosapentaenoic acid, Docosahexaenoic acid).

Fatty acids are also found in numerous other nutritional, vitamin and mineral supplements.

USES

Fatty acid (triglyceride) deficiency.

DOSAGE

One or two capsules, two or three times a day with food.

FORMS

Capsules, liquid.

PRECAUTIONS

Safe in pregnancy, breast feeding and children. Not to be used long term.

SIDE EFFECTS

Common: Increased bleeding time.

INTERACTIONS

Other drugs:

- Anticoagulants.

PRESCRIPTION

No

PERMITTED IN SPORT

Yes

OVERDOSE

Unlikely to have serious effects.

OTHER INFORMATION

Does not cause addiction or dependence.

Felbinac

See NSAID

Felodipine

See CALCIUM CHANNEL
BLOCKERS

Fenbufen

See NSAID

Fenofibrate

TRADE NAME

Lipantil Micro

DRUG CLASS

Hypolipidaemic.

USES

Lowers blood fat (cholesterol) levels.

DOSAGE

 67mg. three times a day with food, or 200 to 267mg. once a day with food.

FORMS

Capsules of 67, 200 and 267mg.

SIDE EFFECTS

Common: Nausea, diarrhoea, rash.

Unusual: Headache, tiredness, dizziness.

Severe but rare (stop medication, consult doctor): Poor libido, muscle pain, liver damage, light sensitivity.

INTERACTIONS

Other drugs:

• Anticoagulants, Phenylbutazone, diabetes medications, other medications to lower cholesterol.

PRECAUTIONS

Not to be used in pregnancy and breast feeding.

May be used in children.

Use with caution in kidney disease.

 Do not take if:

• suffering from gall stones, other gall bladder disease, severe liver or kidney disease.

PRESCRIPTION

Yes

PERMITTED IN SPORT

Yes

OVERDOSE

No specific problems. Exacerbation of side effects likely.

OTHER INFORMATION

Normally only used in patients who are resistant to other medications.

See also Clofibrate, HYPOLIPIDAEMICS

Fenoprofen

See NSAID

Fenoterol

See BETA-2 AGONISTS

Fentanyl

TRADE NAME

Durogesic, Sublimaze.

DRUG CLASS

Narcotic analgesic.

USES

Relief of severe pain.

DOSAGE

 Durogesic - One patch applied every three days. Injection - intramuscular or intravenous as determined by doctor.

FORMS

Skin patches of 25, 50, 75 and 100 µg, injection.

PRECAUTIONS

Not for use in pregnancy (C).

Use with caution in breast feeding and children.

Initial dose of patch should not exceed 25µg.

Use with caution in head injuries, fevers, severe lung, kidney, liver and heart disease.

Lower doses required in elderly.

 Do not take if:

- suffering from intermittent or post-operative pain.
- history of drug abuse

SIDE EFFECTS

Common: Tolerance requiring higher doses, addiction to medication, tiredness, constipation, dry mouth, nausea, sweating.

Unusual: Vomiting, confusion, abdominal pain, hallucinations, reduced breath volume, low blood pressure, itchy rash, local skin reactions at site of patch application, excessive happiness (euphoria).

Severe but rare (stop medication, consult doctor): Retention of urine, irregular heart beat, chest pain (angina).

INTERACTIONS

Other drugs:

- Monoamine oxidase inhibitors (MAOI - used for severe depression), sedatives, ribonavir.

Other substances:

- Alcohol.

PRESCRIPTION

Yes

PERMITTED IN SPORT

No

OVERDOSE

Excessive use of patches may result in worsening of side effects to the point of life threatening lung and heart complications. The effects will persist for up to 24 hours after patches removed. Antidote available. Seek urgent medical attention.

OTHER INFORMATION

Patches introduced in 2000 for the treatment of persistent cancer pain with less constipation and sedation than narcotic pain killers taken by mouth or injection. Injection usually used only during a general anaesthetic.

See also other medications listed under Narcotics

Fenticonazole
See IMIDAZOLES

FERROUS SALTS

(Ferric ammonium citrate, Ferrous fumarate, Ferrous gluconate, Ferrous phosphate, Ferrous sulfate)

See Iron

Fexofenadrine

See **ANTIHISTAMINES, NON-SEDATING**

FIBRE

See **Frangula, Ispaghula, Methylcellulose, Pectin, Psyllium, Sterculia**

FIBRINOLYTICS

TRADE and GENERIC NAMES

Actilyse (Alteplase).

Kabikinase, Streptase (Streptokinase).

Varidase (Streptokinase and Streptodornase).

USES

Lysis (destruction) of blood clots in veins and arteries, particularly in heart, lungs and brain.

Cleaning of wounds full of slough.

DOSAGE

 As administered by doctor.

FORMS

Injection, powder.

PRECAUTIONS

Only used in pregnancy (C) if medically essential. Breast feeding should be ceased if medication used. Not designed for use in children, but may be necessary medically.

 Do not take if:

• recent surgery performed.

SIDE EFFECTS

Common: Minor unusual bleeding, fever.

Unusual: Significant unusual bleeding, allergy reaction.

INTERACTIONS

Other drugs:

• Anticoagulants.

PRESCRIPTION

Yes

PERMITTED IN SPORT

Yes, but no vigorous activity should be undertaken for some time after use.

OVERDOSE

Serious, but antidote available.

OTHER INFORMATION

Injection used only in hospital for seriously ill patients. Topical forms used to clean up wound exudates.

See also Aprotinin.

Finasteride

TRADE NAME

Proscar.

USES

Benign enlargement of prostate gland.

DOSAGE

 One tablet a day for six to twelve months.

FORMS

Tablets (blue) of 5mg.

PRECAUTIONS

Must never be used in pregnancy (X) as severe damage may be caused to foetus.

Must never be used in breast feeding or children.

Must never be used in women.

Pregnant women whose male partner is using Finasteride must avoid sex during pregnancy as contact with semen may cause deformities in foetus.

SIDE EFFECTS

Common: Impotence, decreased libido.

Unusual: Breast enlargement in men, rash.

INTERACTIONS

None significant.

PRESCRIPTION

Yes

PERMITTED IN SPORT

Yes

OVERDOSE

No serious consequences expected.

OTHER INFORMATION

Released in 1993. Extremely dangerous in pregnancy, otherwise safe and effective. May take some months for improvement in symptoms. Does not cause dependence or addiction.

Flavoxate

TRADE NAME

Urispas.

DRUG CLASS

Antispasmodic.

USES

Incontinence of urine, frequency of urination, passing urine excessively at night, pain when passing urine, pain after passing urinary catheter.

DOSAGE

 One tablet three times a day.

FORMS

Tablets of 200mg. (white).

PRECAUTIONS

Use with caution in pregnancy, breast feeding and children.

Exclude urinary obstruction and prostate cancer before use.

Use with caution in glaucoma.

 Do not take if:

• suffering from gut obstruction.

SIDE EFFECTS

Common: Headache, nausea, fatigue, diarrhoea.

Unusual: Blurred vision, dry mouth.

INTERACTIONS

None significant.

PRESCRIPTION

Yes

PERMITTED IN SPORT

Yes

OVERDOSE

Exacerbation of side effects likely.

Flecainide

TRADE NAME

Tambocor.

DRUG CLASS

Antiarrythmic.

USES

Control and prevention of certain types of heart beat irregularity.

DOSAGE

 One to three tablets twice a day.

FORMS

Tablets of 50mg. and 100mg., injection.

PRECAUTIONS

Should be used only if essential and with caution in pregnancy (B3). Should only be used if medically essential in breast feeding and children.

Use with caution in heart failure, if pacemaker implanted, kidney or liver disease.

 Do not take if:

- suffering from recent heart attack, or certain types of heart nerve conduction defects.

SIDE EFFECTS

Common: Noises in ears, palpitations, fainting, chest pains, dizziness, rash, nausea, constipation, diarrhoea, belly pains, visual disturbances, shortness of breath.

Unusual: Angina, slow heart rate, high blood pressure, swelling of tissues, vomiting, fever, sweating, impotence, discomfort on urination, arthritis, leg cramps, muscle aches, dry mouth, twitches, double vision, anxiety, confusion, tiredness.

Severe but rare (stop medication, consult doctor): Jaundice, continued angina, severe shortness of breath, marked tissue swelling.

INTERACTIONS

Other drugs:

- Digoxin, Disopyramide, Verapamil, Amiodarone.

PRESCRIPTION

Yes (restricted to treatment of serious cardiac arrhythmias where treatment is started in hospital).

PERMITTED IN SPORT

Yes

OVERDOSE

Low blood pressure and rapid heart rate likely. Administer activated charcoal or induce vomiting if tablets taken recently. Seek medical assistance.

Flucinolone

TRADE NAME

Synalar.

Synalar C (with Clioquinol).

Synalar N (with Neomycin).

DRUG CLASS

Corticosteroid.

USES

Inflammation of skin (eczema, dermatitis etc.).

DOSAGE

 Apply two or three times a day.

FORMS

Cream, ointment.

PRECAUTIONS

Should be used with caution in pregnancy, breast feeding and children. Avoid eyes. Use for shortest period of time possible.

 Do not take if:

• suffering from any form of skin infection, acne, or broken skin.

SIDE EFFECTS

Common: Minimal.

Unusual: Thinning of skin, itching, burning, stinging, scarring of skin.

INTERACTIONS

None significant

PERMITTED IN SPORT

Yes

OTHER INFORMATION

Lowest dose and shortest possible course should be used.

Flucloxacillin

TRADE NAME

Floxapen.

Magnapen (with Ampicillin).

DRUG CLASS

Penicillin antibiotic.

USES

Treatment of infections caused by susceptible bacteria.

DOSAGE

 One or two capsules every six hours 30 min. before food. Course (usually 7 days) should be completed.

FORMS

Capsules, mixture (store in door of refrigerator), injection.

PRECAUTIONS

May be used in pregnancy (B1), children and breast feeding if medically indicated.

Use with caution in kidney failure, liver disease, premature infants and leukaemia.

Not for use in eyes.

 Do not take if:

• allergic to Penicillin

• suffering from glandular fever

SIDE EFFECTS

Common: Mild diarrhoea, nausea, vomiting.

Unusual: Genital itch or rash.

Severe but rare (stop medication, consult doctor): Itchy rash, hives, severe diarrhoea, yellow skin (jaundice), unusual bleeding or bruising.

INTERACTIONS

Other drugs:

• Probenecid.

PRESCRIPTION

Yes

PERMITTED IN SPORT

Yes

OVERDOSE

Vomiting and diarrhoea only likely effects.

OTHER INFORMATION

Used for more severe infections. Some bacteria can break down simpler forms of Penicillin. Cloxacillin, Dicloxacillin and Flucloxacillin are not able to be broken down this way and so can be effective when other Penicillins fail. Does not cause dependence or addiction.

Fluconazole

TRADE NAME

Diflucan.

DRUG CLASS

Antifungal.

USES

Fungal infections of vagina (thrush), mouth, oesophagus, brain and other areas.

DOSAGE

 Vaginal thrush: Single tablet taken once
More severe infections: One to four tablets a day.

PRECAUTIONS

Not to be used in pregnancy (B3) or children unless medically essential. Cease breast feeding before use.

Use with caution in kidney disease and dehydration.

Ensure adequate fluid intake.

FORMS

Tablet of 50 and 200mg., suspension, infusion.

SIDE EFFECTS

Common: Nausea.

Unusual: Headache, rash, vomiting, diarrhoea, belly discomfort.

INTERACTIONS

Other drugs:

• Warfarin, Phenytoin, Cyclosporin, Hypoglycaemics, Rifampicin, Theophylline.

PRESCRIPTION

Yes

PERMITTED IN SPORT

Yes

OVERDOSE

Hallucinations and mental disturbance may occur. Administer activated charcoal or induce vomiting if medication taken recently. Seek medical attention.

OTHER INFORMATION

Introduced in early 1990s. A single dose by mouth will cure most forms of thrush (Candidiasis) in the vagina, mouth or elsewhere in the body. Very useful in the treatment of fungal complications in AIDS. Very expensive.

Flucytosine

TRADE NAME

Ancotil.

DRUG CLASS

Antifungal.

USES

Generalised fungal infections.

DOSAGE

 As determined by doctor.

FORMS

Injection.

PRECAUTIONS

Not to be used in pregnancy (B3) unless clinically essential. Breast feeding should be ceased before use. May be used with caution in children.

Use with caution in bone marrow disease and kidney disease.

SIDE EFFECTS

Common: Nausea.

Unusual: Vomiting, rash, diarrhoea.

INTERACTIONS

Other drugs:

• Amphoterecin B.

PRESCRIPTION

Yes

PERMITTED IN SPORT

Yes

OVERDOSE

May cause kidney damage. Seek medical advice.

OTHER INFORMATION

Extremely expensive, and so reserved for the most severe fungal infections.

Fludrocortisone

TRADE NAME

Florinef.

DRUG CLASS

Corticosteroid.

USES

Addison's disease, adrenogenital syndrome.

DOSAGE

 Tablets: One to three tablets a day as directed by doctor.

FORMS

Tablets of 0.1mg. (pink).

PRECAUTIONS

Should be used in pregnancy (C), breast feeding and children only on specific medical advice.

Use with caution if under stress, and in patients with under active thyroid gland, liver disease, diverticulitis, high blood pressure, myasthenia gravis, or kidney disease.

Medication should not be ceased abruptly, but dosage should be slowly reduced.

 Do not take if:

• suffering from any form of infection.

• having a vaccination

SIDE EFFECTS

Common: May cause bloating, weight gain, rashes and intestinal disturbances.

Unusual: Biochemical disturbances of blood, muscle weakness, bone weakness, impaired wound healing, skin thinning, tendon weakness, peptic ulcers, gullet ulcers, bruising, increased sweating, loss of fat under skin, premature ageing, excess facial hair growth in women, pigmentation of skin and nails, acne, convulsions, headaches, dizziness, growth suppression in children, aggravation of diabetes, worsening of infections, cataracts, aggravation of glaucoma, blood clots in veins and sleeplessness.

Most significant side effects occur only with prolonged use of tablets.

Severe but rare (stop medication, consult doctor): Any significant side effect should be reported to a doctor immediately.

INTERACTIONS

Other drugs:

• Oral contraceptives, Barbiturates, Phenytoin, Rifampicin.

PRESCRIPTION

Yes

PERMITTED IN SPORT

No

OVERDOSE

Medical treatment is required. Serious effects and death rare.

OTHER INFORMATION

Extremely effective and useful medication if used correctly. Must be used with extreme care under strict medical supervision. Lowest dose possible should be used. Not addictive.

Flumethasone

TRADE NAME

Available only in combination with Clioquinol.

Locacorten Vioform (with Clioquinol).

DRUG CLASS

Corticosteroid.

USES

Eczema and inflammation of ear canal.

DOSAGE

 Two or three drops twice a day for no more than ten days.

FORMS

Ear drops

PRECAUTIONS

Ear preparations safe in pregnancy, breast feeding and children over three years.

Avoid eye contact.

Use for shortest period of time possible.

SIDE EFFECTS

Common: Minimal.

Unusual: Prolonged use - thinning of skin, itching, scarring of skin.

INTERACTIONS

None significant.

PRESCRIPTION

Yes

PERMITTED IN SPORT

Yes

Flunisolide

TRADE NAME

Syntaris.

DRUG CLASS

Corticosteroid.

USES

Prevention of hay fever and chronic nasal drip.

DOSAGE

 Initially once or two sprays in each nostril, twice a day. Reduce dose to lowest possible.

FORMS

Nasal spray.

PRECAUTIONS

Use with caution in pregnancy (B3), breast feeding and children. Use with caution in lung or throat infection and tuberculosis.

SIDE EFFECTS

Common: Nasal irritation.

Unusual: Fungal (thrush) infections of nose, nose bleeds.

INTERACTIONS

None significant

PRESCRIPTION

Yes

PERMITTED IN SPORT

Yes

OVERDOSE

Unlikely to have any serious effects. See also Budesonide, Beclomethasone.

Flunitrazepam

TRADE NAME

Rohypnol.

DRUG CLASS

Sedative/hypnotic, Benzodiazepine.

USES

Severe insomnia (sleeplessness).

DOSAGE

 One or two at bedtime. Quarter to one tablet in elderly.

PRECAUTIONS

Should be used with caution in pregnancy (C), but not at all if delivery of infant imminent as it may decrease desire to breathe in newborn infant. Should be used with caution in breast feeding. Not for use in children.

Lower dose required in elderly.

Should be used intermittently and not constantly as dependency may develop.

Stopping suddenly after prolonged constant use may cause withdrawal symptoms.

Use with caution in glaucoma, myasthenia gravis, heart disease, low blood pressure, kidney or liver disease, psychiatric conditions, schizophrenia, depression and epilepsy.

 Do not take if:

- suffering from severe lung disease, confusion.
- tendency to addiction or dependence.
- operating machinery, driving a vehicle or undertaking tasks that require concentration, coordination or alertness within next 12 hours.

FORMS

Tablet of 1mg. (grey green).

SIDE EFFECTS

Common: Confusion and falls in elderly, impaired alertness, dependency.

Unusual: Dizziness, incoordination, poor memory, headache, hangover in morning, slurred speech, nightmares.

INTERACTIONS

Other drugs:

- Other medications that reduce alertness (eg: Barbiturates, Antihistamines, Antianxiety drugs).

- Disulfiram, Cimetidine, Anticonvulsants, Anticholinergics.

Other substances:

- Reacts with alcohol to cause excessive drowsiness.

PRESCRIPTION

Yes (restricted).

PERMITTED IN SPORT

Yes

OVERDOSE

Seldom life threatening. May cause drowsiness, confusion and coma. Induce vomiting if tablets taken recently. Seek medical assistance.

OTHER INFORMATION

One of the most powerful sleeping tablets available. Risk of dependency is high. Should be used only intermittently and for short periods except in exceptional cases.

Fluocinonide

TRADE NAME

Metosyn

DRUG CLASS

Corticosteroid.

USES

Inflammation of skin, itchy and allergic skin conditions

DOSAGE

 Apply three or four times a day.

PRECAUTIONS

Should be used with caution in pregnancy, breast feeding and children.

Avoid eyes.

Use for shortest period of time possible.

 Do not take if:

- suffering from any form of skin infection, acne, or broken skin.

FORMS

Cream, ointment.

SIDE EFFECTS

Common: Minimal.

Unusual: Thinning of skin, itching, burning, stinging, scarring of skin.

INTERACTIONS

None significant

PRESCRIPTION

Yes

PERMITTED IN SPORT

Yes

OTHER INFORMATION

Lowest dose and shortest possible course should be used.

Fluocortolone

TRADE NAME

Ultalanum.

Ultraproct (with Cinchocaine).

DRUG CLASS

Corticosteroid.

USES

Severe inflammation of anus, piles, anal fissure.

DOSAGE

 Ointment: Apply two times a day Suppositories: Insert one into anus once a day after a bowel motion.

FORMS

Ointment, cream, suppositories.

PRECAUTIONS

Should be used with caution in pregnancy.

May aggravate fungal infections of skin.

Use for shortest period of time possible.

 Do not take if:
- suffering from any form of skin infection, anal ulcer or broken skin.

SIDE EFFECTS

Common: Minimal.

Unusual: Thinning of skin, itching, burning, stinging, scarring of skin.

INTERACTIONS

None significant

PRESCRIPTION

Yes

PERMITTED IN SPORT

No

OTHER INFORMATION

Shortest possible course should be used. Not addictive. One of the older types of steroid cream.

Fluoride

(Sodium fluoride)

TRADE NAME

Endekay, Fluorigard.

Luborant (with Carboxymethylcellulose).

Fluoride is also found naturally in water, and in numerous nutritional supplements and medications, all of which are available without prescription. It is also added artificially to some water supplies.

PRECAUTIONS

Not to be used in pregnancy and breast feeding. May be used with caution in children.

Fluoride supplements should only be used where local water supply is low in fluoride.

 Do not take if:
- suffering from severe kidney disease.

DRUG CLASS

Mineral.

USES

Prevention of tooth decay, in addition to calcium and vitamin D in the treatment of osteoporosis, multiple myeloma, Paget's disease.

DOSAGE

 One to three times a day as directed by packaging or doctor.

FORMS

Tablets, mixture, drops.

SIDE EFFECTS

Common: Nil at correct dose.

Un*Common:* Excess dosage for a long period may cause white flecks or brown stains on teeth.

INTERACTIONS

None significant

PRESCRIPTION

No

PERMITTED IN SPORT

Yes

OVERDOSE

Deliberate or accidental overdosage with a large number of tablets may cause significant poisoning. Administer activated charcoal or induce vomiting if taken recently. Symptoms of acute poisoning include vomiting, diarrhoea, convulsions, rapid weak pulse, difficulty in breathing, coma and possibly death. Seek urgent medical assistance.

OTHER INFORMATION

Since the introduction of fluoride to water supplies, as a supplement, and in tooth paste, the incidence of tooth decay in children has dropped dramatically. In areas with fluoride in the water supply additional supplements are not required.

Fluorometholone

TRADE NAME

FML.

DRUG CLASS

Corticosteroid.

USES

Inflammation of eye, iritis.

DOSAGE

 Insert one or two drops two to four times a day.

FORMS

Eye drops.

PRECAUTIONS

May be used with caution in pregnancy, breast feeding and children.

Use with caution in bacterial eye infections.

Not designed for prolonged use.

 Do not take if:

• suffering from any form of viral or fungal eye infection.

• suffering from tuberculosis of eye.

SIDE EFFECTS

Common: Temporary blurred vision.

Severe but rare (stop medication, consult doctor): Glaucoma (halos around objects), eye pain, permanent blurred vision, weeping eye, pus in eye.

INTERACTIONS

None significant.

PRESCRIPTION

Yes

PERMITTED IN SPORT

Yes

OTHER INFORMATION

Must only be used strictly as directed by doctor. Infection must be excluded before use, or eye damage may result. Prolonged use may result in eye damage. Very useful in controlling severe eye inflammation.

Fluorouracil

TRADE NAME

Efudix.

USES

Skin cancer and sun damaged skin.

DOSAGE

 Apply to affected skin once or twice a day with a metal applicator or using a rubber glove for four to six weeks.

FORMS

Cream.

PRECAUTIONS

Should not be used in pregnancy (D) as the safety of this medication in pregnancy has not been established. Should be used in breast feeding and children only if medically essential.

Cream must not be allowed to come into contact with eyes, mouth, lips, nose, anus or vagina.

Do not use on normal skin.

Avoid using cosmetics or other skin preparations on areas of skin being treated.

Avoid sun exposure to areas of skin being treated.

SIDE EFFECTS

Common: Redness, itch, burning, pigmentation.

Unusual: Scarring, dermatitis, soreness, sun sensitivity.

INTERACTIONS

None significant.

PRESCRIPTION

Yes

PERMITTED IN SPORT

Yes

OVERDOSE

Inflammation and soreness of skin. Very serious if swallowed. Seek urgent medical assistance.

OTHER INFORMATION

Very effective and useful in many forms of skin cancer but must be used carefully.

Fluoxetine

TRADE NAME

Prozac.

DRUG CLASS

SSRI antidepressant.

USES

Depression.

DOSAGE

 One or two tablets, once or twice a day.

FORMS

Capsules of 20mg. (green/yellow) and 60mg. (yellow), liquid.

PRECAUTIONS

Should be used in pregnancy (B2), breast feeding and children with considerable caution.

Should be used with caution in epilepsy, liver and kidney disease.

Use with caution after shock treatment.

Lower doses necessary in elderly.

 Do not take if:

• MAOI antidepressants taken recently.

SIDE EFFECTS

Common: Generally minimal. Nausea, drowsiness, sweating, tremor, tiredness, dry mouth, sleeplessness, impotence.

Unusual: Headache, fever, palpitations, sweating, rash, blurred vision.

INTERACTIONS

Other drugs:

• MAOI

• Anticoagulants, Phenytoin, Tryptophan.

Other substances:

• Use of alcohol is not advised.

PRESCRIPTION

Yes

PERMITTED IN SPORT

Yes

OVERDOSE

Symptoms may include nausea, tremor, dilated pupils, dry mouth and irritability. Death or serious effects unlikely. Administer activated charcoal or induce vomiting if tablets taken recently. Seek medical attention.

OTHER INFORMATION

One of the newer antidepressants released in the early 1990s that has dramatically improved the treatment of depression because of its safety and lack of side effects. May take up to two weeks for patient to notice any improvement in depression.

Flupenthixol

TRADE NAME

Depixol, Fluanxol

DRUG CLASS

Antipsychotic.

USES

Schizophrenia, depression and psychoses.

DOSAGE

 One to three tablets, once or twice a day.
One injection every two to four weeks.

FORMS

Injection, tablets.

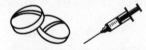

SIDE EFFECTS

Common: Confusion, twitches, tremors, muscle spasms, dry mouth.

INTERACTIONS

Other drugs:

• Tricyclic antidepressants, Phenobarbitone, Carbamazepine, Hypnotics, Lithium, medications that lower blood pressure, Levodopa, MAOI, Metoclopramide.

Other substances:

• Organophosphate insecticides.

• Alcohol

PRECAUTIONS

Use in pregnancy (C) only if medically essential. Use with caution in breast feeding.

Not to be used in children.

Use lower doses in elderly.

Use with caution if taking anti-vomiting drugs.

Use with caution in glaucoma, extreme heat, epilepsy, agitation states, Parkinson,s disease, hardening of arteries, heart disorders, stroke, liver and kidney disease.

 Do not take if:

• suffering from brain damage, blood abnormalities, phaeochromocytoma.

• sensitive to Phenothiazine.

• having surgery.

PRESCRIPTION

Yes

PERMITTED IN SPORT

Yes

OVERDOSE

Causes sedation preceded by agitation, confusion and convulsions. May proceed to collapse, failure of breathing and death. Seek urgent medical attention. Support in hospital necessary.

OTHER INFORMATION

Used long term to prevent symptoms of schizophrenia or other psychiatric disorders.

Fluphenazine

See PHENOTHIAZINES

Flurandrelone

TRADE NAME

Haelan.

DRUG CLASS

Corticosteroid.

USES

Dermatitis, eczema.

PRECAUTIONS

Should be used with caution in pregnancy, breast feeding and children.

Avoid eyes.

Use for shortest period of time possible. Do not use if:

 Do not take if:

• suffering from any form of skin infection, acne, or broken skin.

DOSAGE

 Apply two or three times a day.

FORMS

Cream, ointment.

SIDE EFFECTS

Common: Minimal.

Unusual: Thinning of skin, itching, burning, stinging, scarring of skin.

INTERACTIONS

None significant

PRESCRIPTION

Yes

PERMITTED IN SPORT

Yes

OTHER INFORMATION

Lowest dose and shortest possible course should be used.

Flurazepam

TRADE NAME

Dalmane.

DRUG CLASS

Sedative/hypnotic, Benzodiazepine.

USES

Relieves insomnia (sleeplessness).

DOSAGE

 One or two at bedtime.

FORMS

Capsules of 15mg. (grey/yellow) and 30mg. (black/grey).

PRECAUTIONS

Should be used with caution in pregnancy (C), but not at all if delivery of infant imminent as it may decrease desire to breathe in newborn infant. Should be used with caution in breast feeding. Not for use in children.

Lower dose required in elderly.

Should be used intermittently and not constantly as dependency may develop. Stopping suddenly after prolonged constant use may cause withdrawal symptoms.

Use with caution in glaucoma, myasthenia gravis, heart disease, kidney or liver disease, psychiatric conditions, depression and epilepsy.

 Do not take if:

- suffering from severe lung disease, confusion.

- tendency to addiction or dependence.

SIDE EFFECTS

Common: Confusion and falls in elderly, impaired alertness.

Unusual: Dizziness, incoordination, poor memory, headache, hangover in morning, slurred speech, nightmares.

INTERACTIONS

Other drugs:

- Other medications that reduce alertness (eg: Barbiturates, Antihistamines, Antianxiety drugs).

• Disulfiram, Cimetidine, Anticonvulsants, Anticholinergics.

Other substances:

• Reacts with alcohol to cause excessive drowsiness.

PRESCRIPTION

Yes

PERMITTED IN SPORT

Yes

OVERDOSE

Seldom life threatening. May cause drowsiness, confusion and coma. Administer activated charcoal or induce vomiting if tablets taken recently. Seek medical assistance.

OTHER INFORMATION

Now a rather old fashioned treatment, and mostly superseded by more effective and less addictive drugs.

Flurbiprofen

See NSAIDs

Flutamide

TRADE NAME

Chimax, Drogenil.

USES

Cancer of prostate gland in combination with other medication.

DOSAGE

 One tablet three times a day.

FORMS

Tablets (yellow) of 250mg.

PRECAUTIONS

Not to be used by women or children.

Regular blood tests to check liver function essential.

SIDE EFFECTS

Common: Hot flushes, decreased libido, impotence, diarrhoea, nausea, vomiting, breast enlargement and tenderness.

Severe but rare (stop medication, consult doctor): Yellow skin (jaundice).

INTERACTIONS

Other drugs:

• Warfarin, Paracetamol, Narcotics.

PRESCRIPTION

Yes

OVERDOSE

Exacerbation of side effects only likely result.

OTHER INFORMATION

Not designed to be used alone, but only in combination with other medication for prostate gland cancer.

Fluticasone propionate

TRADE NAME

Cutivate, Flixonase, Flixotide.

Seretide (with Salmeterol).

DRUG CLASS

Corticosteroid.

USES

Prevention of asthma and hay fever, dermatitis.

DOSAGE

 Inhaler: One to four inhalations twice a day
Nose spray: One or two spays in each nostril once a day
Cream: Apply once a day.

FORMS

Inhaler, disc inhaler, nose spray, cream.

PRECAUTIONS

INHALER

Use with caution in pregnancy (B3), breast feeding and children over four years.

Not to be used in children under four years.

Use with caution in lung or throat infection and tuberculosis.

Lung function should be checked regularly to ensure adequate dose is received.

NOSE SPRAY

Use with caution in pregnancy (B3), breast feeding.

Not for use in children under 12 years.

Use with caution in nose infection.

Use lowest effective dose.

CREAM

Use with caution in pregnancy. May be used in breast feeding and children, but not on breasts.

May aggravate fungal infections of skin.

Use for shortest period of time possible.

Do not use if suffering from any form of skin infection, anal ulcer or broken skin.

SIDE EFFECTS

INHALER

Common: Fungal (thrush) infections of mouth, sore throat and mouth, dry mouth.

Unusual: Hoarseness, unusual bleeding and bruising, slowed growth.

NOSE SPRAY

Common: Nose irritation.

Unusual: Nose bleeds, taste and smell disturbances, ulceration.

CREAM

Common: Minimal.

Unusual: Thinning of skin, itching, burning, stinging, scarring of skin.

INTERACTIONS

None significant

PRESCRIPTION

Yes

PERMITTED IN SPORT

Yes

OVERDOSE

Unlikely to have any serious effects. See also Beclomethasone, Budesonide

Fluvastatin

TRADE NAME

Lescol.

DRUG CLASS

Hypolipidaemic.

USES

Treatment of high blood cholesterol level.

DOSAGE

 One or two tablets at night. Maximum 40mg. twice daily.

FORMS

Capsules of 20mg. (brown/yellow) and 40mg. (brown/orange).

PRECAUTIONS

Not for use in pregnancy (C) unless medically essential. Use with caution in children.

Use with caution in muscle, liver and kidney disease.

Use with caution in alcoholics.

Regular blood tests to check cholesterol level and liver function necessary.

Do not take if:

- suffering from liver infection, myopathy.
- Breast feeding.

SIDE EFFECTS

Common: Nausea, diarrhoea.

Unusual: Liver damage, muscle damage.

INTERACTIONS

Other drugs:

- Cimetidine, Cyclosporin, Erythromycin, Gemfibrizol, Glibenclamide, Nicotinic acid, Omeprazole, Ranitidine, Rifampicin, Tolbutamide, Warfarin.

Other substances:

- Excess alcohol.

PRESCRIPTION

Yes

PERMITTED IN SPORT

Yes

OVERDOSE

Induce vomiting or administer activated charcoal if taken recently. seek medical attention.

OTHER INFORMATION

Introduced in 1996 as an effective means of lowering cholesterol when combined with a low cholesterol diet.

Fluvoxamine

TRADE NAME

Faverin.

DRUG CLASS

SSRI antidepressant.

USES

Depression, obsessive compulsive disorder.

DOSAGE

Half to three tablets a day. Increase dose very slowly.

FORMS

Tablets of 50 and 100mg. (white).

PRECAUTIONS

Use with caution in pregnancy (B2), and children.

Use with caution in epilepsy, liver and kidney disease.

Use lower doses in elderly.

Reduce dose slowly before stopping.

Do not take if:

- Breast feeding.
- Taking MAOI.

SIDE EFFECTS

Common: Generally minimal. Nausea, drowsiness, sweating, tremor, tiredness, dry mouth, sleeplessness, impotence.

Unusual: Headache, fever, palpitations, sweating, rash, blurred vision.

INTERACTIONS

Other drugs:

• MAOI, other SSRI, Tryptophan, Tricyclic antidepressants, Lithium, Sumatriptan, Anticoagulants, Theophylline, Clozapine, Propranolol, Terfenadine, Astemizole, Cisapride, Benzodiazepines.

Other substances:

• Alcohol.

PRESCRIPTION

Yes

PERMITTED IN SPORT

No

OVERDOSE

Symptoms may include nausea, tremor, dilated pupils, dry mouth and irritability. Death or serious effects unlikely. Administer activated charcoal or induce vomiting if tablets taken recently. Seek medical attention.

OTHER INFORMATION

Introduced in 1997 as an effective treatment for depression.

Folic acid

TRADE NAMES

Lexpec.

Fefolic FV, Ferrograd Folic, Galfer FA, Lexpec with Iron, Pregaday, Slow-Fe Folic (with Iron).

Folic acid is also found in numerous other vitamin and mineral preparations.

DRUG CLASS

Vitamin.

USES

Some types of anaemia, prevention of anaemia in pregnancy.

DOSAGE

 Tablets and capsules: One or two a day.
Injection: One injection a day.

FORMS

Capsules, tablets, syrup, injection.

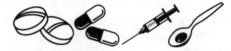

SIDE EFFECTS

Common: Minimal.

Unusual: Nausea, passing excess wind, diarrhoea, irritability, sleep disturbances.

Severe but rare (stop medication, consult doctor): Rash, asthma.

PRECAUTIONS

Safe to use in pregnancy (A), breast feeding and children.

Use with caution in some types of tumours.

 Do not take if:
• suffering from vitamin B12 deficiency.

INTERACTIONS

Other drugs:

• Anticonvulsants (drugs treating epilepsy), Methotrexate, Trimethoprim, Pyrimethamine, Sulfasalazine, Gold.

Other substances:

• Reacts with alcohol.

PRESCRIPTION

No

PERMITTED IN SPORT

Yes

OVERDOSE

No serious effects likely.

OTHER INFORMATION

Folic acid is essential for the formation of certain proteins in the body that are used in the manufacture of haemoglobin. A lack of folic acid causes anaemia. It is found naturally in liver, dark green leafy vegetables, peanuts, beans, whole grain wheat and yeast. It may be considered to be a vitamin.

Folinic acid

See Calcium folinate

Formaldehyde

TRADE and GENERIC NAMES

Veracur.

Also found in other lotions and gels.

DRUG CLASS

Keratolytic.

USES

Plantar warts (veruccae).

DOSAGE

 Apply twice a day and cover with a dressing.

FORMS

Gel, lotion.

PRECAUTIONS

Safe to use on skin in pregnancy, breast feeding and children.

Do not treat warts on face, anus, genitals and other delicate skin.

Try not to apply to normal skin.

SIDE EFFECTS

Common: Skin irritation and redness.

INTERACTIONS

None significant.

PRESCRIPTION

No

PERMITTED IN SPORT

Yes

OVERDOSE

Excessive use may lead to skin damage, burning and pain. Wash off any excess from skin immediately. Very serious if swallowed. Seek urgent medical attention. Do not cause vomiting, but give milk and antacids. See also KERATOLYTICS

Fosfestrol

TRADE NAME

Honvan.

USES

Cancer of prostate gland.

DOSAGE

 Must be determined individually for each patient by doctor depending on response to medication.

FORMS

Tablets (white) of 120mg.

SIDE EFFECTS

Common: Nausea, vomiting, belly cramps, bloating, loss of appetite, fluid retention, breast tenderness and enlargement, headache.

Unusual: Rash, loss of libido, depression, hair loss.

Severe but rare (stop medication, consult doctor): Yellow skin (jaundice), blood clot.

PRECAUTIONS

Not to be used by women or children.

Use with caution in epilepsy, migraine, asthma, depression, diabetes, bone disease, heart or kidney disease.

 Do not take if:

- suffering from liver disease, blood clots.

INTERACTIONS

None significant.

PRESCRIPTION

Yes

PERMITTED IN SPORT

Yes

OVERDOSE

Causes vomiting, diarrhoea, belly cramps, headache and dizziness.

OTHER INFORMATION

Often used in combination with castration and radiotherapy.

Fosinopril

See ACE INHIBITORS

Framycetin

TRADE NAMES

Sofra-Tulle.

Sofradex (with Dexamethasone and Gramicidin).

Soframycin (with Gramicidin).

DRUG CLASS

Antibiotic

USES

Ear and eye infections.

DOSAGE

 Drops: Insert three to six times a day.
Ointment: Insert or apply two or three times a day.
Tulle: Apply to clean wound daily.

FORMS

Eye drops, eye ointment, ear drops, ear ointment, skin ointment, tulle (netting).

PRECAUTIONS

Must be used with caution in pregnancy (D), but damage to foetus unlikely if used only on body surface. May be used in breast feeding and children.

Do not use ear applications if:

- suffering from perforated ear drum

SIDE EFFECTS

Minimal

INTERACTIONS

None significant

PRESCRIPTION

Yes

PERMITTED IN SPORT

Yes

OTHER INFORMATION

Very widely used for treatment of swimmer's ear and conjunctivitis. Tulle useful for infected grazes and ulcers.

Frangula

TRADE NAME

Normacol Plus (with Sterculia).

Also found in other fibre supplements.

DRUG CLASS

Fibre.

USES

Constipation.

DOSAGE

 Take required amount with water two or three times a day.

FORMS

Granules, powder.

SIDE EFFECTS

Common: Minimal

Unusual: Diarrhoea, belly discomfort

INTERACTIONS

Other drugs:

• Thiazide diuretics, Steroids.

Other substances:

• Licorice, high sugar content sweets.

PRECAUTIONS

Safe in pregnancy. Not for use in breast feeding and children under 12 years.

Avoid at bedtime.

Not for prolonged use.

 Do not take if:

• on a salt, potassium or sugar restricted diet

• suffering from severe constipation with impacted faeces.

• suffering from belly pain, nausea or vomiting.

• suffering from ulcerative colitis or acute diverticulitis.

PRESCRIPTION

No

PERMITTED IN SPORT

Yes

OVERDOSE

Take additional water. Belly discomfort and passing excess wind only effects.

Frusemide

TRADE NAME

Frusol, Lasix.

Diumide-K Continus, Lasikal (with Potassium).

Fru-Co, Frumil, Lasoride (with Amiloride).

Frusene (with Triamterene).

Lasilactone (with Spironolactone).

DRUG CLASS

Loop diuretic (increases production of urine).

USES

Excess fluid in body, high blood pressure, heart failure causing build up of fluid in lungs.

PRECAUTIONS

Should only be used in pregnancy (C) if medically essential. Will reduce production of breast milk, and may be used to assist in drying of breast milk in women who have stopped breast feeding. Safe in children and infants.

Should be used with caution in diabetes, diarrhoea and gout.

Regular blood tests to assess levels of chemicals (electrolytes) in blood are recommended if Frusemide used alone.

 Do not take if:

- suffering from severe kidney failure, jaundice, low blood pressure, difficulty in passing urine.

DOSAGE

 One or more tablets in morning to a maximum of 1500mg. Frusemide a day.

FORMS

Tablets, solution, injection.

SIDE EFFECTS

Common: Passing increased amounts of urine.

Unusual: Weakness, dizziness, thirst, muscle cramps, flushing.

Severe but rare (stop medication, consult doctor): Dehydration, blood clots, deafness.

INTERACTIONS

Other drugs:

- Digoxin, Aspirin.
- Medications that lower blood pressure.

PRESCRIPTION

Yes

PERMITTED IN SPORT

No

OVERDOSE

Severe dehydration may result. Induce vomiting if tablets taken recently. Give extra fluids. Seek medical assistance.

OTHER INFORMATION

Widely used, safe, and extremely effective medication that has been available since the 1960s. Potassium supplements may be needed.

Fusafungine

TRADE NAME

Locabiotal.

DRUG CLASS

Antibiotic.

USES

Infections of nose and throat.

DOSAGE

 One spray every four hours in mouth and both nostrils.

FORMS

Spray.

SIDE EFFECTS

Common: Nasal irritation.

INTERACTIONS

None significant.

PRECAUTIONS

Safe in pregnancy, breast feeding
and children.

PRESCRIPTION

Yes

PERMITTED IN SPORT

Yes

OVERDOSE

Diarrhoea only likely effect.

OTHER INFORMATION

Use restricted under the NHS.

Fusidic Acid

See Sodium fusidate and Fusidic acid

Gabapentin

TRADE NAME

Neurontin.

DRUG CLASS

Anticonvulsant.

USES

Epilepsy, particularly epilepsy that affects only part of the body.

DOSAGE

 Slowly increasing dosage until desired result obtained. Taken in two or more doses a day. Maximum 2400mg. a day.

FORMS

Capsules of 100mg. (white), 300mg. (yellow) and 400mg. (orange).

PRECAUTIONS

Use with caution in pregnancy (B1), breast feeding and children under 12 years.

Use with caution in kidney disease, psychiatric disturbances, epilepsy and elderly.

Do not stop suddenly, but reduce dosage slowly.

SIDE EFFECTS

Common: Tiredness, drowsiness, incoordination, nausea, dizziness.

Unusual: Vomiting, blurred vision, tremor, weight gain.

INTERACTIONS

Other drugs:

• Antacids, Cimetidine.

PRESCRIPTION

Yes

PERMITTED IN SPORT

Yes

OVERDOSE

Unlikely to be lethal. Symptoms may include double vision, slurred speech, drowsiness and diarrhoea.

Gamma Globulin (Immunoglobulin)

TRADE NAME

Flebogamma, Gammabulin, Gammagard, Kabiglobulin, Octagam, Sandoglobulin, Vigam.

DRUG CLASS

Immunoglobulin.

PRECAUTIONS

Safe in pregnancy, breast feeding and children.

Use with caution in idiopathic thrombocytopenia.

Do not use high doses.

 Do not take if:

• suffering from IgA deficiency.

USES

Prevention and treatment of hepatitis, polio and measles. Adjunctive treatment for bacterial infections. Low natural levels of immunoglobulin.

DOSAGE

 For injection as determined by doctor for each patient.

FORMS

Injection.

SIDE EFFECTS

Common: Headache, fever, anxiety, flushing, itch.

Unusual: Brain irritation, change in blood pressure, chills, muscle aches.

Severe but rare (stop medication, consult doctor): Allergy reaction.

INTERACTIONS

Other drugs:

• Live virus vaccines (eg: Sabin polio).

PRESCRIPTION

Yes

PERMITTED IN SPORT

Yes

See also IMMUNOGLOBULINS

Gammalinoleic acid (Evening Primrose oil)

See FATTY ACIDS

Gamolenic acid

TRADE NAME

Efamast, Epogam.

USES

Soothes some forms of eczema, breast inflammation.

DOSAGE

 Take four to six capsules twice a day.

FORMS

Capsules.

PRECAUTIONS

Safe to use in pregnancy, breast feeding and children over twelve months.

Use with caution in epilepsy.

SIDE EFFECTS

Common: Minimal

Unusual: Nausea, indigestion, headache.

INTERACTIONS

Other drugs:

• Phenothiazines.

PRESCRIPTION

No

PERMITTED IN SPORT

Yes

OVERDOSE

Unlikely to be serious. Seek medical advice.

OTHER INFORMATION

Does not cause dependence or addiction. Introduced in 1993.

Ganciclovir

TRADE NAME

Cymevene.

DRUG CLASS

Antiviral.

USES

Treatment of cytomegalovirus (CMV) infections of eyes or lungs in patients with AIDS, immunosuppression or transplants.

DOSAGE

 Four tablets three times a day, or by drip into a vein.

FORMS

Tablets, injection.

PRECAUTIONS

Not to be used in pregnancy (D) or breast feeding.

Not for use in infants. Use with caution in children.

Only use in severe cases of CMV.

Use with caution in poor hydration, kidney disease, and elderly.

Regular blood tests to check blood cell levels essential.

SIDE EFFECTS

Common: Low blood white cell count, low blood platelet count (causes abnormal bleeding), anaemia, nausea, diarrhoea, damage to foetus during pregnancy.

Unusual: Vomiting, reduced fertility long term.

Severe but rare (stop medication, consult doctor): Inflamed pancreas (severe belly pain), blood infection..

INTERACTIONS

Other drugs:

• Probenecid, didanosine, zidovudine, cilastin, imipenem.

PRESCRIPTION

Yes

PERMITTED IN SPORT

Yes

OVERDOSE

Highly toxic and may cause severe organ damage. Induce vomiting if taken recently. Seek urgent medical attention.

Gemfibrizol

TRADE NAME

Lopid.

DRUG CLASS

Hypolipidaemic.

USES

Reducing excessive blood levels of cholesterol and triglyceride.

PRECAUTIONS

Use in pregnancy (B3) only if medically essential. Not for use in breast feeding and children.

Regular blood tests to check blood fat levels, liver enzymes and blood cells are recommended.

 Do not take if:

• suffering from gallstones, alcoholism, liver or kidney disease.

• trying to get pregnant as drug may reduce fertility.

DOSAGE

 One tablet twice daily 30min. before meals.

FORMS

Tablet of 600mg. (white), capsules of 300mg. (white/maroon).

SIDE EFFECTS

Common: Heartburn, belly pains, diarrhoea, tiredness, nausea.

Unusual: Vomiting, eczema, rash, dizziness, constipation, headache.

Severe but rare (stop medication, consult doctor): Yellow skin (jaundice).

INTERACTIONS

Other drugs:

• Anticoagulants, Lovostatin.

PRESCRIPTION

Yes

PERMITTED IN SPORT

Yes

OVERDOSE

No significant problems likely.

OTHER INFORMATION

Relatively new medication that is particularly effective and safe in the treatment of excess blood levels of triglycerides.

Gentamicin

TRADE NAME

Cidomycin, Garamycin, Genticin, Minims Gentamicin.

Gentisone HC (with Hydrocortisone).

DRUG CLASS

Aminoglycoside antibiotic.

USES

Severe infections, particularly bone, lung, soft tissue, eye and belly infections.

DOSAGE

 Injection: Every eight hours, or by continuous drip infusion **Eye drops:** Two drops every four hours
Ear drops: Two to four drops, three or four times a day.

FORMS

Injection, eye drops, ear drops.

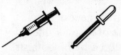

PRECAUTIONS

Not to be used in pregnancy (D) unless absolutely essential for mother's well being. Breast feeding must be ceased before use. Use with caution and only when essential in children.

Eye drops and skin preparations may be used with caution in pregnancy and breast feeding.

Use injection with caution in kidney disease.

Blood tests to check that correct dose is being administered are recommended.

SIDE EFFECTS

Common: Eye and ear drops - Minimal. Injection - Rash, nausea, headache.

Unusual: Ear and kidney damage (dose related), vomiting.

Severe but rare (stop medication, consult doctor): Ear noises or deafness, unusual bleeding or bruising.

INTERACTIONS

Other drugs:

• Penicillin, Cephalosporins, Ethacrynic acid, Frusemide, Vitamin K.

PRESCRIPTION

Yes

PERMITTED IN SPORT

Yes

OVERDOSE

Ear and kidney damage possible. Give copious fluids to increase excretion through kidneys.

OTHER INFORMATION

Very useful for the treatment of severe infections. Little risk of serious side effects if dose monitored by blood tests.

Gestodene

See ORAL CONTRACEPTIVES

Gestrinone

TRADE NAME

Dimetriose.

DRUG CLASS

Sex hormone.

USES

Endometriosis.

DOSAGE

 One capsule twice a day for six months.

FORMS

Capsules (white) of 2.5mg.

PRECAUTIONS

Must not be used in pregnancy (D), breast feeding or children.

Use with caution in elderly.

Use with caution in diabetes and high blood fat (cholesterol or triglycerides) levels.

 Do not take if:

• suffering from significant heart, kidney, liver or metabolic diseases.

• suffering from blood vessel disorders.

• male.

SIDE EFFECTS

Common: Acne, oily skin, hair growth on face, ankle and foot swelling, excess sweating, low libido, leg cramps, headache, nausea, vomiting, loss of appetite, excess hunger, dizziness, tiredness, rash, hot flushes, reduced breast size.

Unusual: Deepening voice, fainting, blurred vision, anxiety, flashing lights in vision, indigestion, diarrhoea, belly pain, weight loss, thirst, muscle cramps, numbness, red face, breast lumps.

INTERACTIONS

Other drugs:

• Epilepsy medications, Rifampicin.

PRESCRIPTION

Yes

PERMITTED IN SPORT

No

OVERDOSE

Serious exacerbation of side effects likely. Induce vomiting and seek urgent medical attention.

Glibenclamide

TRADE NAME

Daonil, Euglucon, Semi-Daonil

DRUG CLASS

Hypoglycaemic.

USES

Diabetes not requiring insulin injections.

DOSAGE

 One or two tablets, one to three times a day before meals. Maximum four tablets a day. Do not vary from prescribed dose without reference to a doctor.

FORMS

Tablets of 2.5 and 5mg.

PRECAUTIONS

Not to be used in pregnancy (C), breast feeding or children.

Use with caution if operating machinery or driving a vehicle.

Use with caution in all forms of kidney disease.

Illness, changes in diet, exercise and stress may change dosage requirements.

Lower doses required in elderly and debilitated patients.

Strict control of carbohydrates and sugars in diet essential.

 Do not take if:

• suffering from severe liver or kidney disease.

SIDE EFFECTS

Common: Minimal.

Unusual: Blurred vision, drowsiness, nausea, heartburn, belly discomfort, rash.

Severe but rare (stop medication, consult doctor): Low blood sugar (see Overdose below), yellow skin (jaundice), unusual bleeding or bruising.

INTERACTIONS

Other drugs:

• ACE inhibitors, Beta blockers, other Hypoglycaemics, Chloramphenicol, Clofibrate, Clonidine, Coumarin, Probenecid, MAOI, Miconazole, Salicylates, Tetracycline, Sulphonamides, Diazoxide, Corticosteroids, Nicotinic acid, Oestrogens, Progestogen, Phenothiazines, Phenytoin, Thyroid hormones, Laxatives.

Other substances:

• Reacts adversely with alcohol.

PRESCRIPTION

Yes

PERMITTED IN SPORT

Yes

OVERDOSE

Serious. Symptoms of low blood sugar (hypoglycaemia) may include tiredness, confusion, chills, palpitations, sweating, vomiting, dizziness, hunger, blurred vision and fainting. Significant overdosage can lead to coma and death. Give sugary drinks or sweets if conscious. Seek emergency medical assistance.

OTHER INFORMATION

Used mainly in elderly patients who develop maturity onset diabetes that is not severe enough to require insulin injections.

Gliclazide

TRADE NAME

Diamicron.

DRUG CLASS

Hypoglycaemic.

USES

Diabetes not requiring insulin injections.

DOSAGE

 Half to two tablets, one or two times a day before meals. Maximum four tablets a day. Do not vary from prescribed dose without reference to a doctor.

FORMS

Tablets of 80mg. (white)

PRECAUTIONS

Not to be used in pregnancy (C), breast feeding or children.

Illness, changes in diet, exercise and stress may change dosage requirements.

Lower doses required in elderly and debilitated patients.

Strict control of carbohydrates and sugars in diet essential.

 Do not take if:

• suffering from severe liver or kidney disease.

SIDE EFFECTS

Common: Uncommon.

Unusual: Blurred vision, drowsiness, nausea, heartburn, belly discomfort, rash.

Severe but rare (stop medication, consult doctor): Low blood sugar (see Overdose below), yellow skin (jaundice), unusual bleeding or bruising.

INTERACTIONS

Other drugs:

• ACE inhibitors, Beta blockers, other Hypoglycaemics, Chloramphenicol, Clofibrate, Clonidine, Coumarin, Probenecid, MAOI, Miconazole, Salicylates, Tetracycline, Sulphonamides, Diazoxide, Corticosteroids, Nicotinic acid, Oestrogens, Progestogen, Phenothiazines, Phenytoin, Thyroid hormones, Laxatives.

Other substances:

• Reacts adversely with alcohol.

PRESCRIPTION

Yes

PERMITTED IN SPORT

Yes

OVERDOSE

Serious. Symptoms of low blood sugar (hypoglycaemia) may include tiredness, confusion, chills, palpitations, sweating, vomiting, dizziness, hunger, blurred vision and fainting. Significant overdosage can lead to coma and death. Give sugary drinks or sweets if conscious. Seek emergency medical assistance.

OTHER INFORMATION

Used mainly in elderly patients who develop maturity onset diabetes that is not severe enough to require insulin injections.

Glimepride

TRADE NAME

Amaryl

DRUG CLASS

Hypoglycaemic.

USES

Diabetes not requiring insulin injections.

DOSAGE

 Initially 1mg. a day at breakfast, increasing very slowly to a maximum of 6mg. a day.

FORMS

Tablets of 1mg. (pink), 2mg. (green), 3mg. (yellow) and 4mg. (blue).

PRECAUTIONS

Not to be used in pregnancy (C), breast feeding or children.

Use with caution if operating machinery or driving a vehicle.

Use with caution in all forms of kidney disease.

Illness, changes in diet, exercise and stress may change dosage requirements.

Lower doses required in elderly and debilitated patients.

Strict control of carbohydrates and sugars in diet essential.

 Do not take if:
- suffering from severe liver or kidney disease.

SIDE EFFECTS

Common: Minimal.

Unusual: Blurred vision, drowsiness, nausea, heartburn, belly discomfort, rash.

Severe but rare (stop medication, consult doctor): Low blood sugar (see Overdose below), yellow skin (jaundice), unusual bleeding or bruising.

INTERACTIONS

Other drugs:

- ACE inhibitors, Beta blockers, other Hypoglycaemics, Chloramphenicol, Clofibrate, Clonidine, Coumarin, Probenecid, MAOI, Miconazole, Salicylates, Tetracycline, Sulphonamides, Diazoxide, Corticosteroids, Nicotinic acid, Oestrogens, Progestogen, Phenothiazines, Phenytoin, Thyroid hormones, Laxatives.

Other substances:

- Reacts adversely with alcohol.

PRESCRIPTION

Yes

PERMITTED IN SPORT

Yes

OVERDOSE

Serious. Symptoms of low blood sugar (hypoglycaemia) may include tiredness, confusion, chills, palpitations, sweating, vomiting, dizziness, hunger, blurred vision and fainting. Significant overdosage can lead to coma and death. Give sugary drinks or sweets if conscious. Seek emergency medical assistance.

Glipizide

TRADE NAME

Glibenese, Minodiab.

DRUG CLASS

Hypoglycaemic.

USES

Diabetes not requiring insulin injections.

DOSAGE

 One or two tablets, one to three times a day before meals. Maximum of 20mg. a day. Do not vary from prescribed dose without reference to a doctor.

FORMS

Tablets of 2.5 and 5mg.

PRECAUTIONS

Not to be used in pregnancy (C), breast feeding or children.

Use with caution in all forms of kidney and liver disease.

Illness, changes in diet, exercise and stress may change dosage requirements.

Strict control of carbohydrates and sugars in diet essential.

 Do not take if:
  • suffering from severe liver or kidney disease.

SIDE EFFECTS

Common: Nausea, diarrhoea, constipation.

Unusual: Blurred vision, drowsiness, dizziness, headache, heartburn, belly discomfort, rash.

Severe but rare (stop medication, consult doctor): Low blood sugar (see Overdose below), yellow skin (jaundice), unusual bleeding or bruising.

INTERACTIONS

Other drugs:

• ACE inhibitors, Beta blockers, other Hypoglycaemics, Chloramphenicol, Clofibrate, Clonidine, Coumarin, Probenecid, MAOI, Miconazole, Salicylates, Tetracycline, Sulphonamides, Diazoxide, Corticosteroids, Nicotinic acid, Oestrogens, NSAIDs, Progestogen, Phenothiazines, Phenytoin, Thyroid hormones, Laxatives.

Other substances:

• Reacts adversely with alcohol.

PRESCRIPTION

Yes

PERMITTED IN SPORT

Yes

OVERDOSE

Serious. Symptoms of low blood sugar (hypoglycaemia) may include tiredness, confusion, chills, palpitations, sweating, vomiting, dizziness, hunger, blurred vision and fainting. Significant overdosage can lead to coma and death. Give sugary drinks or sweets if conscious. Seek emergency medical assistance.

OTHER INFORMATION

Used mainly in elderly patients who develop maturity onset diabetes that is not severe enough to require insulin injections.

Gliquidone

TRADE NAME

Glurenorm.

DRUG CLASS

Hypoglycaemic.

USES

Diabetes not requiring insulin injections.

DOSAGE

 45 to 60mg. a day in divided doses before meals. Maximum 180mg. a day.

FORMS

Tablets of 30mg. (white).

PRECAUTIONS

Not to be used in pregnancy (C), breast feeding or children.

Use with caution if operating machinery or driving a vehicle.

Use with caution in all forms of kidney disease.

Illness, changes in diet, exercise and stress may change dosage requirements.

Lower doses required in elderly and debilitated patients.

Strict control of carbohydrates and sugars in diet essential.

 Do not take if:

• suffering from severe liver or kidney disease.

SIDE EFFECTS

Common: Minimal.

Unusual: Blurred vision, drowsiness, nausea, heartburn, belly discomfort, rash.

Severe but rare (stop medication, consult doctor): Low blood sugar (see Overdose below), yellow skin (jaundice), unusual bleeding or bruising.

INTERACTIONS

Other drugs:

• ACE inhibitors, Beta blockers, other Hypoglycaemics, Chloramphenicol, Clofibrate, Clonidine, Coumarin, Probenecid, MAOI, Miconazole, Salicylates, Tetracycline, Sulphonamides, Diazoxide, Corticosteroids, Nicotinic acid, Oestrogens, Progestogen, Phenothiazines, Phenytoin, Thyroid hormones, Laxatives.

Other substances:

• Reacts adversely with alcohol.

PRESCRIPTION

Yes

PERMITTED IN SPORT

Yes

OVERDOSE

Serious. Symptoms of low blood sugar (hypoglycaemia) may include tiredness, confusion, chills, palpitations, sweating, vomiting, dizziness, hunger, blurred vision and fainting. Significant overdosage can lead to coma and death. Give sugary drinks or sweets if conscious. Seek emergency medical assistance.

Glucagon

TRADE NAME

Glucagen.

USES

Low blood sugar in diabetics.

DOSAGE

 Inject contents of ampoule if patient suffers acute low blood sugar not responding to sugar by mouth.

FORMS

Injection.

PRECAUTIONS

May be used with caution in pregnancy (B2). Safe to use in breast feeding and children.

Use repeatedly only with caution.

Use with caution in blood clots, heart attack, liver and kidney disease.

 Do not take if:

- suffering from phaeochromocytoma, insulinoma.

SIDE EFFECTS

Common: Nausea, vomiting.

INTERACTIONS

Other drugs:

- Warfarin, Beta blockers.

PRESCRIPTION

Yes

PERMITTED IN SPORT

Yes

OVERDOSE

Exacerbation of side effects likely.

OTHER INFORMATION

May be life saving. Family members and associates should be instructed in use. Diabetics who use too much insulin or eat too little may suffer from sudden low blood sugar that can cause them to rapidly lose consciousness. An injection of Glucagon will revive them rapidly by releasing sugar stored in body.

Glucose

TRADE NAME

Glucose Intravenous.

Found in nutritional and electrolyte supplements.

Used as an additive or sweetener in many medications.

DRUG CLASS

Sugar.

USES

Correction of severe nutritional loss, correction of insulin overdose, reduction of excessive pressure in brain fluid.

DOSAGE

 Depends on use. Use as directed by doctor.

PRECAUTIONS

Safe in pregnancy, breast feeding and children.

 Do not take if:

- suffering from diabetes, unless suffering insulin overdose.

FORMS

Lozenges, injection, solutions.

SIDE EFFECTS

Minimal

INTERACTIONS

None significant

PRESCRIPTION

No

PERMITTED IN SPORT

Injection: No
Orally: Yes

OVERDOSE

No serious consequences. Vomiting likely.

OTHER INFORMATION

Glucose is a common form of sugar. Works within a couple of minutes after being taken by mouth.

Glutaraldehyde

TRADE NAME

Glutarol.

DRUG CLASS

Keratolytic.

USES

Removal of warts..

DOSAGE

 Apply twice a day to wart.

FORMS

Liquid.

PRECAUTIONS

Safe to use in pregnancy, breast feeding and children.

Avoid warts on face, anus, genitals and other areas of sensitive skin.

SIDE EFFECTS

Common: Skin inflammation and soreness, skin staining.

INTERACTIONS

None significant.

PRESCRIPTION

No

PERMITTED IN SPORT

Yes

OVERDOSE

Serious. Seek urgent medical attention.

See also KERATOLYTICS

Glycerol

TRADE NAME

Microlette, Relaxit (with Laxatives).

Also used in numerous skin and vaginal preparations.

DRUG CLASS

Lubricant.

PRECAUTIONS

Safe in pregnancy, breast feeding, infants and children.

Should not be used repeatedly for prolonged periods.

USES

Constipation, vaginal dryness, skin dryness.

DOSAGE

 One enema inserted rectally as required.

FORMS

Enema.

SIDE EFFECTS

Minimal

INTERACTIONS

None significant

PRESCRIPTION

No

PERMITTED IN SPORT

Yes

OVERDOSE

Causes diarrhoea only.

OTHER INFORMATION

Very safe ancient remedy.

Glyceryl Trinitrate (GTN, Nitroglycerine)

TRADE NAME

Coro-Nitro, Deponit, Glytrin, Minitran, Nitro-Dur, Nitrocine, Nitrolingual, Nitromin, Percutol, Suscard Buccal, Sustac, Transiderm Nitro.

DRUG CLASS

Antiangina.

USES

Relief or prevention of angina.

DOSAGE

 Tablets: One tablet under tongue every ten minutes as required to a maximum of six a day starting immediately any chest pain experienced. Should not be swallowed
Spray: One spray under tongue every five minutes as required to a maximum of two sprays per attack starting immediately any chest pain experienced
Patches: Apply to skin of trunk, upper arms or thighs once a day for 16 hours a day.

FORMS

Tablets, mouth spray, skin patches, injection. Tablets must not be exposed to light. Should be stored below 25°C. Discard bottle three months after opening.

PRECAUTIONS

Should be used with caution in pregnancy (B2) and breast feeding.

Use with caution with strokes, lung disease and in the elderly.

Apply patches to different areas with each application.

Tolerance may develop if used constantly.

 Do not take if:
• suffering from head injury, recent stroke.

SIDE EFFECTS

Common: Headache, flushing, rapid heart rate.

Unusual: Dizziness, fainting.

INTERACTIONS

Other drugs:

• None significant

Other substances:

• Reacts with alcohol. Smoking may exacerbate disease process.

PRESCRIPTION

Yes

PERMITTED IN SPORT

Yes

OVERDOSE

Fainting and low blood pressure occur. Red blood cells may be damaged. Administer activated charcoal or induce vomiting if tablets taken recently. Remove patches and ointment. Seek medical assistance.

OTHER INFORMATION

Tablets under tongue have been used successfully for many decades, but in the last decade better delivery systems in the form of patches and sprays have been developed. Lipstick sized sprays are more convenient, more stable and easier to use than tablets which can deteriorate with time. Nitroglycerine is an incorrect technical name.

GOLD

TRADE and GENERIC NAMES

Myocrisin (Sodium Aurothiomalate).

Ridaura (Auranofin).

DRUG CLASS

Antirheumatic.

USES

Rheumatoid arthritis.

DOSAGE

 Tablets: One tablet two or three times a day with food. Injections: Weekly injections until condition controlled, then reduce frequency slowly.

FORMS

Injection, tablets (Ridaura).

PRECAUTIONS

Should be used with caution in pregnancy (B2), breast feeding and children.

Use with caution in liver and kidney disease.

Lower doses required in elderly.

Regular blood and urine tests required to assess kidney and liver function, blood cells and effectiveness of treatment.

 Do not take if:

• suffering from severe diabetes, severe high blood pressure, heart failure, systemic lupus erythematosus, Sjøgren's syndrome, eczema, blood diseases or colitis.

SIDE EFFECTS

Common: Dermatitis, itch, mouth ulcers, flushing, fainting.

Unusual: Sweating, dizziness, weakness, feeling unwell.

Severe but rare (stop medication, consult doctor): Severe rash, unusual bleeding or bruising.

INTERACTIONS

Other drugs:

• Phenylbutazone, Hydroxychloroquine, Immunosuppressives.

PRESCRIPTION

Yes

PERMITTED IN SPORT

Yes

OTHER INFORMATION

An unusual but remarkably effective treatment that has been used for over thirty years. Careful monitoring of blood tests and skin reactions essential. Gold is not addictive when swallowed or injected, only when collected!

Gonadotrophin, menopausal, human

See Menopausal gonadotrophin, human

Goserelin acetate

TRADE NAME

Zoladex.

DRUG CLASS

Cytotoxic.

USES

Metastatic and severe prostate cancer. Advanced breast cancer. Fibroids of the uterus. Endometriosis.

DOSAGE

 Implant inserted every one to three months.

FORMS

Implants of 3.6mg.

PRECAUTIONS

Not to be used in pregnancy (D), breast feeding or children.

Use with caution in osteoporosis, spinal or ureter disease.

SIDE EFFECTS

Common: Infertility, impotence, decreased libido, hot flushes, headaches, dry vagina, cessation of menstrual periods, changes in blood pressure, breast formation in males, temporary increase in bone pain.

Unusual: Breast pain, joint pain, rash, reactions at site of implant or injection, decrease in bone density (osteoporosis).

INTERACTIONS

Other drugs:

• Sex hormones.

PRESCRIPTION

Yes

PERMITTED IN SPORT

Yes

Gramicidin

TRADE NAMES

Available only in combination with other medications.

Adcortyl with Graneodin (with Neomycin and Triamcinolone).

Graneodin (with Neomycin).

Neosporin (with Polymyxin B and Neomycin).

Sofradex (with Framycetin and Dexamethasone).

Soframycin (with Framycetin).

Tri-Adcortyl (with Triamcinolone, Neomycin, Nystatin).

DRUG CLASS

Antibiotic

USES

Infections of skin, eyes and ears.

DOSAGE

 Ear ointment: Insert twice a day. Ear drops: Insert two or three times a day (may be used in conjunction with wick in ear).
Cream, ointment: Apply three times a day.
Eye drops: Insert every three or four hours.
Eye ointment: Insert three times a day.

FORMS

Eye ointment, eye drops (keep cool), ointment, cream, ear drops, ear ointment.

PRECAUTIONS

Use with caution in pregnancy. May be used in breast feeding and children.

SIDE EFFECTS

Minimal.

INTERACTIONS

None significant.

PRESCRIPTION

Yes

PERMITTED IN SPORT

Yes

OTHER INFORMATION

Gramicidin is a constituent in some of the most widely used and effective combinations for treating eye, ear and skin infections.

Granisetron

TRADE NAME

Kytril.

DRUG CLASS

Antiemetic

USES

Nausea and vomiting associated with drugs to treat cancer (cytotoxics).

DOSAGE

 One or two tablets, once or twice a day.

FORMS

Tablets of 1 and 2mg. (triangular white), liquid, injection, infusion.

PRECAUTIONS

May be used with caution in pregnancy and children. Not for use in breast feeding.

Use with caution in gut obstruction and liver disease.

SIDE EFFECTS

Common: Headache, constipation.

Unusual: Liver damage.

INTERACTIONS

None significant.

PRESCRIPTION

Yes

PERMITTED IN SPORT

Yes

OTHER INFORMATION

Very useful in overcoming the most serious and distressing side-effect of many forms of cancer treatment.

Griseofulvin

TRADE NAME

Grisovin.

DRUG CLASS

Antifungal.

USES

Fungal infection of skin, hair and nails.

DOSAGE

 One tablet a day after food for several weeks or months.

FORMS

Tablets of 125 and 500mg. (white).

PRECAUTIONS

Should not be used in pregnancy (B3) unless medically essential. Breast feeding should be ceased before use. May be used in children.

Avoid sunlight while using medication.

Use with care if operating machinery or driving a vehicle.

Use with care if allergic to Penicillin.

 Do not take if:

• suffering from liver disease, porphyria, systemic lupus erythematosus (SLE).

• trying to fall pregnant.

SIDE EFFECTS

Common: Headache, nausea, sunburn.

Unusual: Dizziness, confusion, tiredness, vomiting, sore mouth, furry tongue.

INTERACTIONS

Other drugs:

• Anticoagulants, Barbiturates, Oral contraceptives. • Cross reacts with Penicillin.

Other substances:

• Reacts adversely with alcohol.

PRESCRIPTION

Yes

PERMITTED IN SPORT

Yes

OVERDOSE

Unlikely to cause serious effects.

OTHER INFORMATION

Widely and commonly used for fungal infections, but more effective (and expensive) medications have been recently introduced.

Growth Hormone

See Somatropin

GTN

See Glyceryl trinitrate

Guanethidine

TRADE NAME

Ismelin

DRUG CLASS

Vasodilator.

USES

Dilating small arteries in areas where circulation is poor, lowering blood pressure, glaucoma.

DOSAGE

 Injection as determined by doctor. One eye drop twice a day.

FORMS

Injection, eye drops.

PRECAUTIONS

Safe in pregnancy (A), breast feeding and children.

Use with caution in peptic ulcers, low blood pressure tendency, asthma, kidney disease and diabetes.

Regular eye checks essential when using eye drops.

 Do not take if:

• suffering from phaeochromocytoma, heart block or abnormal heart rhythm.

SIDE EFFECTS

EYE DROPS *Common:* Eye discomfort and redness, headache.

Unusual: Skin reaction around eye, pigmentation, drooping eye lid, eye surface damage.

INJECTION *Common:* Drowsiness, low blood pressure, faintness, dizziness, slow heart rate.

Unusual: Angina, heart failure, nausea, diarrhoea, asthma, impotence, dermatitis, hair loss.

Severe but rare (stop medication, consult doctor): Blood cell abnormalities.

INTERACTIONS

Other drugs:

• MAOI, Anticoagulants, Antiarrhythmics, Beta-blockers, Digoxin, Antihypertensives, Sympathomimetics, Antipsychotics, Tricyclic antidepressants, Oral contraceptives, Anaesthetics.

Other substances:

• Alcohol

PRESCRIPTION

Yes

PERMITTED IN SPORT

Yes

H2 RECEPTOR ANTAGONISTS

(Reduce stomach acid)

See Cimetidine, Nizatadine, Ranitidine

Haemophilus influenzae B vaccine (HiB vaccine)

TRADE NAMES

Hibtiter.

ACT-HIB DTP, Infanrix-HIB (with Tetanus, Whooping Cough and Diphtheria vaccines).

DRUG CLASS

Vaccine

USES

Prevention of meningitis and epiglottitis (throat infection) caused by Haemophilus influenzae B in children under 5 years.

DOSAGE

 Three or four doses, two months apart.

PRECAUTIONS

Not recommended for use in pregnancy (B2) or adults, but unlikely to cause problems if given accidentally during pregnancy or breast feeding. Designed for use in children and infants.

Use with caution in fever, acute infection or immune system problems.

FORMS

Injection

SIDE EFFECTS

Common: Redness and soreness at injection site.

Unusual: Irritability, tiredness.

INTERACTIONS

None significant.

PRESCRIPTION

Yes

PERMITTED IN SPORT

Yes

OTHER INFORMATION

Introduced in early 1990s to prevent one type of meningitis, and a rare but potentially fatal infection that can attack the epiglottis at the back of the throat and block the airway preventing breathing. All children should start a course of this vaccine at two months of age, and have follow up injections at four, six and eighteen months. Older children need a shorter course, but greatest risk occurs under twelve months.

HAEMOSTATIC AGENTS

See Phytomenadione

Halcinonide

TRADE NAME

Halciderm.

DRUG CLASS

Corticosteroid.

USES

Inflammation of skin (eczema, dermatitis, psoriasis etc.).

DOSAGE

 Apply two or three times a day.

FORMS

Cream.

PRECAUTIONS

Should be used with caution in pregnancy, breast feeding and children.

Avoid eyes.

Use for shortest period of time possible.

Use with caution on face.

 Do not use if:

- suffering from any form of skin infection or tuberculosis.

SIDE EFFECTS

Common: Minimal.

Unusual: Thinning of skin, itching, burning, stinging, scarring of skin.

INTERACTIONS

None significant

PRESCRIPTION

Yes

PERMITTED IN SPORT

Yes

OTHER INFORMATION

Lowest dose and shortest possible course should be used.

Haloperidol

TRADE NAMES

Dozic, Haldol, Haloperidol, Serenace.

DRUG CLASS

Antipsychotic.

USES

Psychotic disorders, acute alcoholism, Tourette's syndrome, severe vomiting, addition to pain killers.

PRECAUTIONS

Should not be used in pregnancy (C) unless medically essential. Breast feeding should be ceased before use. Not for use in children under three years.

Should be used with caution in epilepsy, thyroid disease, severe heart disease and hardening of arteries.

Lower doses necessary in elderly.

 Do not take if:

- suffering from depression, Parkinson's disease.

- operating machinery, driving a vehicle or undertaking tasks that require concentration and coordination.

DOSAGE

Individualised to patients requirements. Follow doctors instructions carefully.

FORMS

Tablets, mixture, injection.

SIDE EFFECTS

Common: Minimal in low doses. Incoordination, drowsiness, muscle spasms, tremor.

Unusual: Depression, anxiety, restlessness, headache, sleeplessness, confusion, dizziness, loss of appetite, rapid heart rate, enlarged breasts (both sexes), increase or decrease in libido.

Severe but rare (stop medication, consult doctor): Repetitive unwanted movements of face, rigid muscles, fever, coma.

INTERACTIONS

Other drugs:

• Narcotics, Analgesics, Barbiturates, Sedatives, Anticoagulants.

Other substances:

• Reacts adversely with alcohol.

PRESCRIPTION

Yes

PERMITTED IN SPORT

Yes

OVERDOSE

May cause sedation, muscle spasms, twitching, convulsions, coma, reduced breathing and death. Administer activated charcoal or induce vomiting if taken recently and patient alert. Seek urgent medical assistance.

HCG

See Chorionic gonadotrophin, human

HEAVY METALS

See Gold, Silver

Heparin

TRADE NAMES

Canusal, Hepsal, Monoparin, Multiparin, Uniparin.

DRUG CLASS

Anticoagulant.

USES

Prevention and treatment of blood clots.

DOSAGE

As determined by doctor.

PRECAUTIONS

Should only be used in pregnancy (C) if medically essential. Breast feeding should be ceased if Heparin treatment necessary. May be used in children.

Lower doses required in elderly.

Regular blood tests to monitor blood clotting time essential.

 Do not take if:

• suffering from bleeding disorders, threatened abortion, heart infection, peptic ulcer, severe high blood pressure, severe liver or kidney disease.

• due for surgery.

FORMS

Injection, Infusion.

SIDE EFFECTS

Common: Excessive bleeding, bruising.

Unusual: Nose bleeds, vomiting blood, blood in faeces, rash, itch, asthma.

INTERACTIONS

Other drugs:

• Other Anticoagulants, Aspirin.

PRESCRIPTION

Yes

PERMITTED IN SPORT

Yes, but not advised in any active sport.

OVERDOSE

Extremely serious. Massive bleeding may occur. Antidote available.

OTHER INFORMATION

Only administered by doctors by injection or infusion (drip) in hospital, or strictly controlled outpatient basis. Used for many years to very effectively control life threatening blood clots. Once stabilised, patient is usually switched to an anticoagulant tablet such as Warfarin. Available in two forms that vary in their speed and method of action.

See also Dalteparin, Enoxaparin.

Heparinoid

TRADE NAMES

Hirudoid, Lasonil.

Anacal (with Lauromacrogol).

USES

Blood clots in veins close to skin, inflammation of veins, softening of hard scars, bruises, swelling caused by injury to tissue, sprains, haematomas (blood collections under skin), haemorrhoids.

DOSAGE

 Apply and massage in once to four times a day.

FORMS

Cream, gel, ointment.

PRECAUTIONS

Safe in pregnancy, breast feeding and children.

 Do not use on:-

• bleeding areas, infected areas and eye.

SIDE EFFECTS

Common: Skin redness.

INTERACTIONS

Other drugs:

• Heparin, Anticoagulant

PRESCRIPTION

No

PERMITTED IN SPORT

Yes

OTHER INFORMATION

Useful and effective medication. Do not use excessive amounts.

Hepatitis A vaccine

TRADE NAME

Avaxim, Havrix, VAQTA.

Hepatyrix (with Typhoid vaccine).

Twinrix (with Hepatitis B vaccine).

DRUG CLASS

Vaccine

USES

Prevention of hepatitis A.

DOSAGE

 Twinrix: Three injections at intervals of one month and six to twelve months give at least five years, and possibly far longer protection

Avaxim, Havrix, Hepatyrix, VAQTA: Two injections, six to twelve months apart give at least five years protection.

FORMS

Injection

PRECAUTIONS

Not designed to be used in pregnancy (B2), but unlikely to cause serious adverse effects if given inadvertently. May be given with caution in breast feeding and children under five years. May be given to children over five years.

Use with caution if exposed to hepatitis A.

 Do not take if:

• suffering from significant fever.

SIDE EFFECTS

Common: Local reaction at injection site.

Unusual: Headache, fever, tiredness, nausea, loss of appetite, general unwellness.

INTERACTIONS

Other drugs:

• Immunoglobulin.

PRESCRIPTION

Yes

PERMITTED IN SPORT

Yes

OVERDOSE

An inadvertent additional vaccination is unlikely to have any serious effects.

OTHER INFORMATION

Hepatitis A causes liver damage and is caught from eating contaminated food or poor personal hygiene. Hepatitis A is very common in some developing countries.

Hepatitis B vaccine

TRADE NAMES

Engerix B, H-B-Vax II.

Twinrix (with Hepatitis A vaccine).

DRUG CLASS

Vaccine.

USES

Prevention of Hepatitis B.

DOSAGE

 Three injections at intervals of one month and five months gives at least five years protection.

FORMS

Injection.

PRECAUTIONS

Should not be used during pregnancy (B2) unless essential. Accidental vaccination during pregnancy is unlikely to cause any significant problem. Use with caution in breast feeding. May be used in children.

Use with caution if immune system damaged, recently exposed to hepatitis B, or severely ill.

 Do not take if:
- suffering from severe infection or fever.

SIDE EFFECTS

Common: Local soreness, swelling, redness and hardness.

Unusual: Headache, dizziness, fever, muscle aches, tiredness, nausea, diarrhoea, joint pain, rash.

INTERACTIONS

None significant.

PRESCRIPTION

Yes

PERMITTED IN SPORT

Yes

OVERDOSE

No adverse effects likely from an inadvertent additional dose.

OTHER INFORMATION

Hepatitis B is endemic (widely spread) in Aborigines and southeast Asians. It is spread by sex, blood, sharing needles, blood splashes into eye, and possibly by close contact of open wounds.

Heroin

DRUG CLASS

Narcotic.

USES

No current recognised medical uses in Britain. Used in some countries for relief of severe pain. Used illegally as a psychoactive drug to cause euphoria.

FORMS

Injection.

PRECAUTIONS

Should never be used in pregnancy, breast feeding or children.

 Do not take if:
- suffering from liver disease, kidney disease, epilepsy, head injury, diabetes, alcoholism, lung disease (eg: asthma),

- driving a car, operating machinery, swimming or undertaking any activity that requires concentration.

SIDE EFFECTS

*Common:*Constipation, confusion, sweating, contracted pupils, difficulty passing urine, dry mouth, flushing, euphoria (artificial happiness), dizziness, slow heart rate, irregular heart rate, sedation, mood change, rash.

Unusual: Itch, blurred vision, low blood pressure, difficulty in breathing, convulsions.

INTERACTIONS

Other drugs:

• Hypnotics, Sedatives, Marijuana, MAOI, Cocaine.

Other substances:

• Increases the effect of alcohol.

PRESCRIPTION

Illegal.

PERMITTED IN SPORT

No

OVERDOSE

Very serious. May cause convulsions, irregular heart beat, difficulty in breathing, coma and death. Seek emergency medical assistance. Antidote available.

OTHER INFORMATION

Illegal drug of dependence. Highly addictive. Toleration may develop quickly (higher dose required to obtain same effect). Possession may lead to criminal charges. Heroin is closely related to Morphine. it may be preferred to Morphine when available because it is said to produce more calming effects.

Hexachlorophane

TRADE NAME

Ster-Zac.

DRUG CLASS

Antiseptic.

USES

Prevention of bacterial skin infections.

DOSAGE

 Use once or twice a day.

FORMS

Cream, powder.

PRECAUTIONS

Safe to use on skin in pregnancy, breast feeding (not breasts) and children.

Do not use on badly burned or damaged skin.

SIDE EFFECTS

Common: Minimal.

Unusual: Light sensitivity, skin irritation.

INTERACTIONS

None significant.

PRESCRIPTION

Cream, yes. Powder, no.

PERMITTED IN SPORT

Yes

OVERDOSE

Vomiting and diarrhoea possible if swallowed.

OTHER INFORMATION

Often used on the cut stump of the umbilical cord of babies after birth.

Hexamethylmelamine

See Altretamine

Hexamine hippurate

TRADE NAME

Hiprex.

DRUG CLASS

Urinary antiseptic.

USES

Prevention of recurrent urine infections.

DOSAGE

 One tablet twice a day.

FORMS

Tablet (white) of 1g.

PRECAUTIONS

Safe for use in pregnancy (A), breast feeding and children.

Use with caution in vegetarians.

 Do not take if:

- suffering from severe liver or kidney disease, dehydration.

SIDE EFFECTS

Common: Nausea, burning urine.

Unusual: Vomiting, rash, stomach discomfort.

INTERACTIONS

Other drugs:

- Urinary alkalinisers, Sulfonamides.

PRESCRIPTION

No

PERMITTED IN SPORT

Yes

OVERDOSE

Exacerbation of side effects likely.

OTHER INFORMATION

Used mainly in women who have recurrent attacks of cystitis, and in patients with a urinary catheter.

Hexetedine

TRADE NAME

Oraldene.

DRUG CLASS

Antiseptic.

USES

Mouth infections, thrush and ulcers; bad breath.

DOSAGE

 Gargle two or three times a day.

FORMS

Solution.

PRECAUTIONS

Safe to use in pregnancy, breast feeding and children over six years.

SIDE EFFECTS

Common: Minimal.

Unusual: Mouth irritation.

INTERACTIONS

None significant.

PRESCRIPTION

No

PERMITTED IN SPORT

Yes

OVERDOSE

Vomiting and diarrhoea possible if significant amount swallowed.

HiB vaccine

See Haemophilus influenzae B Vaccine

Homatropine hydrobromide

See MYDRIATICS

HORMONES, SEX

See Chorionic gonadotrophin, Cyproterone acetate, Danazol, Dienoestrol, Dydrogesterone, Ethinyloestradiol, Gestrinone, Hydroxyprogesterone hexanoate, Medroxyprogesterone acetate, Mesterolone, Nafarelin, Oestradiol, Oestriol, Oestrogens, Oestrone, ORAL CONTRACEPTIVES, Piperazine oestrone sulfate, Testosterone

Human chorionic gonadotrophin

See Chorionic gonadotrophin, human

Hyaluronidase

TRADE NAME

Hyalase.

USES

Injection that aids diffusion of fluids through tissue.

DOSAGE

As determined by doctor for each patient.

PRECAUTIONS

Safe in pregnancy, breast feeding and children.

Do not use if:-

• suffering from infection or cancer.

• not to be injected into a vein.

FORMS

Injection.

SIDE EFFECTS

Minimal.

INTERACTIONS

None significant.

PRESCRIPTION

Yes

PERMITTED IN SPORT

Yes

Hydralazine

TRADE NAME

Apresoline.

DRUG CLASS

Antihypertensive.

USES

High blood pressure, often in combination with other medications. Particularly useful in the high blood pressure associated with pre-eclampsia of pregnancy.

DOSAGE

One to three tablets four times a day to a maximum of 200mg. per day.

FORMS

Tablets of 25mg. (yellow).

PRECAUTIONS

Should not be used in first seven months of pregnancy (C), and only if medically necessary later in pregnancy. Safe in breast feeding. Should not be used in children.

Take with care if suffering from angina, recent heart attack, other heart diseases, recent stroke, kidney or liver disease.

 Do not take if:

- Suffering from SLE (systemic lupus erythematosus), very rapid pulse, aortic aneurysm.

SIDE EFFECTS

Common: Slowed reactions, rapid heart rate, palpitations, dizziness, flushing, low blood pressure, angina.

Unusual: Headaches, joint pains and swelling, muscle aches, nasal congestion, stomach upsets.

Severe but rare (stop medication, consult doctor): Unusual bleeding, irregular heart beat.

INTERACTIONS

Other drugs:

- Vasodilators, Calcium Channel Blockers, ACE Inhibitors, Diuretics, other medications for high blood pressure, Tricyclic antidepressants, Tranquillisers, Beta blockers, Adrenaline, MAOI (Monoamine Oxidase Inhibitors).

Other substances:

- Reacts adversely with alcohol.

PRESCRIPTION

Yes

PERMITTED IN SPORT

Yes

OVERDOSE

Results in rapid heart rate, low blood pressure, dizziness, nausea, sweating, irregular heart rate, angina, heart attack and death. If taken recently induce vomiting. Seek urgent medical assistance.

OTHER INFORMATION

Only used in the most severe and difficult forms of high blood pressure. Interacts with a wide range of other medications.

Hydrochlorthiazide

See THIAZIDE DIURETICS

Hydrocortisone

(Cortisol)

TRADE and GENERIC NAMES

Colifoam, Dioderm, Efcortelan, Efcortesol, Hydrocortistab, Hydrocortone, Mildison Lipocream, Solu-Cortef.

Locoid (Hydrocortisone-17 butyrate).

Actinac (with Chloramphenicol, Allantoin, Sulpha and other ingredients).

Alphaderm (with Urea).

Alphosyl HC (with Coal tar, Allantoin).

Anugesic HC (with Pramoxine, Zinc oxide, Benzyl benzoate and other ingredients).

Anusol HC (with Benzyl benzoate, Bismuth, Zinc oxide and other ingredients).

Calmurid HC (with Urea, Lactic acid).

Daktacort (with Miconazole).

Econacort (with Econazole).

Eurax-Hydrocortisone (with Crotamiton).

Fucidin H (with Sodium fusidate).

Gentisone HC (with Gentamicin).

Gregoderm (with Neomycin, Nystatin, Polymyxin).

Locoid C (with Chlorquinaldol).

Neo-Cortef (with Neomycin).

Nystaform-HC (with Nystatin, Chlorhexidine).

Otosporin (with Neomycin, Polymyxin).

Perinal (with Lignocaine).

Proctofoam HC (with Pramoxine).

Proctosedyl, Uniroid HC (with Cinchocaine).

Quinocort (with Potassium hydroxyquinolone).

Terra-Cortril Nystatin (with Oxytetracycline).

Terra-Cortril Nystatin (with Oxytetracycline, Nystatin).

Timodine (with Benzalkonium chloride, Dimethicone, Nystatin).

Vioform-Hydrocortisone (with Clioquinol).

Xyloproct (with Lignocaine, Zinc oxide, Aluminium acetate).

DRUG CLASS

Corticosteroid.

USES

Inflammation of skin (eczema, dermatitis, acne etc.), anus (piles), rectum (ulcerative colitis), mouth (mouth ulcers), eyes and other tissues.

DOSAGE

 Cream and ointment: Apply three or four times a day. Rectal foam: Insert twice a day initially, then every two days.
Suppositories: Insert up to three times a day initially, then reduce to once a day for up to three weeks.
Eye drops: Insert every two to four hours.
Eye ointment: Insert two to four times a day.
Tablets: As directed by doctor.
Pellets: One pellet dissolved in mouth four times a day.

FORMS

Cream, ointment, foam, suppository, eye drops, eye ointment, tablets, pellets, injection, spray.

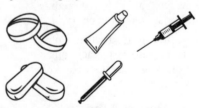

PRECAUTIONS

Tablets, injections and rectal preparations should be used in pregnancy (C), breast feeding and children only on specific medical advice.

Skin and eye preparations safe in pregnancy, breast feeding and children over three years.

Use tablets, injections and rectal preparations with caution if under stress, and in patients with under active thyroid gland, liver disease, diverticulitis, high blood pressure, myasthenia gravis, or kidney disease.

Avoid eyes with all forms except eye drops and ointment.

Do not use skin preparations for long periods in children.

Medication should not be ceased abruptly, but dosage should be slowly reduced.

 Do not take if:

• suffering from infections, peptic ulcer, osteoporosis.

• having a vaccination Do not apply to:-

• infected, fungally affected or ulcerated skin or other tissue.

SIDE EFFECTS

Most significant side effects occur only with prolonged use of tablets, injections or rectal preparations. *Common:* Tablets, injections and rectal preparations - Bloating, weight gain, rashes and intestinal disturbances. Creams and ointments - Rarely cause adverse reactions.

Unusual: Tablets, injections and rectal forms - Biochemical disturbances of blood, muscle weakness, bone weakness, impaired wound healing, skin thinning, tendon weakness, peptic ulcers, gullet ulcers, bruising, increased sweating, loss of fat under skin, premature ageing, excess facial hair growth in women, pigmentation of skin and nails, acne, convulsions, headaches, dizziness, growth suppression in children, aggravation of diabetes, worsening of infections, cataracts, aggravation of glaucoma, blood clots in veins and sleeplessness.

Severe but rare (stop medication, consult doctor): Any significant side effect should be reported to a doctor immediately.

INTERACTIONS

Other drugs:

• Creams do not interact with other drugs.

• Tablets, injections and rectal preparations of Hydrocortisone may be affected by Oral contraceptives, Barbiturates, Phenytoin, and Rifampicin.

PRESCRIPTION

Yes

PERMITTED IN SPORT

Creams and ointments: Yes. Other: No.

OVERDOSE

Medical treatment is required. Serious effects and death rare.

OTHER INFORMATION

Extremely effective and useful medication if used correctly. Safe to use on skin, but other forms must be used with extreme care under strict medical supervision. Lowest dose and shortest possible course should be used. Not addictive.

Hydroflumethazide

See THIAZIDE DIURETICS

Hydrogen peroxide

TRADE NAMES

Crystacide, Hioxyl.

Hydrogen peroxide 6% mouthwash is prepared under numerous locally made trade names.

DRUG CLASS

Antiseptic.

USES

Superficial infections and ulcers of skin and mouth.

DOSAGE

 Apply or gargle two or three times a day.

FORMS

Cream, mouthwash

PRECAUTIONS

Safe to use in pregnancy, breast feeding and children.

Avoid eyes.

Do not use for more than one month.

SIDE EFFECTS

Minimal.

INTERACTIONS

Other drugs:

• Iodine, permanganate.

PRESCRIPTION

No

PERMITTED IN SPORT

Yes

OVERDOSE

Vomiting and diarrhoea only likely effects if swallowed.

OTHER INFORMATION

Very old fashioned, but still effective.

Hydromorphone

TRADE NAME

Palladone.

DRUG CLASS

Narcotic.

USES

Relief of severe cancer pain.

DOSAGE

 One capsule four hourly as required.

FORMS

Capsules of 1.3mg. (orange/clear) and 2.6mg. (red/clear).

PRECAUTIONS

Not for use in pregnancy, breast feeding and children.

Use with caution in underactive thyroid gland, severe lung disease, kidney or adrenal gland disease, and enlarged prostate gland.

Reduce dose in elderly.

 Do not take if:

• suffering from poor lung function, in a coma, severe undiagnosed abdominal disease, head injury, convulsions, alcoholism.

SIDE EFFECTS

Common: Constipation, nausea, vomiting, drowsiness.

Unusual: Tolerance and dependence.

Severe but rare (stop medication, consult doctor): Reduced ability to breathe.

INTERACTIONS

Other drugs:

• MAOI, sedatives.

Other substances:

• Alcohol.

PRESCRIPTION

Yes (very restricted).

PERMITTED IN SPORT

No

OVERDOSE

Serious. Sedation, convulsions, coma and death may occur. Administer activated charcoal or induce vomiting if medication taken recently and patient alert. Seek emergency medical assistance. Antidote available.

OTHER INFORMATION

Highly addictive if used inappropriately. Very effective and unlikely to cause addiction if used appropriately for severe pain. Patients with terminal diseases (eg: cancer) should use dose adequate to control pain, and not be concerned about possibility of addiction. Derived from opium poppy and closely related to heroin.

Hydroxocobalamin (Vitamin B12)

TRADE NAMES

Cobalin-H, Neo-Cytamen.

A large number of other preparations include various forms of Vitamin B12 alone or in combination with other medications.

DRUG CLASS

Vitamin

USES

Pernicious anaemia, pins and needles sensation of feet.

DOSAGE

 Injection: Once every three months, or as determined by doctor. Recommended daily allowance: 2ug a day.

FORMS

Tablets, capsules, mixture, drops, injection.

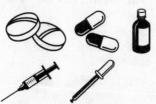

PRECAUTIONS

Safe in pregnancy, breast feeding and children.

Do not take in high doses or for prolonged periods of time.

SIDE EFFECTS

Minimal.

INTERACTIONS

None significant.

PRESCRIPTION

Injection: Yes

Other forms: No

PERMITTED IN SPORT

Yes

OVERDOSE

Unlikely to cause any serious effects.

OTHER INFORMATION

Several chemical variations of Vitamin B12 exist including cyanocobalamin and hydroxycobalamin. They are identical in their actions and use. Cyanocobalamin was the original form of vitamin B12 used medically. Vitamin B12 is a water soluble vitamin found in animal products. It is essential for the formation of red blood cells, normal growth, and normal fat and sugar metabolism. In pernicious anaemia, the body loses the ability to absorb vitamin B12 from the stomach. Remember, vitamins are merely chemicals that are essential for the functioning of the body, and if taken to excess, act as a drug.

See also Cyanocobalamin.

Hydroxyapatite

TRADE NAME

Ossopan.

DRUG CLASS

Electrolyte.

USES

Calcium and phosphorus supplements may be required in osteoporosis, rickets, osteomalacia and during breast feeding.

DOSAGE

 4 to 8 tablets, or one or two sachets a day in divided doses.

FORMS

Tablets, sachets of granules.

PRECAUTIONS

Safe to use in pregnancy and breast feeding.

Use with caution in children.

Use with caution if a history of kidney stones.

 Do not take if:

- suffering from high calcium levels in blood.

- immobilised.

SIDE EFFECTS

Minimal.

INTERACTIONS

None significant.

PRESCRIPTION

No

PERMITTED IN SPORT

Yes

OVERDOSE

Stomach pains, constipation and nausea likely.

Hydroxychloroquine

TRADE NAME

Plaquenil.

DRUG CLASS

Antirheumatic, Antimalarial.

USES

Rheumatoid arthritis, systemic lupus erythematosus (SLE), prevention and treatment of malaria.

DOSAGE

 Rheumatoid and SLE: One tablet two or three times a day with meals
Malaria prevention: Two tablets a week
Malaria treatment: Four tablets at once, two tablets eight hours later, then two tablets a day for a further two days.

PRECAUTIONS

Not to be used in pregnancy (D) as the foetus may be damaged. Use with caution in breast feeding and children.

Use with caution in severe brain disease, severe intestinal disease, porphyria, psoriasis, liver disease and alcoholism.

Exposure to sunlight while taking higher doses may cause excessive sunburn or rash.

Regular eye checks for damage to cornea or retina required if used long term.

FORMS

Tablets (orange) of 200mg.

SIDE EFFECTS

Common: Rash, itching, dry skin, nausea.

Unusual: Vomiting, loss of appetite, belly cramps.

Severe but rare (stop medication, consult doctor): Blurred vision, unusual bleeding or bruising.

INTERACTIONS

Other drugs:

• MAOI

PRESCRIPTION

Yes

PERMITTED IN SPORT

Yes

OVERDOSE

Very serious. Causes severe liver damage. Symptoms include headache, blurred vision, convulsions, heart failure and death. Administer activated charcoal or induce vomiting if medication taken recently. Seek emergency medical treatment.

OTHER INFORMATION

Quinine from the bark of the South American chincona tree has been used to treat malaria for centuries. Hydroxychloroquine is derived from quinine. Found serendipitously to control some rheumatoid conditions, and with most forms of malaria now being resistant to Quinine derivatives, it is now used for this purpose far more often than for malaria. Does not cause addiction or dependence.

Hydroxymethylcellulose

See EYE LUBRICANTS

Hydroxyprogesterone hexanoate

TRADE NAME

Proluton Depot.

DRUG CLASS

Sex hormone.

USES

Failure of menstrual periods, threatened miscarriage.

DOSAGE

Individualised by doctor. Usually one or two ampoules every two weeks.

FORMS

Injection.

PRECAUTIONS

Not to be used in pregnancy (D) unless medically essential to prevent recurrent miscarriage. Not for use in breast feeding or children.

Use with caution in a history of blood clots in veins, eye disease, diabetes, depression, high blood pressure, heart failure.

 Do not take if:

• suffering from blood clot, stroke, liver disease, undiagnosed breast disease.

SIDE EFFECTS

Common: Abnormal vaginal bleeding, headache, reduced fertility.

Unusual: Sleeplessness, nervousness, dizziness, tremor, rash, sweating, nausea, breast tenderness, weight gain.

Severe but rare (stop medication, consult doctor): Blood clot, calf pain, chest pain, yellow skin (jaundice).

INTERACTIONS

Other drugs:

• Anticoagulants, Hypoglycaemics, Insulin.

PRESCRIPTION

Yes

PERMITTED IN SPORT

Yes

OVERDOSE

Exacerbation of side effects likely.

Hydroxyurea

TRADE NAME

Hydrea.

USES

Leukaemia, melanoma, cancer of the ovary.

DOSAGE

 Must be individualised by doctor for each patient depending on disease, severity and weight of patient.

FORMS

Capsules (green/pink) of 500mg.

PRECAUTIONS

Must not be used in pregnancy (D) unless mother's life is at risk as damage to foetus may occur. Breast feeding must be ceased before use. May be used in children if medically essential.

Regular blood and bone marrow tests to check levels of blood and marrow cells and liver function essential.

Adequate contraception must be used by women while Hydroxyurea is being taken.

 Do not take if:
• suffering from anaemia or bone marrow damage.

SIDE EFFECTS

Common: Mouth soreness and ulcers, nausea, loss of appetite, vomiting, diarrhoea, rash.

Unusual: Hair loss.

Severe but rare (stop medication, consult doctor): Yellow skin (jaundice).

INTERACTIONS

Other drugs:

• Other treatments for cancer.

PRESCRIPTION

Yes

PERMITTED IN SPORT

Yes

OVERDOSE

Serious. Induce vomiting if medication taken recently. Seek urgent medical assistance.

Hydroxyzine

See ANTIHISTAMINES, SEDATING

Hylan

TRADE NAME

Synvisc

USES

Pain relief in osteoarthritis of the knee.

DOSAGE

 Weekly injections into knee for three weeks, followed by top up injections every one to six months as necessary.

FORMS

Injection.

PRECAUTIONS

Use with caution in pregnancy and children.

To be injected into joint space only.

 Do not take if:

- suffering from poor lymphatic or blood drainage from leg, infected or inflamed joint, large fluid collection in knee joint.

- allergic to birds.

SIDE EFFECTS

Common: Temporary pain and swelling of knee joint.

INTERACTIONS

None significant.

PRESCRIPTION

No

PERMITTED IN SPORT

Yes

OTHER INFORMATION

Expensive artificial joint fluid released onto market in 1999.

Hyoscine

TRADE NAMES

Buscopan, Scopoderm.

Also found in some locally produced medications for motion sickness and cold remedies.

DRUG CLASS

Anticholinergic (dries secretions). Spasmolytic (eases intestinal spasms). Antiemetic (prevents nausea and vomiting).

USES

Irritable bowel syndrome, gut spasms and colic, prevents motion sickness, dries excess nasal secretions.

DOSAGE

 Tablets - 10 to 20mg. two to four times a day.
Patch - Apply to skin behind ear and leave for up to three days.

FORMS

Tablets, injection, skin patch.

PRECAUTIONS

Should be used with caution in pregnancy (B2) and breast feeding.

 Do not take if:

- suffering from glaucoma, myasthenia gravis, megacolon.

SIDE EFFECTS

Common: Drowsiness, dry mouth, reduced sweating.

Unusual: Rapid heart rate, difficulty in passing urine, dilated pupil.

Severe but rare (stop medication, consult doctor): Hallucinations, confusion, muscle spasm.

INTERACTIONS

Other drugs:

• Dry mouth and drowsiness worsen if used with Tricyclic antidepressants, Amantadine, Quinidine, Antihistamines, Phenothiazines, and Monoamine oxidase inhibitors (MAOI).

• Rapid heart rate worsens if used with Beta blockers.

Other substances:

• Reacts with alcohol to cause excessive drowsiness.

PRESCRIPTION

Yes

PERMITTED IN SPORT

Yes

OVERDOSE

No serious effects reported. Induce vomiting. Doctors would use stomach washout and activated charcoal.

HYPNOTICS AND SEDATIVES

(Sedate and induce sleep)

See BARBITURATES, Chloral hydrate, Chlormethiazole, Flunitrazepam, Midazolam, Nitrazepam, Temazepam, Zaleplon, Zolpidem, Zopiclone

HYPOGLYCAEMICS

(Lower blood sugar level in diabetes)

See Acarbose, Glibenclamide, Glicalazide, Glipizide, INSULINS, Metformin, Repaglinide

HYPOLIPIDAEMICS

(Lower blood fat levels)

See Acipimox, Atorvastatin, Cerivastatin, Cholestyramine, Ciprofibrate, Colestipol, Fenofibrate, Fluvastatin, Gemfibrizol, Pravastatin, Simvastatin

Hypromellose

See EYE LUBRICANTS

Ibuprofen

See NSAID

Ichthammol

TRADE NAMES

Ichthopaste, Icthaband (with Zinc paste).

Also available in numerous locally produced soothing creams and ointments.

USES

Skin inflammation, eczema.

DOSAGE

 Apply two or three times a day.

FORMS

Impregnated bandage, cream, ointment.

PRECAUTIONS

Safe in pregnancy, breast feeding and children.

SIDE EFFECTS

Minimal

INTERACTIONS

None significant

PRESCRIPTION

No

PERMITTED IN SPORT

Yes

Idarubicin

TRADE NAME

Zavedos.

DRUG CLASS

Cytotoxic.

USES

Leukaemia.

DOSAGE

 As determined for each patient by doctor.

PRECAUTIONS

Not to be used in pregnancy (D). Use with caution in breast feeding. May be used in children.

Use with caution in heart disease and bone marrow suppression.

Use with caution if receiving radiotherapy.

Regular blood tests essential to check liver, kidney and blood cell function.

Use with care if driving or operating machinery.

 Do not take if:
- suffering from severe liver or kidney disease, uncontrolled infection.

FORMS

Capsules of 5mg. (orange), 10mg. (red/white) and 25mg. (orange/white). Injection.

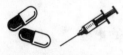

SIDE EFFECTS

Common: Nausea, vomiting, mouth inflammation, belly pain, diarrhoea, loss of hair, rash,

Unusual: Heart damage, itch, redness of palms and soles, kidney and liver damage, ankle swelling.

Severe but rare (stop medication, consult doctor): Abnormal bleeding, abnormal heart rhythm, significant infection.

INTERACTIONS

Other drugs:

• Other medications used to treat leukaemia.

PRESCRIPTION

Yes

PERMITTED IN SPORT

Yes

OVERDOSE

Significant heart damage possible, aggravation of side effects likely. Induce vomiting or administer activated charcoal if capsules taken recently. seek urgent medical attention.

Idoxuridine

TRADE NAME

Herpid (with Dimethyl sulphoxide).

DRUG CLASS

Antiviral.

USES

Herpes infections of eyes and skin, cold sores.

DOSAGE

 Apply four times a day.

FORMS

Solution.

PRECAUTIONS

Use with caution in pregnancy (B3), breast feeding and infants. May be used in children.

Continue eye treatment for five days after cure to prevent recurrence.

Do not take internally.

 Do not use if:-

• suffering from dermographia.

SIDE EFFECTS

Common: Minimal

Unusual: Irritation, pain, itch and swelling of eye.

INTERACTIONS

None significant.

PRESCRIPTION

Yes

PERMITTED IN SPORT

Yes

OTHER INFORMATION

Very effective medication, but must be used immediately any sign of infection present (particularly on cold sores).

Imidapril

See ACE INHIBITORS

IMIDAZOLES

TRADE and GENERIC NAMES

Acnidazil (<u>Miconazole</u> with Benzoyl peroxide).

Canesten, Masnoderm (<u>Clotrimazole</u>).

Canesten HC, Lotriderm (<u>Clotrimazole</u> with Hydrocortisone).

Daktarin, Dumicoat, Gyno-Daktarin (<u>Miconazole</u>).

Daktacort (<u>Miconazole</u> with Hydrocortisone).

Econacort (<u>Econazole</u> with Hydrocortisone).

Ecostatin, Gyno-Pevaryl, Pevaryl (<u>Econazole</u>).

Exelderm (<u>Sulconazole</u>).

Lomexin (<u>Fenticonazole</u>).

Lotriderm (<u>Clotrimazole</u> with Betamethasone).

Pevaryl TC (<u>Econazole</u> with Triamcinolone).

Trosyl (<u>Tioconazole</u>).

NB: Imidazoles are underlined.

USES

Treatment of fungal infections of skin (tinea, athlete's foot, pityriasis versicolor), vagina (thrush), mouth, nails and scalp.

DOSAGE

Skin: Apply two or three times a day
Vagina: Insert once a day at night.

FORMS

Cream, vaginal cream, vaginal pessary, lotion, powder, nail lacquer.

PRECAUTIONS

Safe to use in pregnancy (A), breast feeding and children.

Should not be swallowed.

Use with care on open wounds.

SIDE EFFECTS

Common: Nil

Unusual: Skin irritation, rash.

INTERACTIONS

Nil

PRESCRIPTION

Most forms: No

With Hydrocortisone: Yes

PERMITTED IN SPORT

Yes

OTHER INFORMATION

This class of medication dramatically improved the treatment of fungal infections when introduced in the early 1970s. Very safe and effective.

See also Fluconazole, Itraconazole, Ketoconazole.

Imipenem

See Cilastatin and Imipenem

Imipramine

See TRICYCLICS

Imiquimod

TRADE NAME

Aldara.

DRUG CLASS

Immunomodifier.

USES

Treatment of genital and anal warts, and condyloma acuminata.

DOSAGE

 Apply three times a week at night and leave on for 6 to 10 hours.

FORMS

Cream.

PRECAUTIONS

Use with caution in pregnancy (B1), breast feeding and children.

Use with care in vagina and anal canal.

Avoid inflamed skin.

Remove cream before sexual contact.

Uncircumcised men should wash under foreskin daily.

Do not cover treated warts with a bandage.

Use for no more than four months.

 Do not take if:
- suffering from HIV, AIDS or impaired immunity.

SIDE EFFECTS

Common: Skin irritation and redness, swelling of tissue.

Unusual: Ulceration and scabbing of skin, burning skin pain, headache.

INTERACTIONS

Condoms and diaphragms.

PRESCRIPTION

Yes

PERMITTED IN SPORT

Yes

OTHER INFORMATION

Released in 1999 as a radical and effective new way to treat a very distressing problem that previously often required minor surgery.

IMMUNOGLOBULINS

TRADE and GENERIC NAMES

Immunoglobulins against cytomegalovirus (CMV), hepatitis B, rabies, rhesus factor (anti-D), tetanus and zoster (chickenpox) are available as well as pooled Normal Human Immunoglobulin (see Gamma Globulin)

USES

Prevention and treatment of specific diseases or as a boost to patients with a deficient immune system.

DOSAGE

 Depends on disease and individual patient requirements.

PRECAUTIONS

May be used in pregnancy, breast feeding and children.

Should only be used when strictly medically indicated.

Caution must be used with repeat doses.

FORMS

Injection.

SIDE EFFECTS

Common: Tenderness at injection site.

Unusual: Fever, tiredness, belly discomfort, flush, headache, rash, itch, shortness of breath, nausea.

INTERACTIONS

Other drugs:

• Vaccines.

PRESCRIPTION

Yes

PERMITTED IN SPORT

Yes

OVERDOSE

Inadvertent additional dose may cause allergy reaction (sometimes serious) or exacerbation of side effects.

OTHER INFORMATION

Purified from blood donations.

See also Gamma Globulin.

IMMUNOMODIFIERS

(Modify body's immune system)

See Azathioprine, Cyclosporin, Imiquimod, Interferon

Indapamide

TRADE NAME

Natrilix.

DRUG CLASS

Diuretic (increases urine production).

USES

High blood pressure.

DOSAGE

 One tablet in morning.

FORMS

Tablet of 1.5 and 2.5mg. (white).

PRECAUTIONS

Should only be used in pregnancy (C) and breast feeding if medically essential. Not for use in children.

Regular blood tests necessary to check for irregularities in blood chemistry (electrolytes).

 Do not take if:

• suffering from severe kidney or liver disease.

SIDE EFFECTS

Common: Tiredness, dizziness, headache, muscle cramps, diarrhoea.

Unusual: Rash, impotence, sleeplessness, nausea, gout.

Severe but rare (stop medication, consult doctor): Fainting.

INTERACTIONS

Other drugs:

• Barbiturates, Narcotics, Lithium, other Diuretics.

Other substances:

• Reacts adversely with alcohol.

PRESCRIPTION

Yes

PERMITTED IN SPORT

No

OVERDOSE

No serious effect. Induce vomiting if taken recently.

OTHER INFORMATION

Often used in combination with other blood pressure medications to increase their effect.

Indinavir

TRADE NAME

Crixivan.

DRUG CLASS

Antiviral.

USES

AIDS, HIV infection.

DOSAGE

 Up to 800mg. three times a day. Often combined with other therapy.

FORMS

Capsules of 200mg. and 400mg. (white).

PRECAUTIONS

Use with considerable caution in pregnancy (B3), breast feeding and children.

Use lower dose in elderly.

Use with caution in liver disease and diabetes.

Ensure adequate fluid intake.

SIDE EFFECTS

Common: Nausea, diarrhoea, headache and others.

Unusual: Vomiting, kidney stones, liver damage causing jaundice.

Severe but rare (stop medication, consult doctor): Anaemia.

INTERACTIONS

Other drugs:

- Alprazolam, Astemizole, Calcium channel blockers, Cisapride, Didanosine, Erythromycin, Ketoconazole, Midazolam, Rifabutin, Rifampicin, SSRI, Terfenadine, Triazolam,.

Other substances:

- Grapefruit.

PRESCRIPTION

Yes

PERMITTED IN SPORT

Yes

Indomethacin

See NSAID

Indoramin

TRADE NAMES

Baratol, Doralese.

DRUG CLASS

Alpha blocker.

USES

Controls high blood pressure, relieves difficulty in passing urine caused by enlarged prostate gland.

DOSAGE

Varies from 25mg. to 200mg. a day in divided doses.

FORMS

Tablets of 20mg. (cream triangular), 25mg. (blue) and 50mg. (green).

PRECAUTIONS

May be used with caution in pregnancy, breast feeding and children.

Use with caution in significant heart disease, kidney and liver disease, Parkinson's disease, epilepsy and depression.

 Do not take if:

• suffering from heart failure.

SIDE EFFECTS

Common: Drowsiness, dry mouth, stuffy nose.

Unusual: Weight gain, difficulty in ejaculation.

INTERACTIONS

Other drugs:

• MAOI, other medications for high blood pressure.

PRESCRIPTION

Yes

PERMITTED IN SPORT

Yes

OVERDOSE

Drowsiness and depressed reflexes most likely effects.

Influenza virus vaccine

TRADE NAMES

Begrivac, Fluarix, Fluvirin, Influvac

DRUG CLASS

Vaccine.

USES

Prevention of influenza.

DOSAGE

One injection in Autumn every year. Two injections a month apart for first vaccination if under 18 years.

FORMS

Injection.

PRECAUTIONS

Not designed to be used in pregnancy (B2), but no adverse effects expected if vaccination given inadvertently. May be used in breast feeding. Use in children only if specifically indicated.

 Do not take if:

• suffering from fever.

• allergic to eggs.

SIDE EFFECTS

Common: Local discomfort at injection site.

Unusual: Fever.

INTERACTIONS

Other drugs:

• Theophylline, Warfarin, Phenytoin.

PRESCRIPTION

Yes

PERMITTED IN SPORT

Yes

OVERDOSE

An inadvertent additional dose is unlikely to cause any serious effects.

OTHER INFORMATION

Influenza vaccine gives only limited protection, but this increases with subsequent doses. It should be given to persons over 65 years, persons with debilitating illness, persons with chronic diseases (eg: of the lung, heart, kidneys etc.), persons undergoing immunotherapy, and health and medical personnel.

Inositol nicotinate

See Nicotinic Acid

INSULINS

TRADE and GENERIC NAMES

NEUTRAL INSULIN - Onset of action, 30 - 60 min.; peak action, 4 hours; duration, 6 -10 hours.

Humalog, Human Actrapid, Human Velosulin, Human S, Hypurin Bovine Neutral, Hypurine Porcine Neutral, Insumin Rapid, Novo Rapid, Pork Actrapid.

ISOPHANE INSULIN - Onset of action, 2 - 4 hours; peak action, 4 - 12 hours; duration, 24 hours.

Human Insulatard, Humulin 1, Hypurin Bovine Isophane, Hypurin Porcine Isophane, Insuman Basal, Pork Insulatard.

PROTAMINE ZINC INSULIN - Onset of action, 4 - 8 hours; peak action, 16 hours; duration, 36 hours.

Hypurin Bovine PZI.

LENTE INSULIN (INSULIN zinc SUSPENSION) - Onset of action, 3 hours; peak action, 6 - 10 hours; duration, 24 hours.

Human Monotard, Humulin Lente, Hypurin Bovine Lente, Lente MC.

ULTRALENTE INSULIN (CRYSTALLINE INSULIN ZINC SUSPENSION) - Onset of action, 4 - 6 hours; peak action, 10 - 30 hours; duration, 24 - 36 hours.

Humulin Ultratard, Humulin Zn.

BIPHASIC INSULIN (mixture of Neutral insulin and Isophane insulin)- Onset of action, 30 - 60 min.; peak action, 4 - 12 hours; duration, 24 hours.

Humalog Mix25, Human Mixtard, Humulin M, Hypurin Porcine 30/70, Insuman Comb, Pork Mixtard.

USES

Diabetes mellitus.

DOSAGE

 As determined by doctor or patient depending on blood sugar levels. Varies from one individual to another, and depends on food intake and exercise.

PRECAUTIONS

Safe to use in pregnancy (A), breast feeding and children.

Pregnancy, illness, infections, change in diet, exercise and stress may cause change in insulin requirements.

Regular monitoring of blood sugar levels essential.

Knowledge of dietary requirements by patient essential.

Vary site of insulin injection.

Relatives and close friends should be made aware of symptoms of hypoglycaemia (low blood sugar) and first aid requirements.

FORMS

Injection, injection pens.

SIDE EFFECTS

Common: Minimal.

Unusual: Low blood sugar, loss of fat at site of regular injection.

INTERACTIONS

Other drugs:

• Corticosteroids, Thiazides, Frusemide, Ethacrynic acid, Oral contraceptives, Thyroxine, MAOI, Salicylates, Beta blockers.

PRESCRIPTION

Yes

PERMITTED IN SPORT

Yes

OVERDOSE

Very serious. Symptoms of low blood sugar (hypoglycaemia) may include tiredness, confusion, palpitations, sweating, vomiting, dizziness, hunger, blurred vision and fainting. Significant overdosage can lead rapidly to coma and death. Give sugary drinks or sweets if conscious. Seek emergency medical assistance.

OTHER INFORMATION

Insulin is a natural hormone that is essential for the transport of sugar from the blood stream into the cells of the body. It is produced in the pancreas, which lies in the centre of the belly. Most insulin used is artificially manufactured human insulin which is identical in every way to the insulin produced in the human pancreas. In past years, and in a small number of cases today, pig or cow insulin is used.

Interferon

TRADE NAMES

Intron A, Roferon A, Viraferon (Interferon alpha).

Avonex, Betaferon, Rebif (Interferon beta).

Immukin (Interferon gamma).

DRUG CLASS

Immunomodifier.

USES

Some types of leukaemia, genital warts, some skin cancers, multiple myeloma, AIDS, hepatitis B and C.

DOSAGE

 Depends on disease and patient's condition. Must be individualised by doctor.

FORMS

Injection.

PRECAUTIONS

Should not be used in pregnancy (C) unless medically essential as risk of miscarriage increased.

Breast feeding should be ceased before use. Use with considerable caution in children.

Use with caution in heart disease, psychiatric conditions and psoriasis.

Ensure adequate fluid intake.

Regular medical check ups essential.

 Do not take if:

• suffering from severe liver disease or autoimmune disease.

SIDE EFFECTS

Common: Fever, fatigue, headache, muscle pain, chills, loss of appetite, nausea, backache, joint pains, rash.

Unusual: Dry mouth, altered taste, low blood pressure, vomiting, diarrhoea, dizziness, confusion, sleeplessness, depression, hair loss, sweating.

INTERACTIONS

Other drugs:

• Narcotics, Hypnotics, Sedatives.

PRESCRIPTION

Yes

PERMITTED IN SPORT

Yes

OVERDOSE

Exacerbation of side effects likely.

OTHER INFORMATION

Wide range of uses from serious exotic diseases to use by general practitioners to treat skin cancers. Once hailed as a miracle cure-all drug when introduced in the early 1980s. Very useful when prescribed appropriately.

Iodine

TRADE NAMES

Betadine, Inadine, Poviderm (Povidone-iodine).

Other forms of Iodine found in numerous non-prescription antiseptics, mineral and vitamin supplements.

DRUG CLASS

Antiseptic, mineral.

USES

Prevention and treatment of minor bacterial, viral and fungal infections of skin, mouth and vagina. Iodine deficiency.

DOSAGE

 Recommended daily allowance: 120 to 150 mcg a day.
Skin preparations: Apply several times a day as needed

Vaginal pessaries: Insert two at night
Vaginal douche: Dilute 1 to 30 with water. Douche each morning for seven to 14 days.

FORMS

Cream, gargle, lotion, ointment, pads, paint, powder, scrub, spray, swabs, vaginal gel, vaginal douche, vaginal pessary.

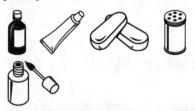

PRECAUTIONS

Safe for use in pregnancy, breast feeding and children.

Vaginal forms should not be used in pregnancy or severe kidney disease.

Not for use on premature infants.

 Do not use if:

• sensitive to Iodine

SIDE EFFECTS

Nil

INTERACTIONS

Other drugs:

• Vaginal preparations may interact with Lithium.

PRESCRIPTION

No

PERMITTED IN SPORT

Yes

OVERDOSE

May cause diarrhoea and stomach upsets if significant amount swallowed.

OTHER INFORMATION

Widely used, safe and effective. Small number of people are excessively sensitive to Iodine.

Ipratropium bromide

TRADE NAMES

Atrovent, Ipratropium Steri-Neb, Respontin, Rinatec.

Combivent (with Salbutamol).

Duovent (with Fenoterol).

DRUG CLASS

Bronchodilator.

USES

Asthma, chronic lung disease, hay fever.

DOSAGE

 Asthma spray: Two inhalations three or four times a day
Nose spray: Two sprays into each nostril two to four times a day.

FORMS

Inhaler, nebuliser solution, nasal spray.

PRECAUTIONS

May be used in pregnancy (B1), breast feeding and children.

Use with caution in glaucoma, enlarged prostate gland, difficulty in passing urine, constipation and irregular heart beat.

Avoid contact with eyes.

SIDE EFFECTS

Common: Dry mouth, throat irritation.

Unusual: Blurred vision, difficulty in passing urine, cough.

Severe but rare (stop medication, consult doctor): Eye pain or halos seen around objects.

INTERACTIONS

Other drugs:

• Sodium cromoglycate.

PRESCRIPTION

Yes

PERMITTED IN SPORT

Yes

OVERDOSE

Exacerbation of side effects only likely consequence.

OTHER INFORMATION

Commonly used in conjunction with other medication for severe asthma, emphysema and chronic bronchitis. May be used alone in some forms (eg: exercise induced) of asthma. Very useful and safe medication.

Irbesartan

See ANGIOTENSIN II RECEPTOR ANTAGONISTS

IRON

TRADE and GENERIC NAMES

Ferfolic SV (Ferrous gluconate with Folic acid).

Ferrograd Folic, Slow-Fe Folic (Ferrous sulphate with Folic acid).

Ferrograd, Slow-Fe (Ferrous sulphate).

Fersaday, Fersamal, Galfer (<u>Ferrous fumarate</u>).

Jectofer (<u>Iron sorbitol</u>).

Lexpec with Iron (<u>Ferrous ammonium citrate</u> with Folic acid).

Plesmet (<u>Ferrous glycine sulphate</u>).

Pregaday (<u>Ferrous fumarate</u> with Folic acid).

Sytron (<u>Sodium iron edetate</u>).

Venofer (<u>Iron-hydroxide sucrose</u>).

Numerous other vitamin and mineral supplements also contain various forms of iron (eg: Ferrous phosphate).

NB: Iron compounds underlined.

DRUG CLASS

Mineral.

USES

Iron deficiency, some types of anaemia.

DOSAGE

One tablet or capsule a day on an empty stomach
Recommended daily intake: 12 to 16 mg a day.

FORMS

Tablets, capsules, mixture, injection.

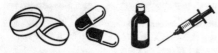

PRECAUTIONS

Safe in pregnancy (A), breast feeding and children.

 ### Do not take if:

• suffering from haemochromatosis, anaemia not due to iron deficiency.

SIDE EFFECTS

Common: Slight stomach upsets.

Unusual: Temporary tooth staining.

INTERACTIONS

None significant.

PRESCRIPTION

No

PERMITTED IN SPORT

Yes

OVERDOSE

Constipation and stomach cramps only likely effects.

OTHER INFORMATION

Iron is absorbed from the gut at a set rate, and using higher doses is unlikely to have any clinical effect. Iron is found in red meats (particularly liver) and green vegetables. Pregnant women are at risk of iron deficiency because the developing baby to build muscle and blood cells.

Isoniazid

TRADE NAMES

Rifater (with Pyrazinamide, Rifampicin).

Rifinah, Rimactizid (with Rifampicin).

USES

Tuberculosis (TB).

DOSAGE

One tablet, two or three times a day. Dosage adjusted carefully to match weight of patient.

FORMS

Tablets.

SIDE EFFECTS

Common: Pins and needles, nausea.

Unusual: Vomiting, diarrhoea, belly discomfort, fever, rash.

Severe but rare (stop medication, consult doctor): Eye damage, unusual bruising or bleeding, yellow skin (jaundice).

INTERACTIONS

Other drugs:

• Phenytoin, Carbamazepine.

Other substances:

• Reacts with alcohol.

PRECAUTIONS

May be used safely in pregnancy (A), breast feeding and children.

Use with caution in liver and kidney disease.

Regular checks of eyes recommended.

Regular blood tests to check liver and kidney function recommended.

Do not take if:

• suffering from severe liver disease.

PRESCRIPTION

Yes

PERMITTED IN SPORT

Yes

OVERDOSE

Serious. May cause vomiting, dizziness, blurred vision, slurred speech, hallucinations, difficulty in breathing, convulsions and coma. Administer activated charcoal or induce vomiting if medication taken recently. Seek urgent medical assistance.

Isophane Insulin

See INSULINS

Isoprenaline

TRADE NAME

Saventrine.

USES

Heart diseases due to the blockage of nerve conduction within the heart and resulting in irregular heart rhythm or stopping of the heart.

Severe lung spasm (bronchospasm - similar to asthma) during surgery.

Sudden severe drop in blood pressure, shock.

DOSAGE

 As determined by doctor.

FORMS

Injection.

PRECAUTIONS

Safe in pregnancy (A) and breast feeding.

Use with caution in some types of heart disease, high blood pressure, diabetes, over active thyroid gland.

Use lower doses in elderly and children.

Patient should be connected to a heart monitor during administration.

Do not take if:

• suffering from rapid heart rate, overdose of digoxin, recent heart attack or angina.

SIDE EFFECTS

Common: Irregular heart beat, nervousness, headache, dizziness, restlessness.

Unusual: Hot flushes, tremor, weakness, muscle tension.

Severe but rare (stop medication, consult doctor): Very high blood pressure.

INTERACTIONS

Other drugs:

• Adrenaline, digoxin, chlorpromazine, MAOI.

PRESCRIPTION

Yes

PERMITTED IN SPORT

No

OVERDOSE

Very serious. Urgent medical attention necessary. See also Adrenaline

Isosorbide

TRADE NAMES

Cedocard-Retard, Elantan, Imdur, Isib 60XL, Ismo, Isodur XL, Isotard XL, MCR-50, Monit, Mono-Cedocard, Monomax (Isosorbide mononitrate).

Isocard, Isoket, Isordil, Sorbid SA (Isosorbide dinitrate and Sorbide nitrate).

Imazin XL (Isosorbide mononitrate with Aspirin).

DRUG CLASS

Antiangina.

USES

Prevention and treatment of angina, some types of heart failure, poor blood supply to heart.

DOSAGE

 Depends on form
Long acting tablets: One or two tablets once a day
Sublingual tablets: One or two tablets under tongue every two or three hours
Normal tablets: One to three tablets three times a day
Spray: One or two sprays to the chest once or twice a day.

FORMS

Tablets, capsules, sublingual (under tongue) tablets, spray.

PRECAUTIONS

Should be used with caution in pregnancy (B1, B2) and breast feeding. Not for use in children.

Tolerance may develop if used long term.

Long acting tablets and capsules not designed for use in acute angina. They should not be ceased suddenly, but withdrawn slowly.

Use with caution in kidney and liver disease, reduced brain blood flow and low blood pressure.

 Do not take if:

• suffering from right heart failure, low blood pressure, constrictive pericarditis, severe anaemia, increased brain pressure.

SIDE EFFECTS

Common: Headache, low blood pressure, rapid heart rate, dizziness, poor appetite, nausea, sleep disturbances.

Unusual: Flushing, swelling of tissues, rash, vomiting, anaemia.

Severe but rare (stop medication, consult doctor): Slow heart rate.

INTERACTIONS

Other drugs:

• Phenothiazines, Tricyclics, Anticholinergics, Beta blockers. • Drugs that lower blood pressure.

PRESCRIPTION

Yes

PERMITTED IN SPORT

Yes

OVERDOSE

Headache, severe low blood pressure, rapid heart rate and collapse may occur. Administer activated charcoal or induce vomiting if tablets taken recently. Seek urgent medical attention.

OTHER INFORMATION

Used for several decades for treatment and prevention of angina. Slow release long acting forms have far fewer side effects and have dramatically improved the life of patients with angina.

See also Glyceryl trinitrate.

Isotretinoin

TRADE NAMES

Isotrex, Roaccutane.

Isotrexin (with Erythromycin).

USES

Severe acne not responding to other medication.

DOSAGE

 Capsules: One or two capsules once or twice a day with food for up to 16 weeks.
Gel: Apply sparingly once a day at night.

FORMS

Capsules of 5mg. and 20mg., gel.

PRECAUTIONS

Absolutely forbidden in pregnancy (X), breast feeding and children under twelve.

Must be used with caution in all patients.

Adequate contraception essential for all women using Isotretinoin.

Use with caution if cholesterol or triglyceride levels high.

Regular blood tests recommended.

Use with caution in diabetes.

Avoid sun exposure during use.

Never exceed recommended dose or length of course.

 Do not take if:

• suffering from liver disease or any form of cancer.

• taking Tetracyclines.

SIDE EFFECTS

Common: Sore mouth and lips, dry eyes, dry mouth, dry skin, nose bleeds, muscle pain, joint pain, joint stiffness, hair thinning, peeling of palms and soles, sun sensitivity.

Unusual: Tiredness, headache, depression, gout, diarrhoea, initial worsening of acne, altered blood test results.

Severe but rare (stop medication, consult doctor): Severe headache, intractable vomiting, visual disturbances.

INTERACTIONS

Other drugs:

• Tetracycline.

Other substances:

• Reacts with alcohol.

PRESCRIPTION

Yes (capsules restricted to specialist dermatologists and consultant physicians in hospitals only).

PERMITTED IN SPORT

Yes

OVERDOSE

May cause headache, vomiting, flushing, mouth soreness and dryness, abdominal pain and incoordination. Seek medical assistance.

OTHER INFORMATION

A very potent and potentially dangerous drug, but if used correctly can dramatically and often permanently cure severe chronic acne. Use in pregnancy will always cause severe damage to foetus.

See also Etretinate

Ispaghula

TRADE NAMES

Fybogel, Fybogest, Isogel, Konsyl, Regulan.

Fybogel Mebeverine (with Mebeverine).

Manevac (with Senna).

DRUG CLASS

Fibre.

USES

Constipation.

DOSAGE

 Take required amount with water twice a day.

FORMS

Granules, powder.

PRECAUTIONS

Safe in pregnancy and breast feeding.

 Do not take if:

• on a salt restricted diet

• suffering from megacolon

SIDE EFFECTS

Common: Minimal.

Unusual: Diarrhoea, belly discomfort.

INTERACTIONS

None significant

PRESCRIPTION

No

PERMITTED IN SPORT

Yes

OVERDOSE

Take additional water. Belly discomfort and passing excess wind only effects.

OTHER INFORMATION

Widely used, natural fibre supplement.

Isradipine

See CALCIUM CHANNEL BLOCKERS

Itraconazole

TRADE NAME

Sporanox.

DRUG CLASS

Antifungal.

USES

Fungal infections of mouth (thrush), skin, vagina and eye.

DOSAGE

 One or two capsules, once or twice a day with food.

FORMS

Capsules (blue/pink) of 100mg.

PRECAUTIONS

Not to be used in pregnancy (B3) unless medically essential. Cease breast feeding before use. Use with caution in children.

Not to be used long term.

Use with caution in liver disease.

SIDE EFFECTS

Common: Nausea, diarrhoea, headache, dizziness.

Severe but rare (stop medication, consult doctor): Yellow skin (jaundice).

INTERACTIONS

Other drugs:

• Digoxin, Cyclosporin, Phenytoin, Rifampicin, H2 Antagonists, Anticoagulants, Isoniazid, Hypoglycaemics, Norethisterone.

Other substances:

• Reacts with alcohol.

PRESCRIPTION

Yes

PERMITTED IN SPORT

Yes

OVERDOSE

May cause liver damage. Administer activated charcoal or induce vomiting if taken recently. Seek medical assistance.

OTHER INFORMATION

Introduced 1994. Expensive.

No medications have a name starting with the letter J.

Kaolin

TRADE NAME

Available alone and in combination with other medications in some locally produced antidiarrhoeal preparations.

DRUG CLASS

Antidiarrhoeal.

USES

Diarrhoea.

DOSAGE

 30 mLs initially, then 15 to 30 mLs every two to four hours as required for condition. Take at least an hour away from other medications.

FORMS

Suspension.

PRECAUTIONS

Safe in pregnancy, breast feeding and children over three years.

 Do not take if:

- suffering from kidney disease
- for prolonged periods.

SIDE EFFECTS

Common: Minimal

Unusual: Constipation.

INTERACTIONS

Other drugs:

- Kaolin markedly affects the absorption of many other drugs including Antibiotics, Anticoagulants, H2 antagonists, Iron, Isoniazid, Phenothiazines and Aspirin.

PRESCRIPTION

No.

PERMITTED IN SPORT

Yes.

OVERDOSE

Causes constipation, nausea and vomiting.

OTHER INFORMATION

Kaolin is a form of clay that has been used for thousands of years to treat diarrhoea, but is now considered to be of only slight benefit and has been superseded by more effective medications. Also used in making fine china.

KERATOLYTICS

TRADE and GENERIC NAMES

Acnecide, Brevoxyl, Panoxyl (Benzoyl peroxide)

Acnidazil (Benzoyl peroxide, Miconazole)

Acnisal, Occlusal, Verrugon (*Salicylic acid*)

Aquasept, Manusept, Ster-Zac Bath (Triclosan)

Aserbine (Benzoic acid, Malic acid, Salicylic acid and other ingredients)

Avoca (Silver nitrate)

Benzamycin (<u>Benzoyl peroxide</u>, Erythromycin)

Brasivol (<u>Aluminium oxide</u>)

Capasal (<u>Salicylic acid</u> with Coal tar and oils)

Cocois (<u>Salicylic acid</u> with Coal tar, Sulphur and oils)

Cuplex (<u>Salicylic acid, Lactic acid</u> with Copper acetate)

Diprosalic (<u>Salicylic acid</u> with Betamethasone)

Duofilm, Salactol, Salatac (<u>Salicylic acid, Lactic acid</u>)

Gelcosal (<u>Salicylic acid</u> with Coal tar)

Hemocane (<u>Benzoic acid</u>, Lignocaine, Zinc oxide, Bismuth oxide, Cinnamic acid)

Ionil T (<u>Salicylic acid</u> with Coal tar, Benzalkonium chloride)

Meted (<u>Salicylic acid</u> with Sulphur)

Monophytol (<u>Salicylic acid</u> with Chlorbutol and other ingredients)

Movelat (<u>Salicylic acid</u> with Mucopolysaccharide polysulphate)

Oilatum Plus (<u>Triclosan</u> with Paraffin, Benzalkonium chloride)

Posalfilin (<u>Salicylic acid</u> with Podophyllum)

Pragmatar (<u>Salicylic acid</u> with Coal tar, Sulphur)

Psorin (<u>Salicylic acid</u> with Coal tar, Dithranol)

Pyralvex (<u>Salicylic acid</u> with Anthraquinone)

Quinoderm, Quinoped (<u>Benzoyl peroxide</u>, Potassium hydroxyquinolone)

Retin-A, Retinova, Vesanoid (<u>Tretinoin</u>)

Skinoren (<u>Azelaic acid</u>)

Stiedex Lotion (Salicylic acid with Desoxymethasone)

NB: Keratolytics are underlined

Formaldehyde, Lactic acid, Isotretinoin and Etretinate (see separate entries) are also Keratolytics.

DRUG CLASS

Keratolytics remove keratin from skin to thin, dry and soften the skin.

Keratin is a protein that creates the horny, hard layers of the skin.

Triclosan and Azelaic acid also have antiseptic properties.

USES

Acne, minor skin infections.

DOSAGE

 Follow directions on packaging, as directions vary with composition, form and strength.

FORMS

Gel, cream, ointment, liquid, wash, foam, wipes, solution, bar, soap, caustic pencil.

PRECAUTIONS

Tretinoin should not be used in pregnancy. Other Keratolytics may be used in with caution in pregnancy, breast feeding and children. Not designed for use in young children.

Avoid eyes, nostrils, mouth, vagina and anus with all preparations.

Avoid open wound contact. Avoid sun exposure after use. Do not exceed recommended dose.

 Do not take if:
- suffering from eczema or sunburn.

SIDE EFFECTS

Common: Stinging, warmth, skin redness.

Unusual: Swelling, peeling, sun sensitivity.

Severe but rare (stop medication, consult doctor): Skin pain, marked swelling, severe peeling.

INTERACTIONS

Other drugs:

• Other Keratolytics, abrasives.

Other substances: • Many cosmetics.

PRESCRIPTION

Trentinoin: Yes.
Other: No.

PERMITTED IN SPORT

Yes

OVERDOSE

Excessive use may lead to skin damage, burning and pain. Wash off any excess from skin immediately.

OTHER INFORMATION

Tretinoin is a vitamin A derivative. All Keratolytics must be used carefully, but if correctly used, may markedly improve acne.

See also SALICYLATES (Salicylic acid), Acitretin, Formaldehyde, Glutaraldehyde, Isotretinoin, Lactic Acid.

Ketoconazole

TRADE NAME

Nizoral.

DRUG CLASS

Antifungal.

USES

Significant fungal infections of skin and internal organs, severe dandruff, tinea.

DOSAGE

 Tablets: One tablet a day with food
Cream: Apply once or twice a day
Shampoo: Apply to wet scalp for five minutes twice a week for four weeks.

FORMS

Tablets (white) of 200mg., cream, shampoo.

PRECAUTIONS

Tablets should not be used in pregnancy (B3) unless medically essential, and breast feeding should be ceased before use. Tablets not to be used in children. Shampoo and cream may be used in pregnancy, breast feeding and children with caution.

Should not be used long term.

Use with caution in older women.

Use with caution in adrenal disease, if allergic to Penicillin or if Griseofulvin taken recently. Avoid eye contact with cream and shampoo.

 Do not take if:

• suffering from liver disease.

• taking Terfenadine or Astemizole.

SIDE EFFECTS

Common: Tablets - Nausea. Shampoo and cream - Skin irritation, itch, rash and redness.

Unusual: Vomiting, diarrhoea, belly pain, rash, itch, headache, dizziness.

Severe but rare (stop medication, consult doctor): Yellow skin (jaundice).

INTERACTIONS

Other drugs:

• Tablets - Astemizole, Terfenadine, Isoniazid, Rifampicin.

• Shampoo - Corticosteroid scalp applications.

PRESCRIPTION
Yes.

PERMITTED IN SPORT
Yes.

OVERDOSE
Induce vomiting if medication taken recently. Seek medical assistance.

OTHER INFORMATION
Introduced in mid 1980s. Very effective, but may cause liver damage if used inappropriately or for long periods.

See also Econazole.

Ketoprofen
See NSAID

Ketorolac trometanol
See NSAID

Ketotifen

TRADE NAME
Zaditen.

DRUG CLASS
Antihistamine.

USES
Allergic conditions, hay fever, allergic conjunctivitis, asthma prevention.

DOSAGE
 1mg. to 2mg. twice a day.

FORMS
Tablets of 1mg. (white), Capsules of 1mg. (white), elixir.

PRECAUTIONS
Not to be used in pregnancy and breast feeding.

May be used in children over two years of age.

Reduce dose slowly over two or more weeks.

SIDE EFFECTS
Common: Drowsiness, dry mouth, slow reactions.

Unusual: Irritability, weight gain, skin reactions.

INTERACTIONS
Other drugs:
• Sedatives, Hypoglycaemics, Antihistamines.

Other substances:
• Alcohol.

PRESCRIPTION
Yes.

PERMITTED IN SPORT
Yes.

OVERDOSE
May result in convulsions, hallucinations, delirium, anxiety, muscle spasms, rapid heart rate, flushing, dry skin, dry mouth and coma. First aid involved inducing vomiting and seeking urgent medical attention.

OTHER INFORMATION
An unusual antihistamine in that it prevents asthma, as well as the more traditional effects of this class of medication.

See also ANTIHISTAMINES, SEDATING

Labetalol

TRADE NAME

Trandate.

DRUG CLASS

Alpha-Beta Blocker, Antihypertensive.

USES

High blood pressure.

DOSAGE

 100mg. to 400mg., two to four times a day to a maximum of 2400mg. per day.

FORMS

Tablets (orange) of 50mg, 100mg. and 200mg.

SIDE EFFECTS

Common: Minimal

Unusual: Slow heart rate, dizziness, headache, tiredness, blurred vision, eye irritation, asthma, rash, difficulty in passing urine.

INTERACTIONS

Other drugs:

- Beta agonists, Calcium channel blockers, drugs for treatment of irregular heart beat.

- Tremor with Tricyclic antidepressants.

- Cimetidine increases blood levels of Labetalol.

PRESCRIPTION

Yes

PERMITTED IN SPORT

No

OVERDOSE

Low blood pressure and slow heart rate. Lay patient flat and raise legs. Administer charcoal or induce vomiting if tablets taken recently. Seek medical assistance.

PRECAUTIONS

Should not be used in pregnancy (C) unless medically essential. Should be used with caution in breast feeding and elderly. Not recommended in children.

Should not be stopped suddenly, but dosage should be slowly reduced over several days.

Use lower doses in elderly.

 Do not take if:

- suffering from heart disease, narrowed arteries, Prinzmetal angina, diabetes, overactive thyroid gland, phaeochromocytoma or liver failure.

- having a general anaesthetic. Discuss with doctor

Lacidipine

See **CALCIUM CHANNEL BLOCKERS**

Lactic acid

TRADE NAMES

Available only in combination with other medications.

Calmurid (with Urea).

Calmurid HC (with Urea, Hydrocortisone).

Cuplex (with Copper acetate).

Duofilm, Salactol, Salatac (with Salicylic acid).

Lacticare (with Sodium pyrrolidone carboxylate).

Available in numerous other creams and lotions.

DRUG CLASS

Acid.

USES

Thickened skin, warts, corns.

DOSAGE

 Apply one or two times a day.

FORMS

Cream, lotion, solution, paint.

PRECAUTIONS

Safe in pregnancy, breast feeding and children.

Avoid eyes, mouth and nostrils.

SIDE EFFECTS

Common: Stinging.

INTERACTIONS

None

PRESCRIPTION

No

PERMITTED IN SPORT

Yes See also KERATOLYTICS

Lactulose

TRADE NAMES

Duphalac, Lactugal.

DRUG CLASS

Laxative.

USES

Severe constipation. Also used in rare form of brain inflammation.

DOSAGE

 30 to 45 mLs. three or four times a day.

FORMS

Solution.

PRECAUTIONS

Safe in pregnancy, breast feeding and children.

Should be used with caution in diabetics.

Should not be used for more than six months without medical checkup.

SIDE EFFECTS

Common: Intestinal cramps, bloating, passing wind.

Unusual: Diarrhoea, nausea, loss of appetite, increased thirst.

INTERACTIONS

Other drugs:

• Interacts with Neomycin and other antibiotics given by mouth.

PRESCRIPTION

No

PERMITTED IN SPORT

Yes

OVERDOSE

Diarrhoea and intestinal cramps only problem.

OTHER INFORMATION

Normally only used for severe constipation when other medications ineffective.

Lamivudine

TRADE NAMES

Epivir, Zeffix.

Combivir (with Zidovudine).

DRUG CLASS

Antiviral.

USES

HIV infection, AIDS, chronic hepatitis B.

DOSAGE

 100 to 150mg., once or twice a day, often in combination with other antivirals.

FORMS

Tablets, mixture.

PRECAUTIONS

Use with considerable caution in pregnancy (B3) and children. Use with caution in breast feeding.

Use with caution in kidney and liver disease, diabetes and pancreas disease.

SIDE EFFECTS

Common: Nausea, headache, tiredness, inability to sleep, rashes.

Unusual: Pancreatitis.

INTERACTIONS

None significant.

PRESCRIPTION

Yes

PERMITTED IN SPORT

Yes

Lamotrigine

TRADE NAME

Lamictal.

DRUG CLASS

Anticonvulsant.

USES

Epilepsy, particularly seizures that affect only one part of the body and are not controlled by other anticonvulsants.

DOSAGE

 Gradually increase dose until control obtained, usually between 200mg. and 400mg. a day taken in two doses. Lower doses used in combination with other anticonvulsants.

FORMS

Tablets (yellow) of 25mg., 50mg., 100mg. and 200mg.

PRECAUTIONS

Use with great caution in pregnancy (B3), breast feeding and children under 12 years.

Use with caution in kidney and liver disease.

Regular blood tests to check liver and kidney function and clotting are necessary.

Do not stop suddenly, but reduce dosage slowly.

SIDE EFFECTS

Common: Rash, dizziness, headache, double vision, incoordination, tiredness, nausea, blurred vision, vomiting.
Unusual: Swelling of tissue, blistering and peeling of skin, blood cell damage.

INTERACTIONS

Other drugs:

• Other Anticonvulsants.

PRESCRIPTION

Yes

PERMITTED IN SPORT

Yes

OVERDOSE

Sedation, incoordination, double vision and vomiting may occur. Administer charcoal or induce vomiting if taken recently. Seek medical assistance.

OTHER INFORMATION

Introduced in 1993 to assist the most severe and difficult to control forms of epilepsy. Unfortunately, cost and side effects limit its usefulness.

Lansoprazole

See PROTON PUMP INHIBITORS

Latanoprost

TRADE NAME

Xalantan.

USES

Glaucoma.

DOSAGE

One drop in affected eye(s) once a day. Apply pressure to tear duct at inner corner of eye for five minutes after application.

FORMS

Eye drops.

PRECAUTIONS

Use with considerable caution in pregnancy (B3). Use with caution in breast feeding and children.

Use with caution in eye inflammation, pigmentary and hereditary glaucoma.

 Do not use if:

• wearing contact lenses.

SIDE EFFECTS

Common: Change in eye colour, irritation of eye surface, redness of eye, blurred vision, eye burning and itching.

Unusual: Swelling of eye surface, ulceration of eye surface.

INTERACTIONS

Other drugs:

• Thiomersal drops, Acetazolamide.

PRESCRIPTION

Yes

PERMITTED IN SPORT

Yes

OVERDOSE

Eye irritation and exacerbation of side effects likely.

OTHER INFORMATION

Introduced for treatment of glaucoma unresponsive to other medications.

LAXATIVES

(Relieve constipation)

See Bisacodyl, Docusate sodium, Fibre, Lactulose, Paraffin, Poloxamer, Senna, Sodium acid phosphate, Sodium phosphate, Sodium picosulfate

L-Dopa

See LEVODOPA COMPOUNDS

Leflunomide

TRADE NAME

Arava.

USES

Treatment of severe rheumatoid arthritis.

DOSAGE

 100mg. a day for three days, then 10mg. to 20mg. once a day.

FORMS

Tablets of 10mg. (white), 20mg. (yellow) and 100mg. (white).

PRECAUTIONS

Never to be used in pregnancy (X) and breast feeding.

May be used with caution in children and the elderly.

Regular blood tests to check liver function and blood cell count necessary.

Use with caution in generalised infection, bone marrow damage, tuberculosis and kidney damage.

 Do not take if:

• suffering from immunodeficiency, low platelet or white cell count, severe infection, Stevens-Johnson syndrome, liver disease or erythema multiforme.

• female partner is pregnant (may be transferred during sex).

SIDE EFFECTS

Common: Skin reactions, nausea, diarrhoea, hair loss.

Unusual: High blood pressure, sore mouth, belly pain, liver and blood cell damage, tendon and muscle pain, headache, dizziness, weight loss, pins and needles sensation, allergy reaction.

Severe but rare (stop medication, consult doctor): Severe skin reaction, blistering and loss of skin.

INTERACTIONS

Other drugs:

• Methotrexate, Phenytoin, Warfarin, Tolbutamide, some vaccines, Rifampicin, charcoal, Cholestyramine.

Other substances:

• Alcohol.

PRESCRIPTION

Yes

PERMITTED IN SPORT

Yes (restricted to specialists).

OVERDOSE

Likely to be serious, but no information available. Seek urgent medical attention.

OTHER INFORMATION

Introduced in 1999 as a last resort, but effective treatment, for the most severe forms of rheumatoid arthritis.

Lente insulin

See INSULINS

Lercanidipine

See CALCIUM CHANNEL BLOCKERS

Letrozole

TRADE NAME

Femara.

DRUG CLASS

Antineoplastic.

USES

Some types of advanced breast cancer in postmenopausal women.

DOSAGE

 One tablet a day.

FORMS

Tablets of 2.5mg. (dark yellow).

PRECAUTIONS

Not to be used in pregnancy (D), breast feeding or children.

Use with caution in kidney and liver disease.

 Do not take if:

• still having menstrual periods.

SIDE EFFECTS

Common: Headache, nausea, diarrhoea, swelling of hands and feet, tiredness, hot flushes, hair thinning, rash, vaginal discharge.

Unusual: Weight change, muscle pain, vaginal bleeding, sweating, dizziness, tiredness, increased appetite, joint pain, urgent desire to pass urine, acne, breast enlargement.

Severe but rare (stop medication, consult doctor): Blood clot in vein (thrombosis).

INTERACTIONS

None yet known in newly released drug.

PRESCRIPTION

Yes

PERMITTED IN SPORT

Yes

OVERDOSE

Effect unknown. Induce vomiting or administer activated charcoal if tablets taken recently. Seek medical attention.

OTHER INFORMATION

Introduced in 1998 for treatment of severe relapses of some types of breast cancer.

LEUKOTRENE RECEPTOR ANTAGONISTS

(Prevent and treat asthma)

See Zafirlukast

Leuprorelin

TRADE NAME

Prostap SR.

DRUG CLASS

Antineoplastic.

USES

Prostate cancer, endometriosis, fibroids of the uterus prior to surgery.

DOSAGE

 Monthly injection.

FORMS

Depot injection.

SIDE EFFECTS

Common: Hot flushes, sweats, swelling of hands and feet, nausea, diarrhoea.

Unusual: Pain at cancer or fibroid sites, shortness of breath, tiredness, headache, emotional instability, palpitations, breast tenderness.

Severe but rare (stop medication, consult doctor): High blood pressure.

PRECAUTIONS

Not to be used in pregnancy (D), breast feeding and children.

Use with caution with metastatic cancer involving the spine, urinary tract obstruction.

 Do not take if:

- suffering from osteoporosis, undiagnosed bleeding from the vagina.

INTERACTIONS

None significant.

PRESCRIPTION

Yes

PERMITTED IN SPORT

Yes

Levobunolol

See BETA BLOCKERS

Levocabastine

TRADE NAME

Livostin.

USES

Allergic conjunctivitis, hay fever.

DOSAGE

 Eye drops: One drop in eye twice a day
Nose drops: Two sprays in each nostril two to four times a day.

FORMS

Eye drops, nose spray.

PRECAUTIONS

Must not be used in pregnancy (D).

Use with caution in breast feeding and kidney disease.

Use with caution if wearing contact lenses.

Do not use continuously for more than eight weeks.

SIDE EFFECTS

Common: Local irritation, headaches.

Unusual: Tiredness, nose bleed.

INTERACTIONS

None significant.

PRESCRIPTION

Yes

PERMITTED IN SPORT

Yes

OVERDOSE

Unlikely to be serious.

See also Emedastine

LEVODOPA COMPOUNDS

TRADE and GENERIC NAMES

Madopar (Levodopa and Benserazide).

Sinemet (Levodopa and Carbidopa).

DRUG CLASS

Antiparkinsonian.

USES

Parkinson's disease.

DOSAGE

 Individualised depending on patient's response. Follow doctor's instructions carefully.

FORMS

Capsules, tablets.

PRECAUTIONS

Should be used in pregnancy (B3) only if medically essential. Breast feeding should be ceased before use. Not for use in children.

Use with caution in psychiatric conditions, heart disease, peptic ulcers, epilepsy, osteoporosis, glaucoma and osteomalacia.

Do not undertake sudden increases in exercise levels.

 Do not take if:

• suffering from severe heart disease, glandular disease, severe lung disease, liver or kidney disease, psychoses, melanoma, tremor, Huntington's chorea.

• under 30 years of age.

SIDE EFFECTS

Common: Nausea, loss of appetite, palpitations, weight gain, constipation, incoordination, twitching, depression, tiredness, hiccups, sleeplessness, muscle cramps, excess excitability, tissue swelling, drowsiness.

Unusual: Vomiting, angina, shortness of breath, reduced libido, irregular heart rhythm, diarrhoea, leg pain, fainting, hallucinations, confusion.

Severe but rare (stop medication, consult doctor): Significant psychiatric disturbances.

INTERACTIONS

Other drugs:

- Drugs acting on the heart.
- Drugs used to treat psychiatric conditions.
- Drugs used in general anaesthetics.

PRESCRIPTION

Yes

PERMITTED IN SPORT

Yes

OVERDOSE

Symptoms include all side effects above, but exaggerated in severity. Administer activated charcoal or induce vomiting if patient alert and medication taken recently. Seek urgent medical assistance.

OTHER INFORMATION

Despite their significant side effects, these medications have dramatically improved the quality of life for many patients with Parkinson's disease. Hailed as a miracle cure when introduced in the late 1960's, levodopa is now accepted as just one part of the treatment for this disease. Unfortunately, its effect tends to decrease the longer it is used. An important brain hormone, dopamine is depleted in Parkinson's disease. Providing extra material from which the brain can make dopamine improves the condition for many years.

Levofloxacin

TRADE NAME

Tavanic.

DRUG CLASS

Quinolone antibiotic.

USES

Bacterial infections including sinusitis, acute bronchitis, pneumonia, kidney and bladder infections, skin infections.

DOSAGE

 250mg. to 500mg. once or twice a day.

FORMS

Tablets (off white) of 250 and 500mg.

PRECAUTIONS

Not to be used in pregnancy and breast feeding. Not recommended in children.

Use with caution in porphyria, severe kidney disease and persistent diarrhoea.

Avoid strong ultraviolet light.

 Do not take if:

- suffering from epilepsy, drug induced tendon disorders.

SIDE EFFECTS

Common: Nausea, diarrhoea.

Unusual: Mild liver damage.

Severe but rare (stop medication, consult doctor): Severe liver damage, tendon damage.

INTERACTIONS

Other drugs:

- Iron, Antacids, Sucralfate, NSAIDs, Fenbufen, Probenecid, Cimetidine.

PRESCRIPTION

Yes

PERMITTED IN SPORT

Yes

OVERDOSE

Exacerbation of side effects most likely result. Induce vomiting if medication taken recently. Maintain adequate fluid intake.

Levonorgestrel

See ORAL CONTRACEPTIVES

Lignocaine

See ANAESTHETICS, LOCAL

Linoleic acid (Evening primrose oil)

See FATTY ACIDS

Liothyronine

See THYROID HORMONES

Lisinopril

See ACE INHIBITORS

Lithium carbonate

TRADE NAME

Camcolit, Li-Liquid, Liskonum, Litarex, Priadel.

Efalith (with Zinc sulphate).

DRUG CLASS

Antipsychotic.

USES

Manic - depressive psychoses, severe depression, aggressive behaviour, other psychiatric conditions. Cream used for oily dermatitis.

DOSAGE

 One or two tablets, two or three times a day. Sustained release tablets taken once or twice a day. Dosage must be individualised for each patient. Follow doctors instructions carefully.
Cream - apply thinly twice a day.

FORMS

Tablets , liquid, cream (Efalith).

PRECAUTIONS

Lithium must not be used in pregnancy (D) except under exceptional circumstances as it may cause malformations of the heart and damage to the thyroid gland of the foetus. Breast feeding must be ceased if Lithium is taken. Not for use in children.

Diet should remain regular during dosage with Lithium as changes in diet and fluid intake can affect blood levels of Lithium.

Regular blood tests to check dosage of Lithium recommended.

 Do not take if:

- suffering from significant heart and kidney disease, Addison's disease, underactive thyroid gland.

SIDE EFFECTS

Common: Weight gain, goitre, swelling of tissues (oedema), dermatitis, loss of appetite, nausea, belly discomfort, diarrhoea, tiredness, slurred speech.

Unusual: Vomiting, tremor, agitation.

INTERACTIONS

Other drugs:

• Steroids, appetite suppressants, other Psychotropic drugs, NSAID.

PRESCRIPTION

Yes

PERMITTED IN SPORT

Yes

OVERDOSE

Extremely serious. Symptoms may include diarrhoea, vomiting, weakness, incoordination, drowsiness, twitching, disorientation, coma and death. Administer activated charcoal or induce vomiting if taken recently and patient alert. Seek emergency medical assistance.

OTHER INFORMATION

Widely used and effective treatment developed in Australia. Used for some specific types of mental illness. Does not cause addiction or dependence.

LOCAL ANAESTHETICS

See ANAESTHETICS, LOCAL

Lodoxamide

TRADE NAME

Alomide.

USES

Allergic conjunctivitis, keratoconjunctivitis.

DOSAGE

One drop in eye four times a day.

FORMS

Eye drops.

PRECAUTIONS

May be used with caution in pregnancy (B1), breast feeding and children. Use with caution if wearing contact lenses.

SIDE EFFECTS

Common: Eye discomfort, eye itch, blurred vision.

Unusual: Crusting of lid margins, dry eye, red eye, excess tears.

INTERACTIONS

None significant.

PRESCRIPTION

Yes

PERMITTED IN SPORT

Yes

OVERDOSE

Unlikely to be serious.

OTHER INFORMATION

Introduced in 1997 as an effective treatment for allergic reaction in the eye unrelieved by simpler medications.

Lofepramine

See TRICYCLIC ANTIDEPRESSANTS

Lofexidine

TRADE NAME

Britlofex.

USES

Control of withdrawal from narcotics (eg. heroin, methadone).

DOSAGE

 Start with one or two tablets a day and slowly increase until symptoms relieved or maximum of 12 tablets a day.

FORMS

Tablets of 0.2mg. (peach).

PRECAUTIONS

Use with caution in pregnancy, breast feeding and children.

Use with caution in severe heart disease, recent heart attack, slow heart rate, history of depression and chronic kidney disease.

SIDE EFFECTS

Common: Drowsiness, dry mouth and nose.

Unusual: Slow heart rate, low blood pressure.

INTERACTIONS

Other drugs:

• Sedatives, Tricyclic antidepressants.

Other substances:

• Alcohol.

PRESCRIPTION

Yes

PERMITTED IN SPORT

Yes

OVERDOSE

Serious. Induce vomiting or administer activated charcoal if swallowed recently. May induce heart attack. Seek urgent medical attention.

Lomefloxacin

TRADE NAME

Okacyn.

DRUG CLASS

Antibiotic.

USES

Bacterial eye infections (conjunctivitis).

DOSAGE

 One drop every five minutes for 20 minutes, then one drop twice a day for seven to ten days.

FORMS

Eye drops.

PRECAUTIONS

Not to be used in pregnancy and breast feeding. May be used in children.

 Do not use if:

• wearing contact lenses.

• under other circumstances

SIDE EFFECTS

Common: Mild eye irritation.

INTERACTIONS

None significant.

PRESCRIPTION

Yes

PERMITTED IN SPORT

Yes

OVERDOSE

Unlikely to have serious effects if swallowed.

OTHER INFORMATION

Introduced in 1999 to treat more difficult infections.

LOOP DIURETICS

(Increase production of urine)

See Bumetanide, Frusemide

Loperamide

TRADE NAMES

Imodium, Loperagen, Norimode.

DRUG CLASS

Antidiarrhoeal.

USES

Diarrhoea.

DOSAGE

 Two capsules at once, then one capsule after each episode of diarrhoea to a maximum of eight capsules a day.

FORMS

Capsules, syrup.

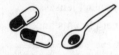

PRECAUTIONS

Should be used in pregnancy (B3) and breast feeding only on medical advice. Not approved for use in children under 12 years.

Do not use for more than 48 hours without medical advice.

 Do not take if:

- suffering from cirrhosis of liver or severe kidney disease.
- suffering from glaucoma or difficulty in passing urine.

SIDE EFFECTS

Common: Excess passage of wind, constipation, nausea, belly pain.

Unusual: Giddiness, rash, vomiting, metallic taste, decreased sexual drive, headache, weakness, tiredness, dry mouth, blurred vision.

INTERACTIONS

Other drugs:

- Interacts with Tranquillisers in some patients.
- May interact with Monoamine oxidase inhibitors (MAOI).

Other substances:

- Do not take Loperamide with alcohol.

PRESCRIPTION

Up to eight capsules no prescription. Prescription required for larger quantities.

PERMITTED IN SPORT

Yes

OVERDOSE

Constipation and vomiting only likely effects.

OTHER INFORMATION

Widely used and relatively safe medication. Acts to sedate bowel muscles without any effect on the brain.

Loratadine

See ANTIHISTAMINES, NON-SEDATING

Lorazepam

See ANXIOLYTICS

Losartan

See ANGIOTENSIN II RECEPTOR ANTAGONISTS

Loxapine

TRADE NAME

Loxapac.

DRUG CLASS

Antipsychotic.

USES

Serious psychiatric disorders, psychoses.

DOSAGE

 20mg. to 250mg. a day in divided doses, increasing dose very slowly from a low level.

FORMS

Capsules of 10mg. (yellow/green), 25mg. (dark green/light green) and 50mg. (dark green/blue).

PRECAUTIONS

Use with caution in pregnancy and breast feeding. Not recommended in children.

Use with caution in epilepsy, heart disease, glaucoma and difficulty in passing urine.

 Do not take if:

• suffering from depressed consciousness, severe depression.

SIDE EFFECTS

Common: Reduced alertness, drowsiness, dizziness, faintness, muscle weakness and twitching.

Unusual: Confusion, dry mouth, rapid heart rate, high or low blood pressure, heart beat alterations, skin reactions, nausea, vomiting, shortness of breath, headache.

Severe but rare (stop medication, consult doctor): Neuroleptic malignant syndrome (high fever, muscle rigidity, coma).

INTERACTIONS

Other drugs:

• Sedatives, Phenytoin, Lithium, Anticholinergics.

Other substances:

• Alcohol.

PRESCRIPTION

Yes

PERMITTED IN SPORT

Yes

OVERDOSE

May be serious. Seek urgent medical attention. Induce vomiting or give activated charcoal if taken recently.

L-Tryptophan

See Tryptophan

Lymecycline

TRADE NAME

Tetralysal.

DRUG CLASS

Tetracycline antibiotic.

USES

Bacterial infections of lungs, ears, skin, sinuses and throat.

DOSAGE

 One capsule, twice a day.

FORMS

Capsules (white).

PRECAUTIONS

Not to be used in pregnancy (D) or children under twelve years as Tetracyclines may cause permanent staining of teeth of foetus or child. Use with caution in breast feeding.

Use with caution in kidney and liver disease.

Never use expired medication as it may become toxic.

 Do not take if:

• suffering from severe kidney disease, systemic lupus erythematosus (SLE), Staphylococcal infection.

SIDE EFFECTS

Common: Loss of appetite, nausea, sore mouth, diarrhoea, difficulty in swallowing, inflamed colon.

Unusual: Vomiting, inflamed pancreas, rash, secondary fungal infection (thrush).

Severe but rare (stop medication, consult doctor): Severe belly pain, severe diarrhoea, tooth discolouration, significant skin rash.

INTERACTIONS

Other drugs:

• Anticoagulants, Penicillin, Antacids, Iron, Oral contraceptives.

Other substances:

• Milk may reduce absorption from gut.

PRESCRIPTION

Yes

PERMITTED IN SPORT

Yes

OVERDOSE

Exacerbation of side effects only likely effect.

See also Chlortetracycline, Demeclocycline, Doxycycline, Methacycline, Minocycline, Tetracycline.

LUBRICANTS, EYE

See EYE LUBRICANTS

Lysine aspirin

See Aspirin

MACROLIDES

See Azithromycin, Clarithromycin, Erythromycin, Roxithromycin

Magnesium

TRADE NAMES

Magnesium, in various forms, is found in numerous vitamin and mineral supplements.

DRUG CLASS

Mineral.

USES

Magnesium deficiency.

DOSAGE

 Recommended daily intake: Females - 270 mg a day; Males - 320 mg a day.

FORMS

Tablets, capsules.

PRECAUTIONS

Safe to use in pregnancy, breast feeding and children.

SIDE EFFECTS

Minimal

INTERACTIONS

None significant

PRESCRIPTION

No

PERMITTED IN SPORT

Yes

OVERDOSE

Stomach and bowel upsets likely.

Magnesium Salts

See ANTACIDS, ELECTROLYTES

Malathion

TRADE NAMES

Derbac-M, Prioderm, Suleo-M.

DRUG CLASS

Insecticide.

USES

Head and pubic lice, scabies.

DOSAGE

 Apply to affected area once and leave for twelve hours. Do not use more than once a week for three weeks.

FORMS

Lotion.

PRECAUTIONS

Safe to use in pregnancy, breast feeding and children.

Not for use in infants under six months.

Avoid eyes, nose, mouth, anus and vagina.

Use with care in asthma.

SIDE EFFECTS

Common: Minor skin irritation.

INTERACTIONS

None significant.

PRESCRIPTION

No

PERMITTED IN SPORT

Yes

OVERDOSE

Serious effects possible if swallowed. Seek urgent medical attention.

MAOI

(Monoamine oxidase inhibitors)

TRADE and GENERIC NAMES

Nardil (Phenelzine).

Parnate (Tranylcypromine).

DRUG CLASS

Antidepressant.

USES

Depression, phobias (fears).

DOSAGE

 One or two tablets, two or three times a day.

FORMS

Tablets

SIDE EFFECTS

Common: Dizziness, constipation, dry mouth, low blood pressure, drowsiness, weakness, fatigue, swelling of tissues (oedema), nausea.

Unusual: Blurred vision, sweating, glaucoma, inability to pass urine.

Severe but rare (stop medication, consult doctor): Agitation.

INTERACTIONS

Other drugs:

• Interacts with a very wide range of medications. Do not take any medication, including non-prescription and supermarket items without consulting a doctor.

Other substances:

• Reacts adversely with alcohol, particularly wine and beer.

• Reacts adversely with cheese, broad beans, pickled herrings, yeast extracts (eg: Vegemite, Marmite) and beef extracts.

PRECAUTIONS

Should be used in pregnancy only if medically essential. Not for use in breast feeding or children.

Use with caution in kidney disease.

Occasional blood tests to check liver function are recommended.

Regular blood pressure checks to detect low blood pressure are recommended.

Possible serious interactions with food and medication. Read literature supplied by doctor or pharmacist carefully and do not take drug unless you understand instructions completely.

 Do not take if:

• suffering from epilepsy, heart disease, stroke, high blood pressure, severe headaches or liver disease.

• over 60 years of age.

PRESCRIPTION

Yes

PERMITTED IN SPORT

Yes

OVERDOSE

Very serious. Faintness, chest pain, headache, low blood pressure, agitation, clammy skin, fits, coma and death may occur. Administer activated charcoal or induce vomiting if tablets taken recently and patient alert. Seek urgent medical assistance.

OTHER INFORMATION

A very useful medication in severely depressed patients, but its usefulness is limited by its side effects and severe potential to interact with other drugs and foods.

Maprotiline

TRADE NAME

Ludiomil.

DRUG CLASS

Tetracyclic antidepressant.

USES

Depression.

DOSAGE

 Usually 25mg. to 75mg. a day. Maximum 150mg.

FORMS

Tablets of 10mg. (cream), 25mg. (red), 50mg. (orange), 75mg. (brown).

PRECAUTIONS

Use with caution in pregnancy and breast feeding. Not recommended in children.

Use with caution in heart disease, low blood pressure, bipolar disorder, over active thyroid gland, schizophrenia, suicidal tendencies and chronic constipation.

Use with care if wearing contact lenses.

Regular blood tests to check liver and kidney function necessary.

Do not stop suddenly, but reduce dose slowly.

 Do not take if:

- suffering from mania, severe liver or kidney disease, epilepsy, glaucoma, difficulty in passing urine, recent heart attack, heart electrical problems, alcoholism.

SIDE EFFECTS

Common: Slow reactions.

Unusual: Skin rash, dry mouth.

Severe but rare (stop medication, consult doctor): Convulsions.

INTERACTIONS

Other drugs:

- MAOI, other anti-depressants, Antihypertensives, Antipsychotics, Anaesthetics, Benzodiazepines, Cimetidine, Coumarin, Anticholinergics, Quinidine, Methylphenidate, diabetic medications.

Other substances:

- Alcohol.

PRESCRIPTION

Yes

PERMITTED IN SPORT

Yes

OVERDOSE

Serious. Symptoms include drowsiness, high blood pressure, rapid heart rate, coma and death. Administer activated charcoal or induce vomiting if tablets taken recently and patient alert. Seek urgent medical assistance. Patients are often observed in intensive care units.

See also Mianserin.

Marijuana

OTHER NAMES:

Pot, cannabis, grass, hash, dope, charas, THC (tetrahydrocannabinol)

DRUG CLASS

Cannabinoid.

USES

No recognised medical uses.

Used experimentally for nausea, vomiting, pain relief, intestinal spasm, sedation, epilepsy, glaucoma, high blood pressure and muscle spasm.

Used illegally as a psychoactive drug to cause euphoria (artificial happiness).

FORMS

Used experimentally as a tablet or mixture. Used illegally in many forms including smoke and cooked in soup or biscuits.

PRECAUTIONS

Should never be used in pregnancy, breast feeding or children. Marijuana may damage the foetus.

 Do not use if:

- suffering from psychiatric disturbances, asthma, chronic lung disease.

- driving a car, operating machinery, swimming or undertaking any activity that requires concentration.

SIDE EFFECTS

Common: Unwanted flash backs, sexual disinhibition, drowsiness, palpitations, rapid pulse, dry mouth, sore and red eyes, dizziness, poor concentration, nausea, poor coordination.

Unusual: Hallucinations, vomiting, panic attacks, blackouts, perceptual changes, impotence, infertility.

Long term: Increased risk of lung cancer (greater risk than with tobacco smoking) and emphysema. Can bring on certain serious mental illnesses.

INTERACTIONS

Other drugs:

- Hypnotics, Sedatives, Heroin.

Other substances:

- Increases the effect of alcohol.

- May lead to desire for stronger psychoactive drugs.

PRESCRIPTION

Illegal

PERMITTED IN SPORT

No

OVERDOSE

May be serious if swallowed in large quantities. Exacerbation of side effects, convulsions and coma may lead rarely to death. Seek urgent medical attention.

OTHER INFORMATION

Illegal drug of dependence. Toleration may develop quickly (higher dose required to obtain same effect). Possession may lead to criminal charges. Derived from the Indian Hemp plant. Used at least once by about one third of population. Metabolised slowly by the liver, and stored in fat. Complete elimination of a single dose may take up to 6 weeks.

Measles vaccine

TRADE NAMES

MMR II, Priorix (with Mumps and Rubella vaccines).

DRUG CLASS

Vaccine.

USES

Prevention of measles (Morbilli).

DOSAGE

 One injection.

FORMS

Injection.

PRECAUTIONS

Should not be used in pregnancy (B2), but unintentional use during pregnancy unlikely to have any serious effect. May be used in breast feeding and children.

Use with caution if history of febrile convulsions or head injury.

 Do not take if:

- suffering from active infection or tuberculosis.
- taking drugs for cancer or leukaemia.
- recent blood transfusion or globulin injection.
- sensitivity to hen eggs.

SIDE EFFECTS

Common: Redness, soreness and lump at injection site; fever.

Unusual: Rash.

INTERACTIONS

Other drugs:

- Some other vaccines.

PRESCRIPTION

Yes

PERMITTED IN SPORT

Yes

OVERDOSE

An unintentional additional dose is unlikely to have any serious effect.

OTHER INFORMATION

Measles has been eradicated in many countries by immunisation. In most cases it is a mild disease, but occasionally it can cause brain damage and death. All children should be vaccinated at one and five years of age. An attenuated live virus vaccine.

Mebendazole

TRADE NAME

Vermox.

DRUG CLASS

Anthelmintic (kills worms).

USES

Threadworm, roundworm, whipworm and hookworm infestations of the intestine.

DOSAGE

 Threadworm: One tablet as a single dose, repeated in two to four weeks.
Other infestations: One tablet twice a day for three days.

FORMS

Tablets, suspension.

PRECAUTIONS

Not for use in pregnancy (B3) unless medically necessary. Breast feeding should be ceased before use. May be used in children over two years.

SIDE EFFECTS

Common: Minimal.

Unusual: Diarrhoea, vomiting, belly pains, drowsiness, itch, headache, dizziness.

Severe but rare (stop medication, consult doctor): Rash, itch.

INTERACTIONS

Other drugs:

• Cimetidine.

PRESCRIPTION

Yes

PERMITTED IN SPORT

Yes

OVERDOSE

Exacerbation of side effects plus possible liver damage. Seek medical attention.

OTHER INFORMATION

Widely, safely and effectively used.

Mebeverine

TRADE NAMES

Colofac.

Fybogel Mebeverine (with Ispaghula).

DRUG CLASS

Antispasmodic.

USES

Spasms of the intestine. Irritable bowel syndrome.

DOSAGE

 One tablet two or three times a day before food. One sachet twice a day in water 30 minutes before meals.

PRECAUTIONS

Safe use in pregnancy has not been established. Should be used with caution in breast feeding.

Do not take if:

• suffering from angina, heart disease, severe liver disease, severe kidney disease, lactose intolerance.

FORMS

Tablets of 200mg. and 135mg., liquid, granules.

SIDE EFFECTS

Common: Minimal

Unusual: Indigestion, heartburn, dizziness, sleeplessness, loss of appetite, constipation.

INTERACTIONS

None significant

PRESCRIPTION

Yes

PERMITTED IN SPORT

Yes

OVERDOSE

No significant problems reported.

OTHER INFORMATION

Very safe, long established and widely used medication.

Medroxyprogesterone acetate (MPA)

TRADE NAMES

Depo Provera, Fartulal, Provera.

Tridestra (with Oestradiols).

Premique (with Oestrogen).

DRUG CLASS

Sex hormone

USES

Endometriosis, cessation of menstrual periods, abnormal bleeding from uterus, breast cancer, cancer of lining of uterus, some types of kidney cancer.

In combination with oestrogen in the treatment of menopause.

Injection used for contraception.

DOSAGE

 Tablets: Half to three or more tablets a day, depending on diagnosis
Injection: One injection every three months for contraception.

FORMS

Tablets, injection.

PRECAUTIONS

Not to be used in pregnancy (D), breast feeding or children.

Use with caution with a history of blood clots in veins, eye disease, diabetes, depression, high blood pressure, heart failure.

 Do not take if:

- suffering from blood clot, stroke, liver disease, undiagnosed breast disease.

- recent abortion performed.

SIDE EFFECTS

Common: Abnormal vaginal bleeding, headache, reduced fertility.

Unusual: Sleeplessness, nervousness, dizziness, tremor, rash, sweating, nausea, breast tenderness, weight gain.

Severe but rare (stop medication, consult doctor): Blood clot, calf pain, chest pain, yellow skin (jaundice).

INTERACTIONS

Other drugs:

- Anticoagulants, Hypoglycaemics, Insulin.

PRESCRIPTION

Yes

PERMITTED IN SPORT

Injection: No
Tablets and capsules: Yes

OVERDOSE

Exacerbation of side effects likely.

OTHER INFORMATION

Injection used for contraception since late 1960s. Tablets very useful for controlling menstrual period problems, and delaying periods that may be due at an awkward time.

Mefenamic Acid

See NSAID

Mefloquine

TRADE NAME

Lariam.

DRUG CLASS

Antimalarial.

USES

Prevention and treatment of malaria.

DOSAGE

 Prevention: One tablet a week for one week before entering, and two weeks after leaving malarious country.
Treatment: Three tablets at once, then two tablets six hours later.

FORMS

Tablets (white) of 250mg.

PRECAUTIONS

May be used in pregnancy (B3) if medically necessary. Breast feeding should be ceased before use. Not designed for use in children under 14 years.

Use with caution in heart disease and epilepsy.

 Do not take if:

• suffering from liver or kidney disease, convulsions, psychiatric disturbances.

SIDE EFFECTS

Common: Dizziness, vomiting.

Unusual: Giddiness, faints, pins and needles, muscle pain, fever.

Severe but rare (stop medication, consult doctor): Psychiatric disturbances.

INTERACTIONS

Other drugs:

• Quinine, Chloroquine, Anticonvulsants, Beta blockers, Typhoid oral vaccine.

PRESCRIPTION

Yes

PERMITTED IN SPORT

Yes

OVERDOSE

Exacerbation of side effects likely. Administer activated charcoal or induce vomiting if medication taken recently. Seek medical assistance.

OTHER INFORMATION

Introduced in the late 1980s to combat the increasing incidence of chloroquine resistant malaria. Effective, easy to use and safe.

Megestrol

TRADE NAME

Megace.

USES

Breast cancer, endometriosis.

DOSAGE

 One tablet four times a day.

FORMS

Tablet (white) of 40mg. and 160mg.

PRECAUTIONS

Not to be used in pregnancy (D) unless mother's life at risk as damage to foetus possible. Breast feeding must be ceased before use. Not for use in children.

Women must use adequate contraception while taking Megestrol.

Regular blood tests to check blood sugar level recommended.

Use with caution in blood clots and diabetes.

SIDE EFFECTS

Common: Nausea, weight gain, fluid retention, abnormal vaginal bleeding.

Unusual: Vomiting, tumour pain, bone pain, hot flushes.

INTERACTIONS

None significant.

PRESCRIPTION

Yes

OVERDOSE

Not likely to be serious. Exacerbation of side effects probable. Seek medical attention.

Meloxicam

See NSAID

Melphalan

TRADE NAME

Alkeran.

USES

Cancer of breast and ovary, sarcoma, melanoma, multiple myeloma, polycythaemia vera.

DOSAGE

 Must be individualised by doctor for each patient depending on disease, severity, age and weight of patient.

FORMS

Tablets of 2mg. and 5mg. (white), injection.

PRECAUTIONS

Must not be used in pregnancy (D) unless medically essential for the life of the woman. Breast feeding must be ceased before use. Not for use in children unless essential for the life of the child.

Regular blood tests to check blood cells essential.

SIDE EFFECTS

Common: Damage to bone marrow and white blood cells, nausea, vomiting, diarrhoea, sore mouth.

Unusual: Hair loss, anaemia, lung damage.

Severe but rare (stop medication, consult doctor): Severe abnormal bleeding or bruising.

INTERACTIONS

Other drugs:

• Cyclosporin, Nalidixic acid, Mephalan.

PRESCRIPTION

Yes

PERMITTED IN SPORT

Yes

OVERDOSE

Very serious. Destruction of bone marrow possible, which may lead to fatal infections. Seek urgent medical attention.

Menopausal gonadotrophin, human

See Menotrophin

Menotrophin

(Menopausal gonadotrophin, human)

TRADE NAME

Menogon.

DRUG CLASS

Hormone.

USES

Male and female infertility. Stimulates production of sperm and eggs.

DOSAGE

 As determined by doctor for each patient.

FORMS

Injection.

PRECAUTIONS

Not to be used in pregnancy, breast feeding and children.

Only for use in specific types of female infertility caused by failure of egg release from the ovaries.

Regular blood tests to measure hormone levels essential.

Regular ultrasound scans to assess size of ovaries essential.

 Do not take if:

• suffering from tumour of ovary, testes or pituitary gland.

SIDE EFFECTS

Common: Ovarian pain, multiple pregnancy, injection site pain.

INTERACTIONS

Other drugs:

• Sex hormones.

PRESCRIPTION

Yes

PERMITTED IN SPORT

Yes

Menthol

TRADE NAMES

Balmosa, Salonpas (with Camphor, Methyl salicylate and other ingredients).

Frador (with Chlorbutol and other ingredients).

Radian B (with Aspirin, Camphor, Methy salicylate).

Also found in numerous other lotions, creams, ointments etc.

USES

Relief of muscular pain, relief of nasal congestion, disguising unwanted aromas.

DOSAGE

 Varies with form. As directed on packaging.

FORMS

Gel, Cream, Ointment, Powder, Inhaler, Mixture, Lotion, Spray.

PRECAUTIONS

Nil

SIDE EFFECTS

Minimal

INTERACTIONS

None significant

PRESCRIPTION

No

PERMITTED IN SPORT

Yes

OVERDOSE

Not a problem.

OTHER INFORMATION

Used primarily for its aroma and ability to dissolve other medications. Clinical effects probably minimal.

Meprobamate

TRADE NAME

Equagesic (with Etoheptazine, Aspirin).

DRUG CLASS

Anxiolytic.

USES

Anxiety, tension, stress, muscle pain, headaches.

DOSAGE

 One or two tablets two or three times a day.

FORMS

Tablet.

PRECAUTIONS

Should not be used in pregnancy (C) unless medically essential. Should be used with caution in breast feeding. Not for use in children under six years.

Should not be stopped suddenly, but dosage should be slowly reduced.

Use with caution in epilepsy, liver and kidney disease.

Lower doses required in elderly.

 Do not take if:

- suffering from porphyria.
- if operating machinery, driving a vehicle, or undertaking tasks that require concentration and alertness.

SIDE EFFECTS

Common: Dependency if used long term, drowsiness, dizziness, incoordination, nausea, palpitations.

Unusual: Slurred speech, headache, weakness, blurred vision, pins and needles sensation, over excitement, vomiting, diarrhoea, rapid heart rate, heart beat irregularities.

Severe but rare (stop medication, consult doctor): Dermatitis, unusual bleeding or bruising.

INTERACTIONS

Other drugs:

• Digoxin, Oestrogen, Oral contraceptive pill.

• Other Anxiolytics.

Other substances:

• Reacts adversely with alcohol.

PRESCRIPTION

Yes (restricted in combination with the narcotic Etoheptazine)

PERMITTED IN SPORT

No

OVERDOSE

Serious. Drowsiness, lethargy, incoordination, coma and death possible. Administer activated charcoal or induce vomiting if tablets taken recently and patient alert. Seek urgent medical attention.

OTHER INFORMATION

Dependency a problem with long term use. Should be used intermittently if possible.

Meptazinol

TRADE NAME

Meptid.

DRUG CLASS

Analgesic.

USES

Moderate pain.

DOSAGE

 One tablet every four hours.

FORMS

Tablets of 200mg. (orange), injection.

PRECAUTIONS

May be used with caution in pregnancy and breast feeding. Not recommended in children.

Use with caution in liver or kidney disease, severe lung disease.

For short term use only.

SIDE EFFECTS

Common: Dizziness, nausea.

INTERACTIONS

None significant.

PRESCRIPTION

Yes

PERMITTED IN SPORT

No

OVERDOSE

Moderately serious. May cause vomiting, drowsiness, convulsions, reduced breathing, coma and very rarely death. Seek urgent medical attention.

Mequitazine

See ANTIHISTAMINES, SEDATING

Mercaptopurine

TRADE NAME

Puri-Nethol.

USES

Leukaemia.

DOSAGE

 Must be individualised for each patient by doctor depending on response.

FORMS

Tablets (fawn) of 50mg.

PRECAUTIONS

Must not be used in pregnancy (D) unless the mother's life is at risk as the foetus may be damaged. Breast feeding must be ceased before use. May be used with caution in children.

Adequate contraception must be used by women taking Mercaptopurine.

Regular blood tests to check blood cells and liver function essential.

SIDE EFFECTS

Common: Liver and bone marrow damage.

Unusual: Loss of appetite, nausea, vomiting, mouth ulcers.

Severe but rare (stop medication, consult doctor): Yellow skin (jaundice), unusual bleeding or bruising.

INTERACTIONS

Other drugs:

• Allopurinol, Warfarin.

PRESCRIPTION

Yes

PERMITTED IN SPORT

Yes

OVERDOSE

May cause fatal damage to liver or bone marrow. Administer activated charcoal or induce vomiting if medication taken recently. Seek urgent medical assistance.

OTHER INFORMATION

Despite serious side effects, Mercaptopurine may save or prolong life in patients with leukaemia.

Meropenem

TRADE NAME

Meronem.

DRUG CLASS

Antibiotic.

USES

Serious bacterial infections.

DOSAGE

 500mg. to 1000mg. by drip into a vein every eight hours.

FORMS

Injection.

PRECAUTIONS

Use with caution in pregnancy (B2), breast feeding and infants.

Use with caution in Pseudomonas infections, liver and kidney disease.

SIDE EFFECTS

Common: Injection site redness and pain, diarrhoea.

Unusual: Liver damage, large bowel damage, growth of resistant bacteria, damage to white blood cells.

Severe but rare (stop medication, consult doctor): Unusual bleeding or bruising.

INTERACTIONS

Other drugs:

• Probenecid.

PRESCRIPTION

Yes

PERMITTED IN SPORT

Yes

OTHER INFORMATION

Used only in hospital.

Mesalazine

TRADE NAMES

Asacol, Pentasa, Salofalk.

DRUG CLASS

Bowel anti-inflammatory.

USES

Ulcerative colitis, Crohn's disease, other forms of bowel inflammation.

DOSAGE

 One or two tablets 30 minutes before meals three times a day with plenty of fluid.

FORMS

Tablet, enema, foam enema, suppositories, granules.

PRECAUTIONS

Should not be used near the end of pregnancy (C). Should not be used in breast feeding.

Not recommended in children.

 Use lower dose in elderly.

Use with caution in patients with liver disease and kidney disease.

 Do not take if:

• allergic to Aspirin or Salicylates.

SIDE EFFECTS

Common: Headache, nausea, rash, belly pains, diarrhoea.

Unusual: Kidney damage, pancreas inflammation.

Severe but rare (stop medication, consult doctor): Unexplained bleeding or bruising, severe belly pain (pancreatitis).

INTERACTIONS

Other drugs:

• Do not use with Lactulose or Anticoagulants.

• Interacts with Sulfonylureas, Methotrexate, and Probenecid

PRESCRIPTION

Yes

PERMITTED IN SPORT

Yes

OTHER INFORMATION

Very effective medication for a number of uncommon diseases.

Mesterolone

TRADE NAME
Pro-viron.

DRUG CLASS
Sex hormone.

USES
Male infertility, male impotence.

DOSAGE
 One tablet, one to three times a day.

FORMS
Tablets of 25mg. (white).

PRECAUTIONS
Not to be used in women or children.

Use with caution in prostate disease.

 Do not take if:
- suffering from prostate cancer or liver tumour.

SIDE EFFECTS
Common: Prolonged penile erection.

INTERACTIONS
None significant.

PRESCRIPTION
Yes

PERMITTED IN SPORT
No

OVERDOSE
Painful, damaging, prolonged penile erection possible. Induce vomiting or administer activated charcoal if taken recently. Seek medical attention.

Mestranol
See ORAL CONTRACEPTIVES

Metformin

TRADE NAME
Glucophage.

DRUG CLASS
Hypoglycaemic.

USES
Diabetes not requiring Insulin injections.

DOSAGE
 One or two tablets, two or three times a day before meals. Do not vary from prescribed dose without reference to a doctor.

FORMS
Tablets of 500mg. (white).

PRECAUTIONS
Not to be used in pregnancy (C), breast feeding or children.

Annual blood tests to check for pernicious anaemia recommended.

Illness, changes in diet, exercise and stress may change dosage requirements.

Lower doses required in elderly and debilitated patients.

Strict control of carbohydrates and sugars in diet essential.

 Do not take if:
- suffering from severe heart disease, blood clot in lungs, pancreatitis, alcoholism, severe liver or kidney disease.
- using Insulin.

SIDE EFFECTS

Common: Uncommon.

Unusual: Nausea, vomiting, belly discomfort, weakness.

Severe but rare (stop medication, consult doctor): Low blood sugar (see Overdose below), yellow skin (jaundice), unusual bleeding or bruising, rash.

INTERACTIONS

Other drugs:

• Cimetidine, other Hypoglycaemics, Beta blockers, Fenclofenac, Anticoagulants, Thiazides, Thyroxine.

Other substances:

• Reacts adversely with alcohol.

PRESCRIPTION

Yes

PERMITTED IN SPORT

Yes

OVERDOSE

Serious. Symptoms of low blood sugar (hypoglycaemia) may include tiredness, confusion, chills, palpitations, sweating, vomiting, dizziness, hunger, blurred vision and fainting. Significant overdosage can lead to coma and death. Give sugary drinks or sweets if conscious. Seek emergency medical assistance.

OTHER INFORMATION

Used mainly in elderly patients who develop maturity onset diabetes that is not severe enough to require insulin injections.

Methadone

TRADE NAME

Physeptone.

DRUG CLASS

Narcotic, Analgesic.

USES

Severe pain, narcotic addiction.

DOSAGE

 One or two tablets every six to eight hours. 2mLs. to 10mLs. of syrup a day.

FORMS

Tablets (white) of 5mg., syrup, injection.

PRECAUTIONS

Not to be used in the last stages of pregnancy (C) as Methadone may cause the newborn infant to have difficulty in breathing. Use with caution in breast feeding and children.

Not designed for prolonged use.

 Do not take if:

• suffering from severe lung disease.

• operating machinery or driving a vehicle.

SIDE EFFECTS

Common: Dizziness, drowsiness, vomiting, mood changes.

Unusual: Difficulty in breathing

INTERACTIONS

Other drugs:

• MAOI

Other substances:

• Alcohol should not be used with Methadone.

PRESCRIPTION

Yes (very restricted)

PERMITTED IN SPORT

No

OVERDOSE

Serious. Symptoms may not appear for some hours after medication taken, and may include drowsiness, difficulty in breathing and coma. Administer activated charcoal or induce vomiting if medication taken recently and patient alert. Seek urgent medical attention. Antidote available.

OTHER INFORMATION

Used in a slowly reducing dose to ease Heroin addicts off their addiction. May itself be addictive if used inappropriately.

Methionine

TRADE NAMES

Methionine.

Paradote (with Paracetamol).

DRUG CLASS

Antidote.

USES

Counteracts overdosage with Paracetamol, liver damage.

Paradote combines Paracetamol and Methionine to prevent liver damage in case of overdose.

DOSAGE

 Paracetamol: Five tablets at once, repeated at four hour intervals for a total of four doses.
Paradote: Two every four hours to a maximum of eight a day.

FORMS

Tablets.

PRECAUTIONS

May be used in pregnancy, breast feeding and children.

Administer activated charcoal or induce vomiting if medication or poison taken recently.

Treatment must be undertaken immediately after vomiting has been successfully induced, before any signs of poisoning are evident.

Medication does not replace hospital care and other treatments.

Hospitals usually measure levels of Paracetamol before starting specific treatment.

SIDE EFFECTS

Minimal

INTERACTIONS

None significant

PRESCRIPTION

No

PERMITTED IN SPORT

Yes

OTHER INFORMATION

Overdosage with paracetamol may cause fatal liver damage. Methionine may prevent this damage if given within ten hours of the overdose being taken.

Methocarbamol

TRADE NAME

Robaxin.

USES

Muscle spasms.

DOSAGE

 Two tablets, four times a day.

FORMS

Tablets (white) of 750mg.

PRECAUTIONS

Use with caution in pregnancy and breast feeding. Not recommended in children.

Use with caution in kidney and liver disease.

 Do not take if:

- suffering from brain damage, epilepsy, myasthenia gravis or in a coma.

SIDE EFFECTS

Common: Drowsiness.

Unusual: Allergic reaction.

INTERACTIONS

Other drugs:

- Sedatives, Stimulants, Anticholinergics.

Other substances:

- Alcohol.

PRESCRIPTION

Yes

PERMITTED IN SPORT

Yes

Methotrexate

TRADE NAME

Maxtrex.

USES

Numerous types of cancer including cancer of breast and uterus, leukaemia, severe psoriasis, severe rheumatoid arthritis.

DOSAGE

 Must be individualised for each patient by doctor depending on disease, severity and weight of patient.

FORMS

Tablets of 2.5 and 10mg. (yellow).

PRECAUTIONS

Must not be used in pregnancy (D) unless mother's life is at risk, as the foetus may be damaged. Breast feeding must be ceased before use. May be used in children if medically essential.

Regular blood tests to check blood cells and liver function are essential.

Adequate contraception must be used by women while Methotrexate is being taken.

Use with caution in infection, peptic ulcer and ulcerative colitis.

 Do not take if:

- suffering from severe liver or kidney disease, significant infection.

SIDE EFFECTS

Common: Mouth ulcers, nausea, belly pains, diarrhoea.

Unusual: Tiredness, chills, dizziness, reduced resistance to infection, rash, infertility.

Severe but rare (stop medication, consult doctor): Yellow skin (jaundice), unusual bleeding or bruising.

INTERACTIONS

Other drugs:

• NSAID, Aspirin, Sulfonamides, Phenytoin, Tetracyclines, Chloramphenicol, Folic acid, Probenecid, Co-trimoxazole.

PRESCRIPTION

Yes

PERMITTED IN SPORT

Yes

OVERDOSE

Serious. Administer activated charcoal or induce vomiting if medication taken recently. Seek urgent medical assistance. Antidote available (see Calcium folinate).

OTHER INFORMATION

Despite risk of significant side effects, methotrexate may save the life, or improve the quality of life, of many patients.

Methotrimeprazine

See PHENOTHIAZINES

Methylcellulose

TRADE NAME

Celevac.

DRUG CLASS

Fibre.

USES

Constipation, fibre supplementation, appetite suppression, diverticulitis.

DOSAGE

Two to five tablets three times a day with water before meals.

FORMS

Tablets (pink).

PRECAUTIONS

Safe in pregnancy and breast feeding.

Ensure adequate fluid intake.

Not recommended in children.

 Do not take if:
• suffering from bowel blockage.

SIDE EFFECTS

Common: Loose bulky motions.

INTERACTIONS

Other drugs:

• May affect the absorption of a wide range of medications.

PRESCRIPTION

No

PERMITTED IN SPORT

Yes

OVERDOSE

No adverse effects likely.

OTHER INFORMATION

Totally inactive in body, and merely acts to add bulk to faeces.

Methyldopa

TRADE NAME

Aldomet.

DRUG CLASS

Antihypertensive.

USES

High blood pressure.

DOSAGE

 One or two tablets two or three times a day to a maximum of 3000mg. a day.

FORMS

Tablets of 125mg., 250mg. and 500mg. (yellow).

PRECAUTIONS

Safe in pregnancy (A), breast feeding and children.

Should be used with caution in patients with a history of depression.

 Do not take if:

- suffering from liver disease.

SIDE EFFECTS

Common: Fever, sedation, headache.

Unusual: Aggravation of angina, swelling of tissues.

Severe but rare (stop medication, consult doctor): Unusual bleeding, severe tiredness.

INTERACTIONS

Other drugs:

- Interacts with some Anaesthetics, Lithium and other medications that lower blood pressure.

Other substances:

- Smoking aggravates high blood pressure.

PRESCRIPTION

Yes

PERMITTED IN SPORT

Yes

OVERDOSE

Causes low blood pressure, sedation, weakness, dizziness, slow heart rate, diarrhoea, nausea and vomiting. Rarely fatal. If taken recently, administer activated charcoal or induce vomiting. If taken more than two hours earlier, give patient additional fluids. Seek medical assistance.

OTHER INFORMATION

An oldie but a goodie. One of the first effective treatments for high blood pressure.

Methylphenidate

TRADE NAMES

Equasym, Ritalin.

DRUG CLASS

Stimulant.

USES

Attention deficit hyperactivity disorder, narcolepsy.

DOSAGE

 Individualised. Start with low dose and gradually increase as determined by doctor until adequate response obtained.

FORMS

Tablets of 5, 10 and 20mg.

PRECAUTIONS

Not for use in pregnancy unless medically essential. Not for use in breast feeding. Not for use in children under 6 years.

Use with caution in high blood pressure and epilepsy.

If possible, should not be used for prolonged periods of time.

 Do not take if:

- suffering from depression, psychoses, anxiety, agitation, twitches, Tourette syndrome, glaucoma, overactive thyroid gland, irregular heart beat or angina.

SIDE EFFECTS

Common: Sleeplessness, irritability, drowsiness, loss of appetite, belly pains, nausea.

Unusual: Vomiting, irregular heart beat, rash, growth retardation, blurred vision, psychiatric disturbances, angina, fever, hair loss.

INTERACTIONS

Other drugs:

- Tricyclic antidepressants, MAOI, Anticoagulants, Anticonvulsants, Phenylbutazone, Guanethidine, medications for treatment of high blood pressure.

PRESCRIPTION

Yes (restricted)

PERMITTED IN SPORT

No

OVERDOSE

Very serious. May cause vomiting, agitation, tremors, twitching, confusion, hallucinations, convulsions, coma and death. Administer activated charcoal or induce vomiting if tablets taken recently. Seek urgent medical attention.

OTHER INFORMATION

May cause dependence if used inappropriately. May make a dramatic improvement in the quality of life for some hyperactive children and their parents.

Methylphenobarbitone

See BARBITURATES

Methylprednisolone

TRADE NAMES

Depo-Medrone, Medrone, Solu-Medrone.

Depo-Medrone with Lidocaine (with Lidocaine).

DRUG CLASS

Corticosteroid.

USES

Severe asthma, rheumatoid and other forms of severe arthritis, auto-immune diseases (eg: Sjøgren's Syndrome), severe allergy reactions, and other severe and chronic inflammatory diseases.

DOSAGE

 Tablets: Strictly as directed by doctor.

FORMS

Tablets, injection.

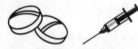

PRECAUTIONS

Should be used in pregnancy (C), breast feeding and children only on specific medical advice.

Use with caution if under stress, and in patients with under active thyroid gland, liver disease, diverticulitis, high blood pressure, myasthenia gravis or kidney disease.

Use for shortest period of time possible.

Medication should not be ceased abruptly, but dosage should be slowly reduced.

 Do not take if:

- suffering from any form of infection, peptic ulcer, or osteoporosis.

- having a vaccination

SIDE EFFECTS

Most significant side effects occur only with prolonged use.

Common: Bloating, weight gain, rashes and intestinal disturbances.

Unusual: Biochemical disturbances of blood, muscle weakness, bone weakness, impaired wound healing, skin thinning, tendon weakness, peptic ulcers, gullet ulcers, bruising, increased sweating, loss of fat under skin, premature ageing, excess facial hair growth in women, pigmentation of skin and nails, acne, convulsions, headaches, dizziness, growth suppression in children, aggravation of diabetes, worsening of infections, cataracts, aggravation of glaucoma, blood clots in veins and sleeplessness.

Severe but rare (stop medication, consult doctor): Any significant side effect should be reported to a doctor immediately.

INTERACTIONS

Other drugs:

- Tablets - Oral contraceptives, Barbiturates, Phenytoin, Rifampicin.

PRESCRIPTION

Yes

PERMITTED IN SPORT

No

OVERDOSE

Medical treatment is required. Serious effects and death rare.

OTHER INFORMATION

Extremely effective and useful medication if used correctly. Tablets must be used with extreme care under strict medical supervision. Lowest dose and shortest possible course should be used. Not addictive.

Methyl salicylate

See SALICYLATES

Methysergide

TRADE NAME

Deseril.

DRUG CLASS

Antimigraine.

USES

Prevention of migraine and cluster headaches.

DOSAGE

 One to four tablets, two or three times a day with food.

FORMS

Tablets of 1mg. (white).

PRECAUTIONS

Should not be used in pregnancy (C), breast feeding or children.

Sudden cessation may cause rebound migraine - reduce dosage slowly when ceasing.

 ### Do not take if:

- suffering from poor circulation to arms and legs, poor circulation to heart, hardening of arteries, vein inflammation, severe infections, high blood pressure, collagen diseases, severe kidney or liver disease, urinary tract disease.

- do not take constantly for more than six months.

SIDE EFFECTS

Common: Nausea, vomiting.

Unusual: Sleeplessness, dizziness, rash, tissue swelling, chest pain, belly pain, pins and needles sensation.

Severe but rare (stop medication, consult doctor): Difficulty in producing urine, backache, pain on passing urine, poor blood supply to legs.

INTERACTIONS

None significant

PRESCRIPTION

Yes

PERMITTED IN SPORT

Yes

OVERDOSE

Administer activated charcoal or induce vomiting if tablets taken recently. Symptoms include vomiting, diarrhoea, thirst, cold skin, itch, rapid weak pulse, tingling, confusion. seek medical assistance.

OTHER INFORMATION

One of several medications that may be used to prevent migraines. Trial and error between these medications if often necessary to find the best one. Because of very rare but serious complications with long term use (retroperitoneal fibrosis - scar tissue forming at back of belly around kidneys), methysergide is often towards the bottom of the list of medications considered.

Metipranolol

See BETA-BLOCKERS

Metoclopramide

TRADE NAMES

Gastrobid Continus, Maxolon.

Migramax (with Aspirin).

Paramax (with Paracetamol).

DRUG CLASS

Antiemetic.

USES

Nausea, vomiting, during investigative procedures.

DOSAGE

One tablet three times a day.

FORMS

Tablets, syrup, injection.

PRECAUTIONS

Safe in pregnancy (A), breast feeding and children.

Use with caution in epilepsy, liver and kidney disease.

Lower doses required in elderly.

Do not persist with medication if vomiting continues, but seek further medical assessment.

 Do not take if:

- suffering from phaeochromocytoma

SIDE EFFECTS

Common: Drowsiness, restlessness, tiredness.

Unusual: Sleeplessness, headache, dizziness, diarrhoea.

Severe but rare (stop medication, consult doctor): Incoordination, twitching, muscle spasms.

INTERACTIONS

Other drugs:

- Narcotics, Sedatives, Anticholinergics, Paracetamol, Tetracycline, L-Dopa, Digoxin.

Other substances:

- Reacts adversely with alcohol.

PRESCRIPTION

Yes

PERMITTED IN SPORT

Yes

OVERDOSE

Abnormal muscle twitching, muscle spasms and incoordination may occur. Seek medical advice.

OTHER INFORMATION

Very widely used, safe and effective medication. Does not cause addiction or dependence.

Metolazone

See THIAZIDE DIURETICS

Metoprolol

See BETA-BLOCKERS

Metronidazole

TRADE NAMES

Anabact, Elyzol, Flagyl, Metrogel, Metrotop, Neutratop, Noritate, Rozex, Zidoval, Zyomet.

Flagyl Compak (with Nystatin).

DRUG CLASS

Antibiotic.

USES

Bacterial infections of gut and vagina, particularly Giardiasis of gut and Trichomonal infections of vagina.

Acne rosacea.

DOSAGE

Tablets: One or two tablets three times a day.
Gel and ointment: Apply thinly twice daily after washing.

FORMS

Tablets, suppository, ointment, gel, suspension, infusion.

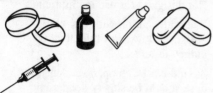

PRECAUTIONS

Use with caution in pregnancy (B2) and breast feeding. Safe to use in children.

Avoid eyes, nostrils, mouth, vagina and anus with skin preparations.

Not designed for long term use.

Use with caution in kidney and liver disease.

 Do not take if:
- suffering from brain disease, blood cell abnormalities.

SIDE EFFECTS

Common: Tablets - Bad taste, nausea, diarrhoea, headache. Skin preparations - Redness, dryness, burning, irritation.

Unusual: Vomiting, loss of appetite, belly discomfort.

INTERACTIONS

Other drugs:

- Warfarin, Cyclophosphamide.

Other substances:

- Reacts adversely with alcohol.

PRESCRIPTION

Yes

PERMITTED IN SPORT

Yes

OVERDOSE

With tablet overdosage disorientation and vomiting only likely effects.

OTHER INFORMATION

Widely used. Very safe and effective. Often used in combination with other antibiotics for infections of female pelvic organs. Most effective treatment for the unusual skin condition of acne rosacea.

Metyrapone

TRADE NAME

Metopirone.

USES

Diagnosis of adrenal gland dysfunction, hyperaldosteronism, Cushing syndrome.

DOSAGE

 Strictly as directed and determined by doctor.

FORMS

Capsules (cream) of 250mg.

PRECAUTIONS

Use with care (B2) in pregnancy, breast feeding and children.

Use with care in liver, pituitary gland and thyroid disease.

 Do not take if:
- suffering from adrenocortical insufficiency.

SIDE EFFECTS

Common: Nausea, diarrhoea, dizziness, sedation, headache.

Unusual: Low blood pressure, belly pain, excess hair growth.

INTERACTIONS

Other drugs:

• May interact with numerous medications.

PRESCRIPTION

Yes

PERMITTED IN SPORT

Yes

OVERDOSE

Very serious damage to numerous glands may occur.

OTHER INFORMATION

Normally only used in hospitals as a diagnostic tool.

Mexilitine

TRADE NAME

Mexitil.

DRUG CLASS

Antiarrhythmic.

USES

Serious heart beat irregularities in the heart ventricles.

DOSAGE

 Complex and variable from one patient to another. Follow doctors instructions carefully.

FORMS

Capsules of 50mg. (red/purple), 200mg. (red) and 360mg. (red/turquoise), injection.

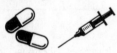

PRECAUTIONS

Should be used with caution in pregnancy (B1) and breast feeding. Not designed for use in children.

Use with caution with low blood pressure, slow heart rate, liver or kidney failure.

Should not be stopped suddenly, but dose should be slowly decreased over several days.

 Do not take if:

• suffering from recent heart attack

• you are hypersensitive to local anaesthetics.

SIDE EFFECTS

Common: Usually only on commencement of medication due to blood concentrations being too high. Minimal on long term use.

Unusual: Nausea, vomiting, hiccups, bad tastes, drowsiness, confusion, dizziness, double vision, tremor, blurred vision, palpitations.

INTERACTIONS

Other drugs:

• Other medications that treat heart rhythm irregularities.

• Theophylline, Narcotics

Other substances:

• Reacts with alcohol and caffeine.

PRESCRIPTION

Yes

PERMITTED IN SPORT

Yes

OVERDOSE

Very serious. Administer activated charcoal or induce vomiting if tablets taken recently. Seek urgent medical assistance. Symptoms may include vomiting, drowsiness, confusion, slow heart rate, heart attack and death.

Miconazole

See IMIDAZOLES

Midazolam

TRADE NAME

Hypnovel.

DRUG CLASS

Sedative/Hypnotic, Benzodiazepine.

USES

Short acting sedation for procedures (eg: Gastroscopy), continuous sedation of acutely ill patients, sedation prior to anaesthesia.

DOSAGE

 As given by doctor.

FORMS

Injection.

PRECAUTIONS

Should be used with caution in pregnancy (C), but not at all if delivery of infant imminent as it may decrease desire to breathe in newborn infant. Should be used with caution in breast feeding and children.

SIDE EFFECTS

Common: Reduces lung and heart activity.

Rare: Hiccups, nausea, vomiting, memory loss of events immediately before and after injection.

INTERACTIONS

Other drugs:

• Cimetidine, Erythromycin, other sedatives.

Other substances:

• Reacts adversely with alcohol.

PRESCRIPTION

Yes

OTHER INFORMATION

Excellent medication to allow many non-painful but uncomfortable and frightening procedures to be performed with minimal risk.

Mifepristone (RU486)

TRADE NAME

Mifegyne.

USES

Termination of pregnancy up to 49 days after last menstrual period.

DOSAGE

 Three tablets taken once. Often followed two days later by a prostaglandin.

FORMS

Tablets of 200mg. (yellow).

PRECAUTIONS

Not to be used in pregnancy (X) unless termination of pregnancy desired.

Not to be used in breast feeding and children.

Follow up visit at 12 to 14 days after taking drug essential to confirm complete abortion.

 Do not take if:

- suffering from bleeding disorders

SIDE EFFECTS

Common: Nausea, vomiting, diarrhoea, chills, fever. Abdominal pain, cramping and vaginal bleeding, from the abortion process.

Unusual: Excessive vaginal bleeding, incomplete abortion,ongoing pregnancy which requires an abortion.

Severe but rare (stop medication, consult doctor): Torrential vaginal bleeding.

INTERACTIONS

None significant.

PRESCRIPTION

Yes

PERMITTED IN SPORT

Yes

OTHER INFORMATION

Introduced in France in 1988, this medication has been surrounded by controversy because of its action, but despite this, it is a safe and effective way of terminating a pregnancy. Usually used in conjunction with misoprostol, which causes contraction of the uterus.

MINERALS

See **Calcium, Fluoride, Iodine, Iron, Magnesium, Phosphorus, Potassium, Selenomethionine(Selenium), Zinc sulphate.**

Minocycline

TRADE NAMES

Aknemin, Minocin.

DRUG CLASS

Tetracycline antibiotic

USES

Infections caused by susceptible bacteria.

DOSAGE

 Treatment: One tablet or capsule a day.
Prevention: One tablet a day.

FORMS

Capsules, tablets, injection.

PRECAUTIONS

Not to be used in pregnancy (D) or children under twelve as Minocycline may cause permanent staining of teeth of foetus or child. Use with caution in breast feeding.

Use with caution in kidney disease.

 Do not take if:

- suffering from severe kidney disease, systemic lupus erythematosus (SLE), Staphylococcal infection.

SIDE EFFECTS

Common: Loss of appetite, nausea, sore mouth, diarrhoea, difficulty in swallowing, inflamed colon.

Unusual: Vomiting, inflamed pancreas, rash, secondary fungal infection (thrush).

Severe but rare (stop medication, consult doctor): Severe belly pain, severe diarrhoea, tooth discolouration.

INTERACTIONS

Other drugs:

• Anticoagulants, Penicillin, Antacids, Iron, Oral contraceptives.

Other substances:

• Milk may reduce absorption from gut.

PRESCRIPTION

Yes

PERMITTED IN SPORT

Yes

OVERDOSE

Exacerbation of side effects only likely effect.

OTHER INFORMATION

Used for a wide range of infections in general practice, including prevention of acne. Does not cause dependence or addiction.

See also Demeclocycline, Doxycycline, Methacycline, Tetracycline.

Minoxidil

TRADE NAMES

Loniten, Ralogaine.

DRUG CLASS

Antihypertensive.

USES

Severe high blood pressure, alopecia (hair loss), baldness.

DOSAGE

 Tablets: 5mg to 50mg a day, usually as a single dose. Solution: Apply twice a day to scalp.

FORMS

Tablets of 2.5, 5 and 10mg., scalp solution.

PRECAUTIONS

Use in pregnancy (C) and breast feeding only if medically necessary.

Should not be used for mild high blood pressure.

Fluid intake must be controlled carefully.

May be necessary to check heart with regular cardiographs (ECG).

 Do not take if:

• suffering from recent heart attack.

SIDE EFFECTS

Common: Excess hair growth on face and scalp, darkening and thickening of fine body hair, weight gain, fluid retention, increased heart rate.

Unusual: Low blood pressure, breast tenderness, rash, nausea, diarrhoea.

INTERACTIONS

None significant.

PRESCRIPTION

Yes

PERMITTED IN SPORT

Yes

OVERDOSE

Low blood pressure only likely effect.

OTHER INFORMATION

Ability to reverse male baldness found by accident in patients taking drug for blood pressure. Success in baldness varies greatly between patients, and long term use is required. Used for only most severe forms of high blood pressure.

MIOTICS

(Medications that contract the pupil in the eye)

See Acetylcholine chloride, Carbachol

Mirtazapine

TRADE NAME

Zispin.

DRUG CLASS

Antidepressant.

USES

Depression.

DOSAGE

 Half to two tablets at night.

FORMS

Tablets of 30mg. (reddish brown).

PRECAUTIONS

Not to be used in pregnancy, breast feeding and children.

Do not stop suddenly, but reduce dose slowly.

Use with caution in kidney and liver disease, epilepsy, low blood pressure, glaucoma, diabetes, prostate gland enlargement, angina and other heart conditions.

SIDE EFFECTS

Common: Weight gain, drowsiness, tissue swelling.

Unusual: Liver damage, low blood pressure, rashes, mania.

Severe but rare (stop medication, consult doctor): Jaundice (yellow skin).

INTERACTIONS

Other drugs:

• MAOI, Sedatives.

Other substances:

• Alcohol.

PRESCRIPTION

Yes

PERMITTED IN SPORT

Yes

Misoprostol

TRADE NAMES

Cytotec.

Arthrotec (with Diclofenac).

Condrotec, Napratec (with Naproxen).

DRUG CLASS

Antiulcerant, Prostaglandin analogue.

USES

Treatment of ulcers of the stomach and duodenum (upper small intestine). Prevention of ulcers in patients who are likely to develop them.

DOSAGE

 Up to 800ug a day divided into two to four doses.

FORMS

Tablets.

PRECAUTIONS

Extremely dangerous in pregnancy (X). Pregnancy must be prevented in any woman using this medication by adequate contraception. May cause miscarriage and serious damage to the foetus. Not recommended in children and breast feeding.

 Do not take if:
- Epileptic, likely to suffer from low blood pressure or asthma.

SIDE EFFECTS

Common: Diarrhoea, belly pains.

Unusual: Belly cramps, menstrual disorders, nausea, headache, passing wind, constipation.

INTERACTIONS

None significant.

PRESCRIPTION

Yes

PERMITTED IN SPORT

Yes

OVERDOSE

The effects of an overdose are unknown.

OTHER INFORMATION

A very potent and effective form of treatment for ulcers that have failed to heal by other methods. Widely used in severely injured or ill patients to prevent stomach ulcers. Must never be used in pregnancy as it causes contraction of the uterus.

Mizolastine

See ANTIHISTAMINES, SEDATING

Moclobemide

TRADE NAME

Manerix.

DRUG CLASS

Antidepressant, RIMA (Reversible inhibitor of monoamine oxidase type A).

USES

Depression.

DOSAGE

 50 to 600mg., once or twice a day after a meal.

PRECAUTIONS

Should be used in pregnancy (B3) and breast feeding only with great caution. Not for use in children.

Use with caution in excited and agitated patients, schizophrenia, high blood pressure, thyroid disease, liver and kidney disease.

Lower doses should be used in elderly.

 Do not take if:
- suffering from schizophrenia and similar psychiatric conditions.

FORMS

Tablets of 150mg. (yellow) and 300mg. (white).

SIDE EFFECTS

Common: Usually minimal. Dizziness, nausea, sleeplessness, headache.

Unusual: Dry mouth, constipation, diarrhoea, anxiety, restlessness.

INTERACTIONS

Other drugs:

• Metoprolol, Cimetidine, Pethidine.

PRESCRIPTION

Yes

PERMITTED IN SPORT

Yes

OVERDOSE

Drowsiness, low blood pressure and rapid heart rate may occur. Not serious. Seek medical advice.

OTHER INFORMATION

Released in the early 1990s it has improved the treatment of depression because of its safety and lack of side effects. May take up to two weeks for patient to notice any improvement in depression.

Modafinil

TRADE NAME

Provigil.

USES

Narcolepsy. Promotes awakening.

DOSAGE

 Two to four tablets, in morning and again at noon if necessary.

FORMS

Tablets of 100mg. (white).

PRECAUTIONS

Not to be used in pregnancy, breast feeding and children.

Ensure adequate contraception used in women.

Use with caution in liver or kidney disease and anxiety disorders.

Blood pressure must be checked regularly.

 Do not take if:

• suffering from high blood pressure, irregular heart beat or other heart disease.

• under other circumstances

SIDE EFFECTS

Common: Excitement, nervousness, aggression, inability to sleep.

Unusual: Personality disorders, loss of appetite, headache, excessive happiness, belly pains, dry mouth, palpitations, high blood pressure, rapid heart rate, tremor, itchy skin.

Severe but rare (stop medication, consult doctor): Facial muscle spasms.

INTERACTIONS

Other drugs:

• Anticonvulsants, oral contraceptives.

PRESCRIPTION

Yes

PERMITTED IN SPORT

No

OVERDOSE

Serious. Seek urgent medical attention. Heart damage likely.

OTHER INFORMATION

Use must be carefully monitored. Addictive.

Moexipril

See ACE INHIBITORS

Mometasone

TRADE NAMES

Elocon, Nasonex.

DRUG CLASS

Corticosteroid.

USES

Severe inflammation of skin (eczema, dermatitis etc.).

Hay fever, allergic rhinitis.

DOSAGE

 Skin: Apply once a day.
Nose: Two sprays in each nostril once a day.

PRECAUTIONS

Should be used with caution in pregnancy (B3), breast feeding and children.

Avoid eyes.

Use for shortest period of time possible.

 Do not use if:

- suffering from any form of skin infection.

FORMS

Cream, ointment, nose spray.

SIDE EFFECTS

Common: Skin - Minimal. Nose spray - Headache, nose bleed, nose irritation.

Unusual: Skin - Thinning of skin, itching, burning, stinging, scarring of skin. Nose - Nasal ulcers.

INTERACTIONS

None significant

PRESCRIPTION

Yes

PERMITTED IN SPORT

Yes

OTHER INFORMATION

Extremely effective and useful skin medication, that is just as effective as other steroid creams that are used two or three times a day. Lowest dose and shortest possible course should be used. Not addictive.

Montelukast

TRADE NAME

Singulair.

USES

Prevention and treatment of chronic asthma.

DOSAGE

 10mg. at bedtime.

FORMS

Tablets of 5mg. (pink) and 10mg. (beige).

PRECAUTIONS

May be used with care in pregnancy (B1), breast feeding and children.

Not for treatment of acute asthma.

Two 5mg. tablets are not equivalent to one 10mg. tablet.

SIDE EFFECTS

Common: Belly pain, headache.

Unusual: Nausea, diarrhoea, rash, insomnia, dizziness, joint and muscle pains, tiredness..

INTERACTIONS

Other drugs:

• Aspirin, NSAID, Phenobarbitone, Phenytoin, Rifampicin.

PRESCRIPTION

Yes

PERMITTED IN SPORT

Yes

OVERDOSE

Exacerbation of side effects likely.

OTHER INFORMATION

Released 1999 for the management of more difficult cases of persistent asthma.

MORNING AFTER PILL

TRADE and GENERIC NAMES

Schering PC4 (Ethinyloestradiol, Levonorgestrel).

Levonelle-2 (Levonorgestrel).

DRUG CLASS

Sex hormone.

USES

Contraception after, but within 72 hours of, unprotected sexual intercourse.

DOSAGE

 Schering PC4: Two tablets immediately, and two more tablets twelve hours later.
Levonelle-2: One tablet immediately, and a second tablet twelve hours later. Often combined with medication to reduce risk of vomiting.

FORMS

Tablets.

PRECAUTIONS

Not for use more than 72 hours after sexual intercourse. Should be kept out of reach of children, and are obviously not for use in children, although accidental usage by children is unlikely to be serious.

Use with caution in heart disease, history of blood clots, epilepsy, migraine, diabetes, severe depression and sickle cell anaemia.

Diarrhoea, vomiting or use of antibiotics may affect action.

 Do not take if:

• suffering from high blood pressure, blood clots, stroke, very high cholesterol blood levels, severe liver disease, Dubin-Johnson syndrome, liver tumour, systemic lupus erythematosus, sex organ or breast cancer, jaundice, otosclerosis or severe skin irritation.

• male

SIDE EFFECTS

Common: Nausea, vomiting, headache, breast tenderness.

Unusual: Break through bleeding.

Severe but rare (stop medication, consult doctor): Severe headache, blood clot, calf or chest pain, severe shortness of breath.

INTERACTIONS

Other drugs:

• Antibiotics, Phenytoin, Primidone, Barbiturates, Rifampicin, Anticoagulants, medications that treat diabetes, Imipramine.

Other substances:

• Smoking increases risk of serious side effects.

PRESCRIPTION

Yes

PERMITTED IN SPORT

Yes

OVERDOSE

Vomiting and abnormal vaginal bleeding only likely effects.

OTHER INFORMATION

Not designed to replace pregnancy prevention by oral contraceptives or other methods. Should not be used repeatedly.

See also ORAL CONTRACEPTIVES

Morphine

TRADE NAMES

Morcap SR, MST Continus, MXL, Oramorph, Sevredol, Zomorph.

Cyclimorph (with Cyclizine).

DRUG CLASS

Narcotic.

USES

Severe pain.

DOSAGE

 Depends on form and level of pain. Follow doctors directions strictly.

FORMS

Tablets, slow release capsules and tablets, mixture, injection.

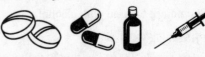

PRECAUTIONS

Should only be used during pregnancy (C) if medically essential. Use with caution in breast feeding. May be used in children.

Use with caution in colic caused by gall stones, pancreatitis, ulcerative colitis, underactive thyroid gland, enlarged prostate gland, head injury and shock.

 Do not take if:

• suffering from heart failure, severe head injury, acute diabetes, severe liver disease, severe alcoholism, poor lung function or convulsions.

• do not operate machinery, drive a vehicle or undertake tasks requiring concentration after use of morphine.

SIDE EFFECTS

Common: Sedation, constipation, confusion, sweating, nausea, loss of appetite.

Unusual: Vomiting, difficulty passing urine, flushing, dizziness, slow heart rate, irregular heart rate, fainting, mood changes.

Severe but rare (stop medication, consult doctor): Difficulty in breathing, convulsions.

INTERACTIONS

Other drugs:

• MAOI, Sedatives, Cimetidine,
  Pentazocine, Thiopentone, Diazepam,
  Doxapam, Barbiturates, Phenothiazines,
  Amphetamines.

Other substances:

• Should not be used with alcohol.

PRESCRIPTION

Yes (very restricted)

PERMITTED IN SPORT

No

OVERDOSE

Serious. Sedation, convulsions, coma and
death may occur. Administer activated
charcoal or induce vomiting if medication
taken recently and patient alert. Seek
emergency medical assistance. Antidote
available.

OTHER INFORMATION

Highly addictive if used inappropriately.
Very effective and unlikely to cause
addiction if used appropriately for severe
pain. Patients with terminal diseases (eg:
cancer) should use dose adequate to
control pain, and not be concerned about
possibility of addiction. Derived from
opium poppy and closely related to
heroin, but not as addictive.

Moxonidine

TRADE NAME

Physiotens.

DRUG CLASS

Antihypertensive.

USES

High blood pressure (hypertension).

DOSAGE

 200 to 600 mcg. a day.

FORMS

Tablets of 200mcg. (pink) and 400mcg.
(red).

PRECAUTIONS

Use with caution in pregnancy and
breast feeding. Not recommended in
children.

Use with caution in kidney and liver
disease, Raynaud's disease, epilepsy,
Parkinson's disease, glaucoma and
depression.

Do not stop suddenly, but reduce
dose gradually.

 Do not take if:

• suffering from
  angioneurotic oedema,
  some types of irregular
  heart beat, unstable
  angina, slow heart beat,
  heart failure, narrowed
  coronary (heart) arteries,
  severe liver or kidney
  disease.

SIDE EFFECTS

Common: Dry mouth, headaches,
tiredness.

Unusual: Dizziness, nausea, insomnia,
dilation of blood vessels.

INTERACTIONS

Other drugs:

• Sedatives.

Other substances:

• Alcohol.

PRESCRIPTION

Yes

PERMITTED IN SPORT

Yes

OVERDOSE

Serious heart effects possible. Seek urgent medical attention.

MPA

See **Medroxyprogesterone acetate**

MUCOLYTICS

(Break down thick mucus)

See **Carbocisteine**

Mumps vaccine

TRADE NAMES

MMR II, Priorix (with Measles and Rubella vaccines).

DRUG CLASS

Vaccine.

USES

Prevention of mumps.

DOSAGE

 Single injection at twelve months or older.

FORMS

Injection.

PRECAUTIONS

Not designed for use in pregnancy (B2), but unlikely to cause adverse effects if given inadvertently. May be used in children and breast feeding.

Use with caution in history of febrile convulsions or brain injury.

 Do not take if:

- suffering from allergy to eggs or poultry.
- significant fever, immune system disease.
- blood transfusion within three months.

SIDE EFFECTS

Common: Burning at site of injection.

Unusual: Fever, enlarged glands, itch, rash.

Severe but rare: Brain inflammation.

INTERACTIONS

None significant.

PRESCRIPTION

Yes

PERMITTED IN SPORT

Yes

OVERDOSE

An additional inadvertent dose is unlikely to have any serious side effects.

OTHER INFORMATION

Mumps is usually a mild disease, but may rarely cause infertility, brain damage and death. Vaccination with rubella, measles and mumps routine in childhood.

Mupirocin

TRADE NAME

Bactroban.

DRUG CLASS

Antibiotic.

USES

Bacterial skin infections, school sores (impetigo).

DOSAGE

 Apply three times a day.

FORMS

Ointment, nasal ointment.

PRECAUTIONS

Use with caution in pregnancy and breast feeding. May be used in children.

Not for use in eyes or mouth.

SIDE EFFECTS

Common: Minimal.

Unusual: Skin irritation.

INTERACTIONS

None significant.

PRESCRIPTION

Yes

PERMITTED IN SPORT

Yes

OTHER INFORMATION

Excellent and safe medication for treating minor skin infections. Introduced in late 1980s.

MUSCLE RELAXANTS

See Baclofen, Botulinum toxin, Carisoprodol, Dantrolene sodium, Orphenadrine, Tizanidine

Mycophenolate

TRADE NAME

Celicept.

DRUG CLASS

Immune system modifier.

USES

Prevention of rejection of kidney or heart transplant.

DOSAGE

 1000mg. twice a day.

FORMS

Capsules of 250mg. (blue/brown), tablet of 500mg. (lavender), infusion.

PRECAUTIONS

Must not be used in pregnancy (D). May be used with caution in children and breast feeding.

Regular blood tests to monitor blood cell function essential.

Use with caution in stomach, intestine and severe kidney disease.

SIDE EFFECTS

Common: Skin cancer incidence increased, infection, low white blood cell count, diarrhoea, bleeding from intestine.

Unusual: Severe abdominal pain.

Severe but rare (stop medication, consult doctor): Cancer of lymph nodes, perforation of intestine.

INTERACTIONS

Other drugs:

• Aciclovir, magnesium salts and aluminium salts (eg: in antacids), oral contraceptives, probenecid, drugs secreted in kidney, cholestyramine. Check with doctor before using any other medication.

Other substances:

• Alcohol.

PRESCRIPTION

Yes

PERMITTED IN SPORT

Yes

OVERDOSE

Extremely serious organ damage may occur. Induce vomiting or administer activated charcoal if taken recently. Seek emergency medical attention.

OTHER INFORMATION

Introduced in 1997.

MYDRIATICS

TRADE and GENERIC NAMES

Mydrilate (Cyclopentolate).

Minims Mydriatics (Atropine, Cyclopentolate, Homatropine hydrobromide, Phenylephrine, Tropicamide).

Mydriacyl (Tropicamide).

DRUG CLASS

Anticholinergic.

USES

Dilates pupil for examination and surgery.

DOSAGE

 Use drops as directed by doctor. Often used by doctors in their surgery or operating theatre.

FORMS

Eye drops.

PRECAUTIONS

May be used in pregnancy and breast feeding. Use with caution in children.

Not designed for prolonged use.

 Do not take if:

• suffering from glaucoma.

SIDE EFFECTS

Common: Irritation of eye with prolonged use, sensitivity to bright light.

Unusual: Disorientation, blurred vision, dry mouth, incoordination, rapid heart rate.

INTERACTIONS

None significant

PRESCRIPTION

Yes

PERMITTED IN SPORT

Yes

OTHER INFORMATION

Mainly used before eye examinations, and before and during eye surgery.

See also Atropine.

Nabumetone

See NSAID

Nadolol

See BETA-BLOCKERS

Naferelin

TRADE NAME

Synarel.

DRUG CLASS

Sex hormone.

USES

Treatment of endometriosis. Preliminary treatment to stimulate ovary before in vitro fertilisation (IVF).

DOSAGE

 One or two sprays into different nostrils, twice a day commencing two to four days after menstrual period starts.

FORMS

Nasal spray.

PRECAUTIONS

Must never be used in pregnancy (D), breast feeding or children.

Use with caution in osteoporosis, polycystic ovaries and hay fever.

 Do not use if:

• suffering from unusual vaginal bleeding.

SIDE EFFECTS

Common: Ovarian pain, ovarian cysts, belly pain, dry vagina, breast shrinkage, hot flushes, poor libido, headaches, acne.

Unusual: Emotional changes, muscle pains, nasal irritation.

INTERACTIONS

Other drugs:

• Other sex hormones.

PRESCRIPTION

Yes

PERMITTED IN SPORT

No

OVERDOSE

Unlikely to be serious.

OTHER INFORMATION

Introduced in the mid 1990s as a radically new and effective treatment for endometriosis via a novel route which overcomes the necessity for injections, and side effects caused by swallowing tablets.

Naftidrofuryl oxalate

TRADE NAME

Praxilene.

DRUG CLASS

Vasodilator.

USES

Poor circulation of blood to brain and other tissues.

DOSAGE

 One or two capsules three times a day.

FORMS

Capsules of 100mg. (pink).

PRECAUTIONS

Use with caution in pregnancy and breast feeding. Not recommended in children.

SIDE EFFECTS

Common: Nausea.

Unusual: Belly pain, rash.

Severe but rare (stop medication, consult doctor): Jaundice (yellow skin) from liver damage.

INTERACTIONS

None significant.

PRESCRIPTION

Yes

PERMITTED IN SPORT

No

Nalbuphine

TRADE NAME

Nubain.

DRUG CLASS

Narcotic.

USES

Moderate to severe pain (eg. heart attack).

DOSAGE

 One or two ampoules in injection as determined by doctor.

FORMS

Injection.

PRECAUTIONS

Use with caution in pregnancy, breast feeding and children.

Use with caution if lung function reduced (eg. emphysema, asthma), head injury, kidney and liver disease.

Beware of use in patients with a history of narcotic abuse.

SIDE EFFECTS

Common: Sedation, sweating, dry mouth.

Unusual: Dizziness, fainting.

INTERACTIONS

Other drugs:

• Sedatives, other narcotics.

PRESCRIPTION

Yes

PERMITTED IN SPORT

No

OVERDOSE

May be serious. Symptoms may not appear for some hours after injection given, and may include drowsiness, difficulty in breathing and coma. Seek urgent medical attention. Antidote available.

OTHER INFORMATION

May be addictive if used inappropriately.

Nalidixic acid

TRADE NAMES

Negram, Uriben.

Mictral (with Sodium bicarbonate, Citric acid and Sodium citrate).

DRUG CLASS

Antibiotic.

USES

Bacterial infections of urine.

DOSAGE

 One or two tablets four times a day.

FORMS

Tablets (beige) of 500mg., granules, suspension.

PRECAUTIONS

Safe to use in pregnancy (A) and breast feeding. Use with caution in children.

Use with caution in epilepsy, hardening of arteries, liver and kidney disease.

 Do not take if:

• suffering from convulsions.

SIDE EFFECTS

Common: Drowsiness, headache, dizziness, sensitivity to bright light, nausea, belly discomfort, rash.

Unusual: Vomiting, diarrhoea, itch, sun sensitive skin.

Severe but rare (stop medication, consult doctor): Yellow skin (jaundice).

INTERACTIONS

Other drugs:

• Nitrofurantoin, Anticoagulants, Antacids, Cyclosporin.

Other substances:

• Reacts with caffeine.

PRESCRIPTION

Yes

PERMITTED IN SPORT

Yes

OVERDOSE

Exacerbation of side effects likely.

OTHER INFORMATION

Often used long term to prevent infections of urine (eg: cystitis). Does not cause dependence or addiction.

Naloxone

TRADE NAME

Narcan.

DRUG CLASS

Antidote.

USES

Reversal of effects of overdosage with narcotics (eg: Morphine, Heroin).

DOSAGE

 Repeated injections at intervals of two or three minutes until desired effect achieved.

FORMS

Injection

PRECAUTIONS

May be used in pregnancy (B1), breast feeding and children of all ages.

Use with caution in narcotic addicts, heart disease.

Exclude other poisons that may be responsible for symptoms.

Patient must be monitored closely by doctors.

SIDE EFFECTS

Common: High blood pressure, irregular heart beat, shortness of breath, convulsions.

Unusual: Heart attack.

INTERACTIONS

None significant

PRESCRIPTION

Yes

PERMITTED IN SPORT

Yes

OTHER INFORMATION

Often life saving in addicts who taker heroin overdose, or in newborn infants of mothers who are heroin addicts. May precipitate withdrawal in narcotic addicts.

Naltrexone

TRADE NAME

Nalorex.

USES

Narcotic drug and alcohol dependence.

DOSAGE

 50mg. once or twice a day for 3 to 12 months. Half dose given initially in narcotic drug addiction.

FORMS

Tablet of 50mg. (yellow).

PRECAUTIONS

Use with caution in pregnancy (B3) and breast feeding.

Use with caution in children.

Use with caution in liver and kidney disease.

Patients must have a negative urine test for narcotics before first dose given, and must never use narcotics.

 Do not take if:

- taking any narcotic or opiate medications (eg. codeine, morphine) or illegal drugs (eg. heroin). May result in fatal reaction.

- suffering from acute hepatitis or liver failure.

SIDE EFFECTS

Common: Severe withdrawal effects if not previously completely withdrawn from alcohol or narcotics, diarrhoea, nausea, dizziness, tiredness.

Unusual: Liver damage, nervousness, fatigue, anxiety, joint and muscle pains.

INTERACTIONS

Other drugs:

- All narcotic drugs (eg. codeine, pethidine, morphine, heroin, opium - may result in death), thioridazine.

Other substances:

- Alcohol.

PRESCRIPTION

Yes

PERMITTED IN SPORT

Yes

OVERDOSE

Exacerbation of side effects likely. Seek medical attention.

OTHER INFORMATION

Should be combined with a drug or alcohol withdrawal program.

See also Acamprosate

Nandrolone decanoate

TRADE NAME

Deca Durabolin.

DRUG CLASS

Anabolic steroid.

USES

Kidney failure, inoperable breast cancer, severe osteoporosis, aplastic anaemia, suppression of white cells, in addition to corticosteroids used long term. Used dangerously and in an unapproved manner by body builders and athletes.

DOSAGE

 As directed and determined by doctor. Usually one injection a week.

FORMS

Injection.

PRECAUTIONS

Must not be used in pregnancy (D) or breast feeding. Use with caution in children as growth suppression may occur.

Use with caution in heart disease, enlarged prostate gland, diabetes.

 Do not take if:
- suffering from prostate and testicular cancer, breast cancer, liver and kidney disease.

SIDE EFFECTS

Common: Increased hairiness and decreased breast size in women, voice deepening in women, acne, frequent unwanted erections, infertility.

Unusual: Anaemia, enlargement of clitoris in women, cessation of menstrual periods, decrease in testicular size, impotence, breast enlargement in males, baldness in females, reduced libido.

Severe but rare (stop medication, consult doctor): Unusual bruising or bleeding, calcium deposits (lumps) in tissue, jaundice (yellow skin).

INTERACTIONS

Other drugs:

- Insulin.

PRESCRIPTION

Yes

PERMITTED IN SPORT

No. Although increasing muscle bulk, there is no evidence that this medication enhances athletic ability. Long term inappropriate use may cause permanent damage to the body.

OVERDOSE

Exacerbation of side effects likely.

OTHER INFORMATION

Does not cause dependence or addiction. Short term gains in muscle bulk when used inappropriately by body builders, may result in long term permanent body damage that may lead to early heart attacks, infertility, bone weakness, liver disease and premature death. Bottom line is - don't use it except under strict medical supervision when indicated for specific diseases.

Naproxen

See NSAID

Naratriptan

TRADE NAME

Naramig.

DRUG CLASS

Antimigraine.

USES

Treatment of acute migraine.

DOSAGE

Take one tablet at onset of migraine. Repeat after four hours if necessary.

FORMS

Tablets of 2.5mg. (green).

SIDE EFFECTS

Common: Tiredness, fatigue, dizziness,tingling, heat sensation.

Unusual: Chest heaviness, pressure, tightness, slow or rapid heart rate, disturbed vision.

INTERACTIONS

Other drugs:

• Other migraine treatments, Methysergide.

PRECAUTIONS

May be used with caution in pregnancy (B3), breast feeding, the elderly and children.

Use with caution in paralysis and visual disturbances due to migraine (exclude other serious causes).

Use with caution in heart disease, kidney and liver disease.

May cross react in patients with a sulphur allergy.

 Do not take if:

• suffering from angina, heart attack, stroke, poor circulation, uncontrolled high blood pressure, severe liver or kidney disease.

PRESCRIPTION

Yes

PERMITTED IN SPORT

Yes

OVERDOSE

Causes high blood pressure and may affect heart. Recovery within eight hours usual unless heart damaged. Seek medical attention.

OTHER INFORMATION

Introduced in 1998. Not addictive.

NARCOTICS

(Pain killing drugs derived from opium)

See Alfentanil, Buprenorphine, Codeine, Dextromoramide, Dextropropoxyphene, Ethoheptazine, Fentanyl, Heroin, Hydromorphone, Methadone, Morphine, Nalbuphine, Oxycodone, Pentazocine, Pethidine, Phenazocine

Nebivolol

See BETA-BLOCKERS

Nedocromil

TRADE NAME

Rapitil, Tilade.

USES

Prevention of asthma, allergic conjunctivitis.

DOSAGE

Inhaler: Two puffs, two to four times a day.
Drops: One drop in each eye, two to four times a day.

FORMS

Inhaler, eye drops.

PRECAUTIONS

Safe to use with caution in pregnancy (B1), breast feeding and children over 12 years.

Not to be used for the relief of acute asthma attacks.

 ## Do not take if:

- sensitive to aerosol propellants. Do not use eye drops
- if wearing contact lenses

SIDE EFFECTS

Common: Inhaler - Unpleasant taste. Eye drops - Temporary irritation.

Unusual: Headache, nausea, cough.

INTERACTIONS

None significant.

PRESCRIPTION

Yes

PERMITTED IN SPORT

Yes

OVERDOSE

Unlikely to cause any serious problems.

OTHER INFORMATION

A very effective preventer of inflammation in the lungs.

Nefazodone

TRADE NAME

Dutonin.

DRUG CLASS

Antidepressant.

USES

Moderate to severe depression, anxiety.

DOSAGE

Start with 100mg. twice a day, increase slowly until effective result obtained. Maximum dose 600mg. a day.

FORMS

Tablets of 50mg. (pink), 100mg. (white), and 200mg. (yellow).

PRECAUTIONS

May be used with caution in pregnancy (B3), breast feeding and children.

Use with caution in brain, kidney, liver, heart and blood vessel disease.

Use with caution in mania, epilepsy, suicidal tendencies, recent surgery and history of priapism (prolonged painful erection of penis).

 Do not take if:

- MAOI (Phenelzine, Tranylcypromine) used within two weeks.

SIDE EFFECTS

Common: Nausea, diarrhoea, low blood pressure, fainting, drowsiness.

Unusual: Vomiting, painful erection of penis.

INTERACTIONS

Other drugs:

- MAOI, terfenadine, astemizole, medications that lower blood pressure, carbamazepine, propranolol, fluoxetine, alprazolam, cisapride, triazolam.

Other substances:

- Alcohol.

PRESCRIPTION

Yes

PERMITTED IN SPORT

Yes

OVERDOSE

May be very serious. Induce vomiting or give activated charcoal if taken recently. Seek urgent medical attention.

OTHER INFORMATION

Introduced in 1997 as an effective treatment for more difficult cases of depression. Not addictive or dependence forming.

Nefopam

TRADE NAME

Acupan.

DRUG CLASS

Analgesic.

USES

Pain, particularly after surgery.

DOSAGE

 One tablet up to three times a day.

FORMS

Tablets of 30mg. (white).

PRECAUTIONS

Use with caution in pregnancy. May be used in breast feeding. Not recommended in children.

Use with caution in liver and kidney disease, and difficulty in passing urine.

 Do not take if:

- suffering from epilepsy or recent heart attack.
- under other circumstances

SIDE EFFECTS

Common: Nausea, nervousness, dry mouth, dizziness.

INTERACTIONS

Other drugs:

- MAOI, Anticholinergics, Sympathomimetics, Tricyclic antidepressants.

Other substances:

- Alcohol.

PRESCRIPTION

Yes

PERMITTED IN SPORT

No

Neisseria meningitidis vaccine

TRADE NAME

Mengivac.

DRUG CLASS

Vaccine.

USES

Prevention of meningitis caused by Neisseria meningitidis in travellers to countries where the disease occurs, close contacts of a victim.

DOSAGE

 Single injection.

FORMS

Injection.

PRECAUTIONS

Not designed to be used in pregnancy (B2), but inadvertent administration is unlikely to cause any serious adverse effect.

Use with caution in malaria or impaired immunity.

 Do not take if:

• suffering from significant fever.

SIDE EFFECTS

Common: Local pain, redness, firmness and swelling at injection site.

Unusual: Enlarged lymph glands, fever, headache, sore throat, unwell feeling.

INTERACTIONS

None significant.

PRESCRIPTION

Yes

PERMITTED IN SPORT

Yes

OVERDOSE

An inadvertent additional vaccination is unlikely to have any serious side effects.

OTHER INFORMATION

Not routinely used.

Neomycin

TRADE and GENERIC NAMES

Minims Neomycin, Nivermycin.

Adcortyl with Graneodin, Tri-Adcortyl Otic (with Triamcinolone, Gramicidin).

Audicort (with Triamcinolone).

Betnesol-N (with Betamethasone).

Cicatrin (with Bacitracin).

Dermovate NN (with Nystatin, Clobetasol).

Graneodin (with Gramicidin).

Gregoderm, Otosporin (with Polymyxin B, Hydrocortisone).

Maxitrol (with Dexamethasone, Polymyxin B).

Naseptin (with Chlorhexidine).

Neo-Cortef (with Hydrocortisone).

Neosporin (with Polymyxin B, Gramicidin).

Otomize (with Dexamethasone, Acetic acid).

Predsol-N (with Prednisolone).

Synalar-N (with Fluocinolone).

Tri-Adcortyl (with Triamcinolone, Gramicidin, Nystatin).

DRUG CLASS

Aminoglycoside antibiotic.

USES

Infections of eye, ear, skin and bowel.

DOSAGE

 Tablets: Two tablets every four hours.
Skin: Apply two or three times a day.
Eye drops: Two drops four times a day.
Eye and ear ointment: Apply twice a day.

FORMS

Tablets, irrigation solution, ear drops, ear ointment, eye drops, eye ointment, cream, lotion, powder.

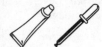

PRECAUTIONS

Skin, eye and ear preparations may be used with caution in pregnancy, breast feeding and children.

Tablets must not be used in pregnancy (D) or breast feeding.

Use tablets with caution in kidney disease and hearing damage.

Tablets are designed for very short term use.

Avoid eye contact with forms not designed for use in eye.

Skin preparations should not be used on viral infections.

SIDE EFFECTS

Common: Tablets - diarrhoea. Other forms - minimal.

Unusual: Tablets - ear and kidney damage.

INTERACTIONS

Other drugs:

• Tablets - Penicillin, Cephalosporins.

PRESCRIPTION

Yes

PERMITTED IN SPORT

Yes

OVERDOSE

Tablets may cause severe diarrhoea, ear and kidney damage.

OTHER INFORMATION

Widely used for superficial mild infections. Available for over forty years.

Netimicin

TRADE NAME

Netilin.

DRUG CLASS

Antibiotic.

USES

Severe bacterial infections.

DOSAGE

 By injection into a muscle, or slow infusion by a drip into a vein, dosage as determined by doctor for each patient.

FORMS

Injection.

SIDE EFFECTS

Common: Adverse effects on ear, nerve and kidney function.

Unusual: Resistant infection.

INTERACTIONS

Other drugs:

• Frusemide, other diuretics, anaesthetics, cephalosporins, numerous other medications.

Other substances:

• Some forms of blood transfusion.

PRECAUTIONS

Must not be used in pregnancy (D). Use with caution breast feeding and children.

Use with caution in kidney disease, myasthenia gravis and low blood calcium levels.

Beware of dehydration.

Reduce dose in elderly.

Not for prolonged use.

PRESCRIPTION

Yes

PERMITTED IN SPORT

Yes

OTHER INFORMATION

Introduced in 1996 for the treatment of more difficult and severe infections.

Neutral insulin

See INSULINS

Nevirapine

TRADE NAME

Viramune.

DRUG CLASS

Antiviral.

USES

AIDS, HIV infection.

DOSAGE

One or two tablets a day in combination with other antiviral treatment.

FORMS

Tablets of 200mg. (white).

PRECAUTIONS

Use with caution in pregnancy (B3), breast feeding and children.

Use with caution in kidney and liver disease.

SIDE EFFECTS

Common: Rash, itch, fever, nausea, headache.

Unusual: Severe skin reactions, vomiting, liver damage.

Severe but rare (stop medication, consult doctor): Jaundice (yellow skin).

INTERACTIONS

Other drugs:

• Rifampicin, rifabutin, sex hormones, oral contraceptives.

PRESCRIPTION

Yes

PERMITTED IN SPORT

Yes

OVERDOSE

May cause serious organ damage. Induce vomiting or give activated charcoal if taken recently. Seek urgent medical attention.

OTHER INFORMATION

Introduced in 1997 as an additive medication for the management of HIV (Human Immunodeficiency Virus) infection.

Niacin

See Nicotinic acid

Nicardipine

See CALCIUM CHANNEL BLOCKERS

Niclosamide

TRADE NAME

Yomesan.

DRUG CLASS

Anthelmintic.

USES

Tapeworm.

DOSAGE

 Four tablets as a single dose.

FORMS

Tablets (yellow) of 500mg.

PRECAUTIONS

May be used with caution in pregnancy (B1). May be used safely in breast feeding and children.

Use with caution in constipation.

SIDE EFFECTS

Common: Minimal

Unusual: Nausea, vomiting.

INTERACTIONS

Other drugs:

• None significant.

Other substances:

• Avoid alcohol during treatment.

PRESCRIPTION

No

PERMITTED IN SPORT

Yes

Nicorandil

TRADE NAME

Ikorel.

DRUG CLASS

Antiangina.

USES

Angina (heart pain).

DOSAGE

 5mg. to 20mg. twice a day. Use minimum effective dose.

FORMS

Tablets of 10mg. and 20mg. (white).

PRECAUTIONS

Use with caution in pregnancy (B3), breast feeding and children.

 Do not take if:

• suffering from low blood pressure or heart failure.

• sensitive to Nicotinic acid.

SIDE EFFECTS

Common: Headache, muscle pain, tiredness, palpitations, dizziness, nausea.

Unusual: High blood pressure, diarrhoea, shortness of breath.

Severe but rare (stop medication, consult doctor): Low blood pressure.

INTERACTIONS

None significant.

PRESCRIPTION

Yes

PERMITTED IN SPORT

Yes

OVERDOSE

Low blood pressure, rapid heart rate and collapse may occur. Induce vomiting or administer activated charcoal if tablets taken recently. Seek medical assistance.

OTHER INFORMATION

Introduced in 1998. Does not cause addiction or dependence.

Nicotinamide

See Nicotinic acid

Nicotine

TRADE NAMES

Nicorette, Nicotinell, Niquitin CQ.

Nicotine is also one of the active chemicals in tobacco.

DRUG CLASS

Stimulant

USES

Assists in stopping smoking.

DOSAGE

 Chewable gum: Chew one or two at a time when urge to smoke is felt. Maximum 60mg a day. Reduce frequency of use over time.

Skin patches: Apply to different place on non-hairy skin of trunk or upper arm once a day in morning. Instructions vary with brands. Follow doctors directions. Progressively reduce strength of patch over ten to twelve weeks

Under tongue dissolvable tablets: One or two tablets placed under tongue every hour

Inhaler: Six to twelve cartridges inhaled a day

Nasal spray: One spray into each nostril every 30 minutes as required. Slowly reduce dose of all forms over several months.

FORMS

Chewable gum, skin patches, under tongue dissolvable tablets, inhaler, nasal spray.

SIDE EFFECTS

Common: Patches - Rash at application site.

INTERACTIONS

Other drugs:

• Cessation of smoking may result in altered availability of many medications, and may require alteration in their doses.

Other substances:

• Continued smoking while using Nicotine may cause significant serious adverse effects.

PRECAUTIONS

Not to be used in pregnancy (D) (NB: Smoking is also harmful to the foetus in pregnancy). Breast feeding should be ceased before use. Not designed for use in children under 14 years.

Not designed for long term use.

Use chewable gum with caution if:

• wearing dentures or having dental work.

• suffering from mouth ulcers or inflammation,

• suffering from peptic ulcer or inflamed stomach.

Use all forms in caution with heart disease.

Use patches with caution in dermatitis and eczema.

 Do not take if:

• suffering from recent heart attack, angina, irregular heart rate or recent stroke.

• continuing to smoke.

PRESCRIPTION

No

PERMITTED IN SPORT

Yes

OVERDOSE

Nausea and vomiting only likely effects.

OTHER INFORMATION

Nicotine medications work best if used with an appropriate smoking cessation program. Will only work if the patient wants to stop smoking, and is prepared to use nicotine as assistance to his or her own determination. Nicotine by itself will not stop someone from smoking.

Nicotine medications may cause dependence. Nicotine is highly addictive.

See also Buproprion.

Nicotinic Acid

(Niacin, Nicotinyl and Nicotinamide)

(Vitamin B3)

TRADE NAMES

Nicotinic Acid.

Hexopal (Inositol nicotinate).

Papulex (Nicotinamide).

Ronicol (Nicotinyl alcohol).

Also found in numerous vitamin and mineral supplements.

DRUG CLASS

Vitamin, Hypolipidaemic, Vasodilator.

USES

High levels of blood cholesterol and triglycerides, pellagra, poor circulation, acne.

DOSAGE

 Pellagra: 500mg a day. High cholesterol/triglyceride: 250mg to 1500mg three times a day after meals.

Poor circulation: One or two tablets, three or four times a day.

Acne: Apply sparingly twice a day.

FORMS

Tablets, capsules, gel.

SIDE EFFECTS

Common: Rashes, itchy skin, changes in heart function, stomach upsets, nervousness.

Unusual: Dry skin, skin pigmentation.

Severe but rare (stop medication, consult doctor): Yellow skin.

INTERACTIONS

Other drugs:

- Drugs used to treat high blood pressure.

- Steroids, Hallucinogens, Reserpine, Chlordiazepoxide.

- Other vitamins may affect nicotinic acid absorption.

PRECAUTIONS

Use with caution in pregnancy (B2) and breast feeding.

Blood tests to check liver function, uric acid levels and blood fat levels recommended.

Use with caution with low blood pressure and poor liver function.

 ### Do not take if:

- suffering from peptic ulcer, stomach upsets, recent heart attack, severe liver disease, diabetes, gout, heart disease, gall bladder disease, glaucoma, tendency to bleed easily.

PRESCRIPTION

No

PERMITTED IN SPORT

Yes

OVERDOSE

Causes flushing, itch, vomiting, diarrhoea, heartburn, belly cramps, fainting. Induce vomiting if tablets taken recently. Seek medical assistance.

OTHER INFORMATION

Used as a starting point in the treatment of high cholesterol blood levels and poor circulation. Remember, vitamins are merely chemicals that are essential for the functioning of the body, and if taken to excess, act as a drug.

See also Acipimox

Nicotinyl alcohol

See Nicotinic Acid

Nicoumalone

TRADE NAME

Sinthrome.

DRUG CLASS

Anticoagulant.

USES

Prevention and treatment of blood clots in arteries and veins.

DOSAGE

 Dosage carefully adjusted by doctor on a regular basis depending on blood test results.

FORMS

Tablets of 1mg. (white).

SIDE EFFECTS

Common: Abnormal bleeding and bruising.

Severe but rare (stop medication, consult doctor): Allergy reactions, hair loss, liver damage (jaundice - yellow skin), skin damage.

INTERACTIONS

Other drugs:

- NSAID, Aspirin, Hypoglycaemics, Sulphonamides, Quinidine, Antibiotics, Phenformin, Cimetidine, Corticosteroids.

- Many other drugs may affect dosage levels.

PRECAUTIONS

Must not be used in pregnancy (D) as it may cause foetal damage and death. Breast feeding should be ceased if use is medically necessary. Not recommended in children.

Regular blood tests to check blood clotting time essential.

Other illnesses (eg: infection) may require an adjustment of dosage.

Read literature accompanying medication very carefully. Ask questions of doctor about anything you do not understand.

Use with caution in high blood pressure and heart failure.

Do not undertake any activity that may result in falls, bruising or extreme exertion.

Do not take if:

- suffering from bleeding tendency, peptic ulcer, dementia, mental diseases, severe high blood pressure, significant liver or kidney disease, endocarditis, abnormal blood cells.
- due to have essential surgery, including dental surgery.
- unable to cooperate with doctor and instructions.

PRESCRIPTION

Yes

PERMITTED IN SPORT

Yes

OVERDOSE

Extremely serious. Administer activated charcoal or induce vomiting only if tablets taken very recently. Seek emergency medical assistance. Massive internal bleeding may cause sudden death. Antidote (Vitamin K) available. Blood transfusion may be necessary.

See also Warfarin

Nifedipine

See **CALCIUM CHANNEL BLOCKERS**

Nimodipine

See **CALCIUM CHANNEL BLOCKERS**

Nisoldipine

See **CALCIUM CHANNEL BLOCKERS**

Nitrazepam

TRADE NAMES

Mogadon, Nitrazepam.

DRUG CLASS

Sedative/hypnotic, Benzodiazepine.

USES

Relieves insomnia (sleeplessness).

DOSAGE

 One or two at bedtime.

FORMS

Tablet of 5mg. (white).

SIDE EFFECTS

Common: Confusion and falls in elderly, impaired alertness.

Unusual: Dizziness, incoordination, poor memory, headache, hangover in morning, slurred speech, nightmares.

INTERACTIONS

Other drugs:

- Other medications that reduce alertness (eg: Barbiturates, Antihistamines, Antianxiety drugs).
- Disulfiram, Cimetidine, Anticonvulsants, Anticholinergics.

Other substances:

- Reacts with alcohol to cause excessive drowsiness.

PRECAUTIONS

Should be used with caution in pregnancy (C), but not at all if delivery of infant imminent as it may decrease desire to breathe in newborn infant. Should be used with caution in breast feeding. Not for use in children.

Lower dose required in elderly.

Should be used intermittently and not constantly as dependency may develop. Stopping suddenly after prolonged constant use may cause withdrawal symptoms.

Use with caution in glaucoma, myasthenia gravis, heart disease, kidney or liver disease, psychiatric conditions, depression and epilepsy.

 Do not take if:

- suffering from severe lung disease, confusion.

- tendency to addiction or dependence.

PRESCRIPTION

Yes

PERMITTED IN SPORT

Yes

OVERDOSE

Seldom life threatening. May cause drowsiness, confusion and coma. Administer activated charcoal or induce vomiting if tablets taken recently. Seek medical assistance.

OTHER INFORMATION

In use for almost thirty years. Very safe and effective, but dependence (inability to sleep or function without medication) a problem if used regularly.

Nitrofurantoin

TRADE NAMES

Furadantin, Macrobid, Macrodantin.

DRUG CLASS

Antibiotic.

USES

Bacterial infections of urine.

DOSAGE

 One or two capsules four times a day with food.

PRECAUTIONS

Safe to use in pregnancy (A), breast feeding and children. Not for use under one month of age.

Not designed for long term use.

Use with caution in kidney function disorders.

 Do not take if:

- suffering from severe kidney failure.

FORMS

Capsules and tablets of 50 and 100mg.

SIDE EFFECTS

Common: Nausea, vomiting.

Severe but rare (stop medication, consult doctor): Numbness or tingling, yellow skin (jaundice).

INTERACTIONS

Other drugs:

• Barbiturates, Antacids, urinary acidifiers and alkalinisers.

PRESCRIPTION

Yes

PERMITTED IN SPORT

Yes

OVERDOSE

Exacerbation of side effects likely. Give additional fluids by mouth to increase rate of excretion.

OTHER INFORMATION

Useful and effective medication.

Nitroglycerine

See Glyceryl Trinitrate

Nizatadine

TRADE NAMES

Axid, Zinga.

DRUG CLASS

Antiulcerant, H2 receptor antagonist.

USES

Prevention and treatment of ulcers of the stomach, oesophagus (gullet) and duodenum (upper small intestine). Prevention of acid reflux into the oesophagus (heartburn).

DOSAGE

 300mg a day in one or two doses.

FORMS

Capsules of 150 and 300mg.

PRECAUTIONS

Care should be taken with use in pregnancy (B3) and breast feeding. Safety in children not established.

 Do not take if:

• suffering from severe kidney disease or phenylketonuria.

• suffering from stomach cancer.

SIDE EFFECTS

Common: Anaemia, tiredness, drowsiness, rash.

Unusual: Constipation, breast enlargement and tenderness (both sexes).

Severe but rare (stop medication, consult doctor): Hepatitis (jaundice), rapid or irregular heart beat.

INTERACTIONS

None significant

PRESCRIPTION

Yes

PERMITTED IN SPORT

Yes

OVERDOSE

No serious effects reported.

OTHER INFORMATION

H2 receptor antagonist that may be more effective in reflux oesophagitis than others in this class.

See also Cimetidine, Famotidine, Ranitidine.

Nonoxynol 9

TRADE NAMES

Delfen, Double Check, Durex Duragel, Gynol II, Ortho-Creme, Ortho-Forms.

DRUG CLASS

Contraceptive, Spermicide.

USES

For use in combination with a diaphragm or condom to prevent pregnancy, kills sperm.

DOSAGE

 Varies with form and product. Use strictly in accordance with directions on packaging.

PRECAUTIONS

Safe if used accidentally in pregnancy (A). Safe in breast feeding. Not designed for use in children.

Wait six to eight hours after sex before removing diaphragm or using douche.

Do not retain diaphragm for more than 24 hours.

Ensure hands and diaphragm are completely clean before insertion.

FORMS

Cream, foam, gel

SIDE EFFECTS

Common: Minimal

Unusual: Irritation of vagina or penis.

INTERACTIONS

None

PRESCRIPTION

No

PERMITTED IN SPORT

Yes

OTHER INFORMATION

Not a reliable form of contraception if used alone. Even in combination with a diaphragm or condom, spermicides have a failure rate of about 5% (ie: five out of 100 women using this method of contraception for a year will fall pregnant). Do not protect against venereal disease.

Norethisterone

TRADE and GENERIC NAMES

Micronor, Noriday, Noristerat, Primolut-N, Utovlan.

Climagest, Climesse, Elleste Duet, Estracombi, Evorel, Kliofem, Kliovance, Nuvelle, Trisequens (with Oestradiol).

Used in numerous Oral Contraceptives (eg: **BiNovum, Brevinor, Loestrin, Norimin, Norinyl, Synphase, TriNovum**) - see separate entry.

DRUG CLASS

Sex hormone.

USES

Abnormal bleeding from uterus, failure of menstrual period, premenstrual tension, breast tenderness, endometriosis, as an addition to oestrogen in menopausal hormone replacement therapy (HRT). Contraception.

DOSAGE

 Tablets: One or two tablets, one to three times a day with fluid. Patches: Apply once or twice a week.

FORMS

Tablets, patches.

PRECAUTIONS

Not for use in pregnancy (D), breast feeding or children.

Use with caution in diabetes.

 Do not take if:

- suffering from severe liver disease, jaundice or blood clots.
- male

SIDE EFFECTS

Common: Abnormal vaginal bleeding, headache.

Unusual: Sleeplessness, nervousness, dizziness, tremor, rash, sweating, nausea, breast tenderness, weight gain.

Severe but rare (stop medication, consult doctor): Blood clot, calf pain, chest pain, yellow skin (jaundice).

INTERACTIONS

Other drugs:

- Other Sex hormones.

Other substances:

- Smoking increases risk of serious side effects.

PRESCRIPTION

Yes

PERMITTED IN SPORT

Yes

OVERDOSE

Unlikely to be serious. Vomiting and abnormal vaginal bleeding likely.

OTHER INFORMATION

Widely used and safe medication. Useful for delaying menstrual period that may be due at an awkward time, or as an additive to menopausal treatments to prevent over stimulation of the uterine lining. Does not cause addiction or dependence. Often used as a contraceptive in women who are breast feeding, when they must be taken at the same time each day to be reliable.

See also Oral Contraceptives

Norfloxacin

TRADE NAME

Utinor.

DRUG CLASS

Quinolone antibiotic.

USES

Urinary infections.

DOSAGE

 One tablet twice a day.

FORMS

Tablet (white) of 400mg.

SIDE EFFECTS

Common: Nausea, headache, dizziness.

Unusual: Tiredness, rash, belly pain, depression, sleeplessness, constipation, excess wind, constipation.

Severe but rare (stop medication, consult doctor): Bloody diarrhoea, unusual bruising or bleeding.

INTERACTIONS

Other drugs:

• Antacids, Nitrofurantoin, Theophylline, Cyclosporin, Probenecid, Anticoagulants.

Other substances:

• Reacts with caffeine.

PRECAUTIONS

Not to be used in pregnancy (B3) and breast feeding unless medically essential. Not for use in children.

Ensure adequate fluid intake.

Use with caution in epilepsy and kidney disease.

Avoid excessive sun exposure while taking medication.

PRESCRIPTION

Yes

PERMITTED IN SPORT

Yes

OVERDOSE

Exacerbation of side effects most likely result. Induce vomiting if medication taken recently. Maintain adequate fluid intake.

OTHER INFORMATION

Introduced in late 1980s. Very effective in treating the more difficult infections of the bladder and kidneys.

Norgestimate
See ORAL CONTRACEPTIVES

Norgestrel
See ORAL CONTRACEPTIVES

Normal Immunoglobulin
See Gamma globulin

Nortriptyline
See TRICYCLICS

NSAID (NONSTEROIDAL ANTI-INFLAMMATORY DRUGS)

TRADE and GENERIC NAMES

Acular, Toradol (Ketorolac trometanol).

Arthrotec (Diclofenac with Misoprostol).

Brexidol, Feldene (Piroxicam).

Brufen, Deep Relief, Fenbid, Ibugel, Ibumousse, Ibuspray, Motrin, Proflex (Ibuprofen).

Butacote (Phenylbutazone).

Clinoril (Sulindac).

Clotam (Tolfenamic acid).

Codafen Continuous (Ibuprofen with Codeine).

Condrotec, Napratec (Naproxen with Misoprostol).

Dicloflex, Diclomax, Motifene, Volraman, Volsaid Retard, Volarol (Diclofenac).

Dolobid (Diflunisal).

Emflex (Acemetacin).

Fenopren (Fenoprofen).

Flexin, Indocid, Indomod
(Indomethacin).

Froben, Ocufen, Strefen (Flurbiprofen).

Keral (Dexketoprofen).

Lederfen (Fenbufen).

Lodine (Etodolac).

Ketocid, Orudis, Oruvail, Powergel
(Ketoprofen).

Mobic (Meloxicam).

Mobiflex (Tenoxicam).

Naprosyn, Nycopren, Synflex
(Naproxen).

Ponstan (Mefenamic acid).

Preservex (Aceclofenac).

Reliflex (Nabumetone).

Rheumox (Azapropazone).

Surgam (Tiaprofenic Acid).

Traxam (Felbinac).

Aspirin and Salicylic acid are also an NSAIDs - See separate entry.

USES

All forms of arthritis, inflammatory disorders, gout, back pain, ankylosing spondylitis, bone pain, period pain, migraine, general pain relief, prevention of blood clots, prevention of miosis (eye contraction) during eye surgery, dermatitis (creams only), correction of heart defect (patent ductus arteriosus) in premature infants (Indomethacin only).

DOSAGE

 Tablets and capsules: One or two tablets, one to four times a day with food. Some preparations are long acting and only require one or two doses a day
Suppository: One or two inserted a day
Mixture: Three or four times a day with food
Ointments, creams, gels: Rub into affected area three or four times a day for up to two weeks

Spray: Seven sprays to affected area three times a day
Eye drops: As directed by eye doctor.

FORMS

Tablets, capsules, mixture, suppository, injection, spray, ointment, gel, cream, mousse, eye drops.

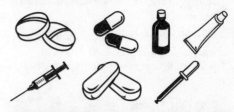

PRECAUTIONS

Should not be used in pregnancy (C) unless medically essential. Breast feeding should be ceased if necessary to use NSAID. Not for use in children under two. Creams safe in pregnancy.

Use tablets and capsules with caution in psychiatrically disturbed patients, epilepsy, severe infection, heart failure and kidney disease.

Lower doses required in elderly, who may suffer more side effects.

Phenylbutazone only used in extenuating circumstances as serious side effects possible.

 Do not take if:

- suffering from peptic ulcer at present or in recent past.

- due for surgery (including dental surgery).

- suffering from bleeding disorder or anaemia.

- suffering from proctitis (suppository only).

SIDE EFFECTS

Common: Creams, gels, sprays etc. - Minimal Other forms - Stomach discomfort, diarrhoea, constipation, heartburn, nausea, headache, dizziness.

Unusual: Blurred vision, stomach ulcer, ringing noise in ears, retention of fluid, swelling of tissue, drowsiness, itch, rash, shortness of breath.

Severe but rare (stop medication, consult doctor): Vomit blood, pass blood in faeces, other unusual bleeding, asthma induced by medication.

INTERACTIONS

Other drugs:

• Must never be used with Anticoagulants.

• Probenecid, Diuretics, Lithium, Methotrexate, Beta Blockers, ACE inhibitors.

• Creams, gels, sprays etc. have minimal interactions.

PRESCRIPTION

Low strength preparations and skin applications: No

High strength preparations: Yes.

PERMITTED IN SPORT

Yes

OVERDOSE

Causes nausea, vomiting, severe headache, dizziness, confusion and convulsions. Administer activated charcoal or induce vomiting if taken recently. Seek medical assistance.

OTHER INFORMATION

Extensively used to give excellent relief to a wide variety of inflammatory conditions. Significant side effects (particularly on the stomach) in about 5% of patients limit their use. Specially coated forms reduce side effects. Minimal side effects with creams, ointments, gels and sprays, but they are less effective.

See also Aspirin, Celecoxib, Salicylates.

Nystatin

TRADE and GENERIC NAMES

Nystan.

Dermovate-NN (with Clobetasol, Neomycin).

Flagyl Compak (with Metronidazole).

Gregoderm (with Neomycin, Polymyxin B, Hydrocortisone).

Nystadermal (with Triamcinolone).

Nystaform (with Chlorhexidine).

Nystaform-HC (with Chlorhexidine, Hydrocortisone).

Terra-Cortril Nystatin (with Oxytetracycline, Hydrocortisone).

Timodine (with Hydrocortisone, Benzalkonium chloride, Dimethicone).

Tinaderm-M (with Tolnaftate).

Tri-Adcortyl (with Triamcinolone, Neomycin and Gramicidin).

Trimovate (with Clobetasone, Oxytetracycline).

DRUG CLASS

Antifungal.

USES

Treatment and prevention of fungal infections of skin (tinea), mouth, vagina (thrush) and intestine (candidiasis).

DOSAGE

 Tablets: One or two, three times a day.
Skin preparations: Apply three times a day.
Vaginal preparations: One pessary or applicator of cream at night for 14 days.

FORMS

Tablets, cream, ointment, suspension, lozenges, vaginal cream, vaginal pessary.

PRECAUTIONS

Safe to use in pregnancy, breast feeding and children.

Applicator of vaginal preparations must be used with care in pregnancy.

SIDE EFFECTS

Minimal

INTERACTIONS

None significant

PRESCRIPTION

Yes

PERMITTED IN SPORT

Yes

OVERDOSE

Diarrhoea, nausea and vomiting only likely effects.

OTHER INFORMATION

Does not cause dependence or addiction. Available for over thirty years. Very safe. Use decreasing in recent years with introduction of more potent antifungals (eg: Imidazoles). Often combined with other medications (particularly steroids) in skin preparations.

OBESITY DRUGS

See Methylcellulose, Orlistat

Octreotide

TRADE NAME

Sandostatin.

USES

Acromegaly (bone overgrowth caused by tumour of pituitary gland), relief of carcinoid tumour symptoms.

DOSAGE

 One or more injections a day as determined by doctor.

FORMS

Injection.

PRECAUTIONS

Must not be used in pregnancy (C) or breast feeding. Use in children only when medically essential.

Use with caution in diabetes.

Regular checks on gall bladder and pituitary gland necessary.

Designed for short term or intermittent use.

SIDE EFFECTS

Common: Pain at injection site, nausea, vomiting, loss of appetite, bloating, excess wind, diarrhoea.

Unusual: Headache, dizziness, fatigue, flushing.

INTERACTIONS

Other drugs:

• Cyclosporin, Cimetidine.

PRESCRIPTION

Yes

PERMITTED IN SPORT

Yes

Oestradiol

(Estradiol)

TRADE and GENERIC NAMES

Climaval, Dermestril, Elleste Solo, Estraderm, Estrapak, Estring, Evorel, Fematrix, Femseven, Menorest, Oestrogel, Progynova, Sandrena, Vagifem, Zumenon.

Climagest, Climesse, Elleste Duet, Estracombi, Evorel Conti, Evorel Sequi, Evorel-Pak, Kliofem, Kliovance, Nuvelle Continuous, Oestradiol, Trisequens (with Norethisterone).

Cyclo-Progynova, Nuvelle, Nuvelle TS (with Levonorgestrel).

Femapak, Femoston (with Dydrogesterone).

Hormonin (with Oestrone, Oestriol).

Tridestra (with Medroxyprogesterone acetate).

DRUG CLASS

Sex hormone

USES

Oestrogen (female hormone) replacement in menopause.

DOSAGE

 Tablets: Dosage individualised by doctor. Usually one tablet once a day.
Patch: Apply once or twice a week.
Pessary: One pessary in vagina every night initially, reducing to twice a week.

FORMS

Tablets, patches, vaginal pessary, vaginal cream, injection, implant.

PRECAUTIONS

Not to be used in pregnancy (B1), breast feeding or children.
Accidental usage in these situations unlikely to be harmful.

Use with caution in epilepsy, migraine, heart failure, high blood pressure, kidney disease, diabetes, porphyria or uterine disease.

 Do not take if:

- suffering from liver disease, breast or genital cancer, blood clots.

SIDE EFFECTS

Common: Abnormal uterine bleeding, vaginal thrush, nausea, fluid retention, weight gain, breast tenderness.

Unusual: Rash at site of patch application, blurred vision, vomiting, bloating, intestinal cramps, pigmentation of skin on face.

Severe but rare (stop medication, consult doctor): Blood clots, calf or chest pain, yellow skin (jaundice).

INTERACTIONS

Other drugs:

- Other Sex hormones.

Other substances:

- Smoking increases risk of serious side effects.

PRESCRIPTION

Yes

PERMITTED IN SPORT

Yes

OVERDOSE

Vomiting and abnormal vaginal bleeding only likely effects.

OTHER INFORMATION

Does not cause addiction or dependence. Very useful in managing the effects of menopause, and reduces the risk of osteoporosis and heart disease after the menopause.

Oestriol

TRADE NAMES

Ortho-Gynest, Ovestin.

Hormonin (with Oestradiol, Oestrone).

DRUG CLASS

Sex Hormone.

USES

Oestrogen (female hormone) replacement in menopause.

DOSAGE

 Tablets: Dosage individualised by doctor. Usually one tablet once a day
Vaginal cream and pessaries:
Use daily at bed time initially, reduce to once or twice a week long term.

FORMS

Tablets (white) of 1mg., vaginal cream, vaginal pessaries.

SIDE EFFECTS

Common: Abnormal uterine bleeding, vaginal thrush, nausea, fluid retention, weight gain, breast tenderness.

Unusual: Rash, blurred vision, vomiting, bloating, intestinal cramps, pigmentation of skin on face.

Severe but rare (stop medication, consult doctor): Blood clots, calf or chest pain, yellow skin (jaundice).

INTERACTIONS

Other drugs:

• Other Sex hormones.

Other substances:

• Smoking increases risk of serious side effects.

PRECAUTIONS

Not to be used in pregnancy (B1), breast feeding or children.
Accidental usage in these situations unlikely to be harmful.

Use with caution in epilepsy, migraine, heart failure, high blood pressure, kidney disease, diabetes, porphyria or uterine disease.

 Do not take if:

• suffering from liver disease, breast or genital cancer, blood clots.

PRESCRIPTION

Yes

PERMITTED IN SPORT

Yes

OVERDOSE

Vomiting and abnormal vaginal bleeding only likely effects.

OTHER INFORMATION

Does not cause addiction or dependence. Very useful in managing the effects of menopause, and reduces the risk of osteoporosis and heart disease after the menopause.

Oestrogen

TRADE NAME

Premarin, Prempak-C.

Premique (with Medroxyprogesterone).

DRUG CLASS

Sex hormone.

USES

Female hormone replacement in menopause.

DOSAGE

 Tablets: Dosage individualised by doctor. Usually one tablet once a day.
Vaginal cream: Insert daily, three weeks per month.

PRECAUTIONS

Not to be used in pregnancy (B1), breast feeding or children.
Accidental usage in these situations unlikely to be harmful.

Use with caution in epilepsy, migraine, heart failure, high blood pressure, kidney disease, diabetes, porphyria or uterine disease.

 Do not take if:

• suffering from liver disease, breast or genital cancer, blood clots.

FORMS

Tablets, vaginal cream, injection.

SIDE EFFECTS

Common: Abnormal uterine bleeding, vaginal thrush, nausea, fluid retention, weight gain, breast tenderness.

Unusual: Rash, blurred vision, vomiting, bloating, intestinal cramps, pigmentation of skin on face.

Severe but rare (stop medication, consult doctor): Blood clots, calf or chest pain, yellow skin (jaundice).

INTERACTIONS

Other drugs:
• Other Sex hormones.
Other substances:
• Smoking increases risk of serious side effects.

PRESCRIPTION

Yes

PERMITTED IN SPORT

Yes

OVERDOSE

Vomiting and abnormal vaginal bleeding only likely effects.

OTHER INFORMATION

Does not cause addiction or dependence. Very useful in managing the effects of menopause, and reduces the risk of osteoporosis and heart disease after the menopause.

See also Estropipate

Oestrone

TRADE NAME

Only used in combination with other forms of oestrogen.

Hormonin (with Oestradiol, Oestriol).

DRUG CLASS

Sex Hormone.

USES

Oestrogen (female hormone) replacement in menopause.

DOSAGE

 One or two tablets a day, continuously or cyclically.

FORMS

Tablets (pink).

PRECAUTIONS

Not to be used in pregnancy (B1), breast feeding or children. Accidental usage in these situations unlikely to be harmful.

Use with caution in epilepsy, migraine, heart failure, high blood pressure, kidney disease, diabetes, porphyria or uterine disease.

 Do not take if:
• suffering from liver disease, breast or genital cancer, blood clots.

SIDE EFFECTS

Common: Abnormal uterine bleeding, vaginal thrush, nausea, fluid retention, weight gain, breast tenderness.

Unusual: Rash, blurred vision, vomiting, bloating, intestinal cramps, pigmentation of skin on face.

Severe but rare (stop medication, consult doctor): Blood clots, calf or chest pain, yellow skin (jaundice).

INTERACTIONS

Other drugs:

• Other Sex hormones.

Other substances:

• Smoking increases risk of serious side effects.

PRESCRIPTION

Yes

PERMITTED IN SPORT

Yes

OVERDOSE

Vomiting and abnormal vaginal bleeding only likely effects.

Ofloxacin

TRADE NAMES

Exocin, Tarivid.

DRUG CLASS

Quinolone antibiotic.

USES

Severe bacterial infections.

DOSAGE

 Tablets: One tablet three times a day.
Eye drops: One drop in affected eye(s) every four to six hours for maximum of ten days.

FORMS

Tablets of 200mg. (off white), 400mg. (yellow), eye drops.

PRECAUTIONS

Use with caution in pregnancy (B3), breast feeding and children.

Use with caution in diabetes, syphilis, tuberculosis, epilepsy, brain disorders, liver and kidney disease.

Ensure adequate hydration.

Not for prolonged use.

SIDE EFFECTS

Common: Fever, rash, inflammation of veins, inflammation of lungs, liver and kidney stress, dizziness, drowsiness,

Unusual: Psychosis, brain pressure and stimulation, persistent diarrhoea, sensitivity to light, weakening of tendons, vomiting.

Severe but rare (stop medication, consult doctor): Seizures, jaundice.

INTERACTIONS

Other drugs:

• Antacids, zinc, cyclosporin, cimetidine, NSAIDs, probenecid, warfarin, theophylline, other antibiotics.

PRESCRIPTION

Yes

PERMITTED IN SPORT

Yes

OVERDOSE

Serious exacerbation of side effects likely. Administer activated charcoal or induce vomiting if tablets taken recently. Seek urgent medical attention.

OTHER INFORMATION

Introduced in 1997 for the treatment of serious infections unresponsive to other antibiotics.

See also Ciprofloxacin.

Olanzapine

TRADE NAME

Zyprexa.

DRUG CLASS

Antipsychotic.

USES

Schizophrenia, psychoses, dementia, other psychiatric conditions.

DOSAGE

 2.5 to 20mg. once a day. Increase dose slowly.

FORMS

Tablets of 2.5mg., 5mg., 7.5mg. and 10mg.

PRECAUTIONS

Use with caution in pregnancy (B3), breast feeding and children.

Use with caution in enlarged prostate gland, glaucoma, poor small bowel function, epilepsy, kidney and liver disease.

Regular blood tests to check function of blood cells and bone marrow necessary.

 Do not take if:

- leukaemia, bone marrow disease.

SIDE EFFECTS

Common: Sleepiness, tiredness, weight gain, dizziness, low blood pressure, swelling of feet and hands, dry mouth.

Unusual: Liver damage, poor coordination, breast milk production.

Severe but rare (stop medication, consult doctor): Severe infection, jaundice (yellow skin).

INTERACTIONS

Other drugs:

- Drugs affecting heart function, drugs acting on the brain, carbamazepine.

Other substances:

- Alcohol, smoking.

PRESCRIPTION

Yes

PERMITTED IN SPORT

Yes

OVERDOSE

Serious exacerbation of side effects likely. Induce vomiting or administer activated charcoal if taken recently. Seek urgent medical attention.

OTHER INFORMATION

Extraordinarily effective drug introduced in 1997 for the treatment of the more difficult forms of schizophrenia and behaviour problems associated with dementia.

Olsalazine

TRADE NAME

Dipentum.

USES

Treatment of complicated cases of ulcerative colitis.

PRECAUTIONS

Should be used with caution in pregnancy (B2) and breast feeding.

Should be used with caution in severe kidney disease.

DOSAGE

 250 to 1000mg. three times a day after meals.

FORMS

Capsule of 250mg. (light brown), tablets of 500mg. (yellow).

SIDE EFFECTS

Common: Diarrhoea (very common), nausea, belly pains.

Unusual: Rash, headache, joint pains.

Severe but rare (stop medication, consult doctor): Many rare and serious effects reported including blood cell abnormalities and liver damage.

INTERACTIONS

Other drugs:

• Anticoagulants.

PRESCRIPTION

Yes

PERMITTED IN SPORT

Yes

OTHER INFORMATION

Used in only very special circumstances in the uncommon condition of ulcerative colitis.

Omeprazole

See PROTON PUMP INHIBITORS

Ondansetron

TRADE NAME

Zofran.

USES

Stops nausea and vomiting caused by cancer treating drugs, radiotherapy or surgery.

DOSAGE

 One to four tablets twice a day.

FORMS

Tablets (yellow) of 4mg., syrup, soluble tablet of 4mg., suppositories, injection.

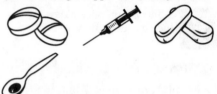

PRECAUTIONS

May be used with caution in pregnancy (B1), breast feeding and children over 4 years.

Use with caution in liver disease.

SIDE EFFECTS

Common: Hot flush, headache, upper belly discomfort.

Unusual: Dry mouth, constipation.

INTERACTIONS

None significant.

PRESCRIPTION

Yes

PERMITTED IN SPORT

Yes

OVERDOSE

Exacerbation of side effects likely.

OTHER INFORMATION

Introduced in 1993 to relieve the severe vomiting that may be caused by some anti-cancer drugs. More effective if given by injection.

OPIATES (Narcotics)

(Pain killing drugs derived from opium)

See Alfentanil, Buprenorphine, Codeine, Dextromoramide, Dextropropoxyphene, Ethoheptazine, Fentanyl, Heroin, Hydromorphone, Methadone, Morphine, Nalbuphine, Oxycodone, Pentazocine, Pethidine, Phenazocine

ORAL CONTRACEPTIVES (CONTRACEPTIVE PILLS)

TRADE and GENERIC NAMES

In this section, the various oral contraceptive pills are divided into groups, depending on:

Whether they contain:-
• two hormones (combined Oestrogen and Progestogen).

• one hormone (Progestogen only mini pill) .

Whether the dosage:
• does not vary (monophasic) during the month

• varies twice (biphasic) during the month

• varies three times (triphasic) during the month.

MONOPHASIC COMBINED OESTROGEN AND PROGESTOGEN PILLS:

Brevinor, Loestrin, Norimin, Ovysmen (Ethinyloestradiol, Norethisterone).

Cilest (Ethinyloestradiol, Norgestimate).

Femodene, Femodette, Minulet (Ethinyloestradiol, Gestodene).

Dianette (Cyproterone acetate, Ethinyloestradiol).

Eugynon 30, Microgynon 30, Ovran, Ovranette (Ethinyloestradiol, Levonorgestrol).

Marvelon, Mercilon (Desogestrel, Ethinyloestradiol).

Norinyl-1 (Mestranol, Norethisterone).

BIPHASIC COMBINED OESTROGEN AND PROGESTOGEN PILLS:-
Binovum (Ethinyloestradiol, Norethisterone).

TRIPHASIC COMBINED OESTROGEN AND PROGESTOGEN PILLS:
Synphase, Trinovum (Ethinyloestradiol, Norethisterone).

Logynon, Trinordiol (Ethinyloestradiol, Levonorgestrol).

Triminulet, Triadene (Gestodene, Ethinyloestradiol).

PROGESTOGEN ONLY (MINI) PILLS:
Femulen (Etynodiol diacetate).

Microval, Norgeston (Levonorgestrol).

Micronor, Noriday (Norethisterone).

Neogest (Norgestrel).

DRUG CLASS

Sex hormones

USES

Prevention of pregnancy, control of irregular or painful menstrual cycle (combined forms only), control of acne in women (**Dianette** particularly).

DOSAGE

 One tablet a day on the day indicated on the pack for 21 or 28 days a month. May fail as a contraceptive if Progestogen only pill missed by more than three hours of normal time of taking, if low dose combined pill missed by more than eight hours of normal time, if medium dose combined pill missed by more than twelve hours of normal time, or if high dose combined pill missed for more than 24 hours of normal time.

FORMS

Tablets.

PRECAUTIONS

Not for use in pregnancy (B3), but serious effects from taking oral contraceptive accidentally during pregnancy are unlikely. Progestogen only pills are recommended during breast feeding, but low dose combined pills may be used if necessary. Should be kept out of reach of children, and are obviously not for use in children, although accidental usage by children is unlikely to be serious.

Use with caution in heart disease, history of blood clots, epilepsy, migraine, diabetes, severe depression and sickle cell anaemia.

Not to be used in pubertal girls until menstruation well established.

Diarrhoea, vomiting or use of antibiotics may affect contraceptive action.

Do not take if:

- suffering from high blood pressure, blood clots, stroke, very high cholesterol blood levels, severe liver disease, Dubin-Johnson syndrome, liver tumour, systemic lupus erythematosus, sex organ or breast cancer, jaundice, otosclerosis or severe skin irritation..

- male.

SIDE EFFECTS

Common: Nausea, pigmentation of facial skin and nipples, headache, breast tenderness, weight change (up or down).

Unusual: Depression, increased sex drive, break through bleeding.

Severe but rare (stop medication, consult doctor): Severe headache, blood clot, calf or chest pain, severe shortness of breath, yellow skin (jaundice).

INTERACTIONS

Other drugs:

- Antibiotics, Phenytoin, Primidone, Barbiturates, Rifampicin, Anticoagulants, medications that treat diabetes, Imipramine.

Other substances:

- Smoking increases risk of serious side effects.

PRESCRIPTION

Yes

PERMITTED IN SPORT

Yes

OVERDOSE

Vomiting and abnormal vaginal bleeding only likely effects.

OTHER INFORMATION

Introduced in the late 1950s, the oral contraceptive has revolutionised sexual mores and liberated women from unwanted pregnancies. Very safe and effective if taken as directed. Regular gynaecological examinations, Pap smears, breast checks and blood pressure checks recommended. If a contraceptive pill is missed, take the missed pill with the next remembered pill, continue taking the pill, but use other forms of contraception (eg: condoms) for the next seven days, but if this seven day period extends into the inactive (sugar) pill section of the pack or into the pill free days of a 21 day pack, do not take the inactive pills or have a break, but continue with the next active pill in a new pack.

See also Morning After Pill

Orciprenaline

TRADE NAME

Alupent.

DRUG CLASS

Bronchodilator.

USES

Asthma, bronchitis.

DOSAGE

 Inhaler: One or two inhalations three or four times a day.
Tablets: One four times a day.

FORMS

Inhaler, tablet of 20mg. (off white), syrup.

PRECAUTIONS

Safe to use in pregnancy (A), breast feeding and older children.

Use with caution in high blood pressure, heart disease, diabetes and labour of pregnancy.

Tolerance may develop with overuse.

 Do not take if:

- suffering from irregular or rapid heart beat, aortic disease or overactive thyroid gland.

SIDE EFFECTS

Common: Palpitations, tremor, restlessness, flush, headache.

Unusual: Nausea, giddiness, sleeplessness.

Severe but rare (stop medication, consult doctor): Chest pain (angina).

INTERACTIONS

Other drugs:

- Sympathomimetics, Beta-Blockers, MAOI.

Other substances:

- Caffeine and alcohol.

PRESCRIPTION

Yes

PERMITTED IN SPORT

No

OVERDOSE

Exacerbation of side effects likely. These may become distressing and may be serious in patients with heart disease or high blood pressure.

OTHER INFORMATION

One of the early treatments for asthma that is no longer widely used.

Orlistat

TRADE NAME

Xenical.

USES

Treatment of obesity.

PRECAUTIONS

Use with caution in pregnancy (B1) and children.

Use with caution with peptic ulcers, psychiatric disturbances, adhesions in belly, kidney stones, serious heart, liver and kidney disease.

 Do not take if:

- breast feeding

- suffering from pancreatitis or some types of gall bladder disease.

- normal or under weight.

DOSAGE

 One tablet three times a day with meals.

FORMS

Capsules (turquoise) of 120mg.

SIDE EFFECTS

Common: Diarrhoea (worse if fat eaten), flatulence, liquid faeces, headache.

Unusual: Incontinence of faeces, nausea, indigestion, bowel noises, anal irritation, dizziness, muscle pains.

Severe but rare (stop medication, consult doctor): Liver damage.

INTERACTIONS

Other drugs:

• Cyclosporin, pravastatin.

PRESCRIPTION

Yes

PERMITTED IN SPORT

Yes

OVERDOSE

Unlikely to be serious.

OTHER INFORMATION

Introduced 2000 as a totally new type of anti-obesity drug that acts by preventing the absorption of fat from the intestine.

See also Methylcellulose.

Orphenadrine

TRADE NAMES

Biorphen, Disipal.

DRUG CLASS

Antiparkinsonian, Muscle relaxant.

USES

Parkinsonism, severe dizziness, other movement disorders, muscle spasm.

DOSAGE

 One to three tablets, three times a day with food.

FORMS

Tablets, solution.

PRECAUTIONS

Should be used with caution in pregnancy (B2) and breast feeding. Not for use in children.

Use with caution with rapid heart rate and heart disease.

Use short term if possible.

 Do not take if:

• suffering from glaucoma, myasthenia gravis, enlarged prostate gland.

SIDE EFFECTS

Common: Minimal. Dry mouth, blurred vision, light headedness.

Unusual: Excitation.

INTERACTIONS

None significant.

PRESCRIPTION

Yes

PERMITTED IN SPORT

Yes

OVERDOSE

May cause excitement, confusion, convulsions, rapid heart rate, inability to pass urine and coma. Administer activated charcoal or induce vomiting if medication taken recently. Seek medical assistance.

OTHER INFORMATION

Does not cause addiction or dependence.

Oxazepam

See ANXIOLYTICS

Oxcarbazepine

TRADE NAME

Trileptal.

DRUG CLASS

Antiepileptic.

USES

Partial epileptic seizures.

DOSAGE

 300 to 1200mg. twice a day.

PRECAUTIONS

Not to be used in pregnancy or breast feeding.

May be used in children over six years of age.

Use with caution in kidney and heart disease.

Use lower doses in elderly.

Regular blood tests to measure sodium levels necessary.

Reduce dosage slowly, do not stop suddenly.

FORMS

Tablets of 150, 300 and 600mg.

SIDE EFFECTS

Common: Tiredness, nausea.

Unusual: Bowel disturbances, visual disturbances, skin rashes.

Severe but rare (stop medication, consult doctor): Altered blood sodium levels.

INTERACTIONS

Other drugs:

• Diuretics, NSAID's, oral contraceptives, phenytoin, phenobarb, MAOI, Lithium.

Other substances:

• Alcohol.

PRESCRIPTION

Yes

PERMITTED IN SPORT

Yes

OTHER INFORMATION

Introduced in 1999 to treat more difficult cases of epilepsy.

Oxerutin

TRADE NAME

Paroven.

PRECAUTIONS

Safe in all but first three months of pregnancy. Safe in breast feeding. Not recommended in children.

Eat diet high in fibre and protein.

USES

Poor arterial and venous circulation, swelling of ankles and other tissue, varicose veins, piles, night cramps.

DOSAGE

 Two capsules twice a day.

FORMS

Capsules of 250mg. (yellow).

SIDE EFFECTS

Common: Minimal

Unusual: Nausea, indigestion, constipation, diarrhoea, flushes, headache.

INTERACTIONS

None significant

PRESCRIPTION

No

PERMITTED IN SPORT

Yes

OVERDOSE

Constipation only likely effect.

OTHER INFORMATION

Successfully used for for many years to prevent tired aching legs, particularly in women who must stand for a long period of time in their work. Very safe. Does not cause dependence.

Oxethazine

See ANTACIDS

Oxitropium

TRADE NAME

Oxivent.

DRUG CLASS

Anticholinergic.

USES

Asthma, emphysema, chronic obstructive airways disease.

DOSAGE

 Two inhalations, two or three times a day.

FORMS

Inhaler, autohaler.

PRECAUTIONS

Not for use in pregnancy, breast feeding and children.

Use with caution in glaucoma, prostate enlargement.

Avoid eyes.

Cease if wheeze or cough worsens.

SIDE EFFECTS

Common: Local mouth irritation.

Unusual: Nausea, dry mouth.

INTERACTIONS

None significant.

PRESCRIPTION

Yes

PERMITTED IN SPORT

Yes

OVERDOSE

Exacerbation of side effects only likely consequence.

OTHER INFORMATION

Not addictive.

See also Ipratropium.

Oxpentifylline

TRADE NAME

Trental.

USES

Poor arterial circulation to legs and arms.

DOSAGE

 One tablet three times a day with meals and liquid.

FORMS

Tablet of 400mg. (pink).

SIDE EFFECTS

Common: Nausea, heartburn, burping, dizziness, headache, flushing, palpitations.

Unusual: Vomiting, tremor, shortness of breath, loss of appetite, anxiety, nose bleed, brittle finger nails, blurred vision, bad taste.

Severe but rare (stop medication, consult doctor): Unusual bleeding.

INTERACTIONS

Other drugs:

• Warfarin, Hypoglycaemics.

PRESCRIPTION

Yes

PERMITTED IN SPORT

Yes

PRECAUTIONS

Should be used with caution in pregnancy, breast feeding and in children.

Should be used with caution in low blood pressure, kidney and liver disease.

Lower dose may be required in elderly.

 Do not take if:

• suffering from heart attack, peptic ulcer or excessive bleeding.

OVERDOSE

Flushing, low blood pressure, convulsions, fever and coma may occur. No deaths reported. Seek medical assistance.

OTHER INFORMATION

Unique drug that works by making cells slip more easily through the smallest capillaries. Introduced in the 1980s, it has had only limited use because of its cost, despite excellent clinical results.

Oxprenolol
See BETA BLOCKERS

Oxybuprocaine
See ANAESTHETICS, LOCAL

Oxybutinin

TRADE NAMES

Cystrin, Ditropan.

DRUG CLASS

Anticholinergic.

USES

Relieves some forms of difficulty in passing urine caused by muscle spasm.

DOSAGE

 One tablet two or three times a day.

FORMS

Tablet of 2.5, 3 and 5mg., elixir.

PRECAUTIONS

Use with caution in pregnancy (B1), and children under five years. Not to be used in breast feeding, as breast milk production may be reduced.

Use with caution in hot climates.

Avoid vigorous exercise while using Oxybutinin.

Use with caution in ulcerative colitis, reflux oesophagitis, over active thyroid gland, heart disease, high blood pressure, enlarged prostate gland, liver and kidney disease.

Regular consultations with doctor necessary to monitor bladder function.

 Do not take if:

• suffering from glaucoma, gut obstruction, megacolon, myasthenia gravis, acute bleeding.

SIDE EFFECTS

Common: Palpitations, rapid heart rate, decreased sweating, constipation, dry mouth, nausea, dizziness.

Unusual: Impotence, rash, drowsiness, hallucinations, dry eyes.

INTERACTIONS

Other drugs:

• Sedatives, other Anticholinergics.

Other substances:

• Reacts adversely with alcohol.

PRESCRIPTION

Yes

PERMITTED IN SPORT

Yes

OVERDOSE

Serious. Symptoms may include restlessness, irrational behaviour, flushing, low blood pressure, difficulty in breathing, paralysis, coma and death. Administer activated charcoal or induce vomiting if medication taken recently and patient alert. Seek urgent medical assistance.

OTHER INFORMATION

Does not cause addiction or dependence. Released in 1994.

Oxycodone

TRADE NAMES

OxyContin, OxyNorm.

DRUG CLASS

Narcotic, Analgesic.

USES

Moderate to severe pain.

DOSAGE

 One tablet every six to twelve hours with food.

FORMS

Tablets, solution.

PRECAUTIONS

Should be used in pregnancy (C) only if medically essential as use of Oxycodone immediately before birth may cause difficulty in breathing for the infant. Use with caution in breast feeding. Not for use in children.

Not designed for prolonged use except in patients with terminal disease.

Do not stop suddenly, but reduce dosage slowly.

Use with caution in severe lung disease, myasthenia gravis, underactive thyroid gland, liver and kidney disease, enlarged prostate gland, shock or bowel obstruction.

Lower doses necessary in elderly and debilitated patients.

Do not take if:

- suffering from severe asthma, irregular heart beat, brain tumour, alcoholism, head injury, convulsions.
- operating machinery or driving a vehicle.

SIDE EFFECTS

Common: Nausea, constipation, drowsiness, confusion.

Unusual: Vomiting, difficulty in passing urine, dry mouth, sweating, flushing, faintness, loss of appetite, dizziness, slow heart rate, mood changes.

Severe but rare (stop medication, consult doctor): Severe headache, convulsions, difficulty in breathing.

INTERACTIONS

Other drugs:

- MAOI, Amphetamines, Chlorpromazine, Sedatives, Antihistamines, Beta blockers, Anticoagulants.

Other substances:

- Do not use alcohol with Oxycodone.

PRESCRIPTION

Yes (restricted)

PERMITTED IN SPORT

No

OVERDOSE

Very serious. Symptoms may include drowsiness, difficulty in breathing, muscle weakness, coma, heart failure and death. Administer activated charcoal or induce vomiting if medication taken recently and patient alert. Seek urgent medical attention. Antidote available.

OTHER INFORMATION

May cause addiction if taken inappropriately for long periods of time.

Oxymetholone

DRUG CLASS

Anabolic steroid.

USES

Used dangerously and in an unapproved manner by body builders and athletes.

PRECAUTIONS

Must not be used in pregnancy (D) or breast feeding.

Use with caution in heart disease, enlarged prostate gland, diabetes.

Do not take if:

- suffering from prostate and testicular cancer, breast cancer, liver and kidney disease.

SIDE EFFECTS

Common: Increased hairiness and decreased breast size in women, voice deepening in women, acne, frequent unwanted erections, infertility.

Unusual: Anaemia, enlargement of clitoris in women, cessation of menstrual periods, decrease in testicular size, impotence, breast enlargement in males, baldness in females, reduced libido.

Severe but rare (stop medication, consult doctor): Unusual bruising or bleeding, calcium deposits (lumps) in tissue, jaundice (yellow skin).

INTERACTIONS

Other drugs:

• Anticoagulants.

PRESCRIPTION

Not legally available.

PERMITTED IN SPORT

No. Although increasing muscle bulk, there is no evidence that this medication enhances athletic ability. Long term inappropriate use may cause permanent damage to the body.

OVERDOSE

Exacerbation of side effects likely.

OTHER INFORMATION

Illegal drug, but imported and used by some body builders and sportsmen. Does not cause dependence or addiction. Short term gains in muscle bulk when used inappropriately may result in long term permanent body damage that may lead to early heart attacks, infertility, bone weakness, liver disease and, premature death. Bottom line is - don't use it.

Oxytetracycline

See TETRACYCLINES

Oxytocin

TRADE NAMES

Syntocinon.
Syntometrine (with Ergometrine).

USES

Starting labour in pregnancy, stopping abnormal bleeding after delivery.

DOSAGE

 As determined by doctor. May be given by drip infusion.

FORMS

Injection.

PRECAUTIONS

Safe to use for induction of labour in pregnancy (A), but should not otherwise be used in pregnancy. Safe for use in breast feeding. Not for use in children.

Use with caution in heart disease.

Do not take injection if:

• previous Caesarean section.

SIDE EFFECTS

Common: Rapid heart rate, retention of fluid.

PRESCRIPTION

Yes

PERMITTED IN SPORT

Yes

OVERDOSE

Unlikely to have serious effects.

OTHER INFORMATION

Injection commonly used to increase intensity of labour and immediately after delivery to reduce bleeding.

Paclitaxel

TRADE NAME

Taxol.

DRUG CLASS

Antimetabolite.

USES

Cancer of the breast and ovaries.

DOSAGE

 As determined by doctor for each patient.

FORMS

Injection.

PRECAUTIONS

Must not be used in pregnancy (D) or children. Use with caution in breast feeding.

Regular blood tests to check function of blood cells essential.

Use with caution in neuropathy (nerve disease).

SIDE EFFECTS

Common: Flushes, rash, shortness of breath, chest pain, fainting, joint and muscle pain

Unusual: Low blood pressure, slow heart rate, damage to nerves Pins and needles sensation, numbness), damage to liver.

Severe but rare (stop medication, consult doctor): Jaundice (yellow skin).

INTERACTIONS

Other drugs:

• Sex hormones.

PRESCRIPTION

Yes

PERMITTED IN SPORT

Yes

OVERDOSE

Serious damage to bone marrow and nerves likely.

Pamidronate

(Disodium pamidronate)

TRADE NAME

Aredia.

DRUG CLASS

Bisphosphonate.

USES

High blood calcium levels, Paget's disease, bone secondary cancer, multiple myeloma.

DOSAGE

 As determined by doctor.

FORMS

Intravenous infusion.

PRECAUTIONS

Use with caution in pregnancy (B3) and breast feeding. Not for use in children.

Not to be injected into muscle or quickly into vein.

Use with caution in hyperparathyroidism, kidney and heart disease.

Regular blood tests to check calcium, and phosphate levels, and kidney function, necessary.

SIDE EFFECTS

Common: Low blood calcium, fever, other biochemical abnormalities, muscle pain, nausea, diarrhoea.

Unusual: Vomiting, headache, drowsiness.

Severe but rare (stop medication, consult doctor): Seizures, damaged blood cells, fluid in lungs, high or low blood pressure, heart failure, kidney failure.

INTERACTIONS

Other drugs:

• Other bisphosphonates.

PRESCRIPTION

Yes

PERMITTED IN SPORT

Yes

Pancreatin

TRADE NAMES

Creon, Nutizym, Pancrease, Pancrex.

USES

Deficiency of pancreatic enzymes due to disease (eg: cystic fibrosis, chronic pancreatitis) or surgery.

DOSAGE

 Taken with each meal in sufficient quantity to adequately digest food. Dosage varies for each person.

FORMS

Capsules, tablets, pellets.

PRECAUTIONS

Safe in pregnancy, breast feeding and children.

 Do not take if:

• suffering from acute pancreatitis.

SIDE EFFECTS

Common: Minimal. Usually dose related.

Unusual: Nausea, diarrhoea, passing excess wind, mouth soreness.

INTERACTIONS

Other drugs:

• Antacids.

PRESCRIPTION

No

PERMITTED IN SPORT

Yes

OVERDOSE

Diarrhoea only likely effect.

OTHER INFORMATION

Totally natural products used to replace a missing digestive enzyme.

See also Tilactase.

Panthenol

See Pantothenic Acid

Pantoprazole

See PROTON PUMP INHIBITORS

Pantothenic acid

(Panthenol, Vitamin B5)

TRADE NAMES

A large number of preparations include Pantothenic acid (Vitamin B5) or its derivative Panthenol, alone or in combination with other vitamins and minerals.

DRUG CLASS

Vitamin.

USES

Vitamin B deficiency.

Cream used for mild burns, nappy rash and sore nipples.

DOSAGE

 Recommended daily allowance: 4 to 7 mg a day.
Apply creams several times a day as required.

FORMS

Tablets, capsules, mixtures, drops, creams.

PRECAUTIONS

Safe in pregnancy, breast feeding and children.

Do not take in high doses or for prolonged periods of time.

SIDE EFFECTS

Minimal.

INTERACTIONS

None significant.

PRESCRIPTION

No

PERMITTED IN SPORT

Yes

OVERDOSE

Unlikely to have serious adverse effects.

OTHER INFORMATION

Pantothenic acid is a water soluble vitamin. Remember, vitamins are merely chemicals that are essential for the functioning of the body, and if taken to excess, act as a drug.

Paracetamol

(Acetaminophen)

TRADE and GENERIC NAMES

Alvedon, Calpol, Disprol, Infadrops, Medinol.

Distalgesic (with Dextropropoxyphene).

Domperamol (with Domperidone).

Fortagesic (with Pentazocine).

Kapake, Solpadol, Tylex (with Codeine).

Midrid (with Isometheptene).

Migraleve (with Buclizine, Codeine).

Paradote (with Methionine).

Paramax (with Metoclopramide).

Remedeine (with Dihydrocodeine).

DRUG CLASS

Analgesic.

USES

Mild to moderate pain relief, fever.

DOSAGE

 One or two tablets every three or four hours. Other forms as directed by directions on packaging, doctor or pharmacist.

FORMS

Tablets, capsules, soluble tablets, chewable tablets, mixture, drops, suppository, powder.

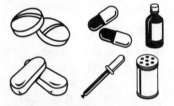

PRECAUTIONS

Safe in pregnancy (A), breast feeding, children and infants over one month of age.

Use with caution in severe liver and kidney disease.

SIDE EFFECTS

Common: Minimal.

Unusual: Nausea, rash.

INTERACTIONS

Other drugs:

• Anticoagulants, Metoclopramide, Propantheline, Antidepressants, Narcotics, Anticonvulsants.

PRESCRIPTION

No.

Prescription required in some forms combined with narcotics.

PERMITTED IN SPORT

Yes

OVERDOSE

Very serious, particularly in children. Symptoms may include vomiting, belly pain and sweating. Delayed effect can be serious liver damage that may cause liver failure, jaundice and death. Administer activated charcoal or induce vomiting if medication taken recently. Seek urgent medical attention. Antidote is methionine.

OTHER INFORMATION

The most widely used pain killer in the world. Very effective, and often underrated in its effectiveness. Extremely safe if taken according to directions. Up to eight tablets a day can be taken for years on end. Found in a wide variety of cold and flu preparations. Paracetamol is given the generic name Acetaminophen in the United States.

Paraffin

TRADE NAME

Alcoderm, E45 Wash, Keri, Oilatum Emollient, Oilatum Gel.

Diprobath, Epaderm, Hydromol, Ultrabase, Unguentum M (with other ingredients).

E45 Bath Oil (with Dimethicone).

Alpha Keri, E45 Cream, E45 Lotion (with Lanolin).

Polytar (with Tar, Arachis oil and other ingredients).

Dermol (with Chlorhexidine, Bezalkonium chloride and other ingredients).

Diprobase (with Cetomacrogol and other ingredients).

Emulsiderm (with Benzalkonium chloride and other ingredients).

Imuderm, Infaderm (with Almond oil).

Lipobase (with Cetomacrogol).

Lacri-Lube, Lubri-Tears (with wool fat).

Oilatum Plus (with Triclosan, Benzalkonium chloride).

Also used as a lubricant in many other skin and eye preparations.

DRUG CLASS

Lubricant, moisturiser, laxative.

USES

Skin dryness, skin itch, eye dryness, vaginal dryness, constipation.

DOSAGE

 Use externally as often as necessary.

FORMS

Cream, oil, lotion, wash, liquid.

PRECAUTIONS

May be used in pregnancy (B2), breast feeding and children.

Should be used long term as a laxative only under medical advice.

SIDE EFFECTS

Minimal.

INTERACTIONS

None significant.

PRESCRIPTION

No

PERMITTED IN SPORT

Yes

OVERDOSE

Diarrhoea only effect if swallowed.

OTHER INFORMATION

Safe and widely used laxative that has been available for thousands of years. White soft paraffin and liquid paraffin are used in many creams as a vehicle for other medications.

See also EYE LUBRICANTS

Paroxetine

TRADE NAME

Seroxat.

DRUG CLASS

SSRI antidepressant.

USES

Depression.

DOSAGE

 One or two tablets a day in morning with food.

FORMS

Tablet of 20mg. (white) and 30mg. (blue), liquid.

PRECAUTIONS

Should be used in pregnancy (B3) with considerable caution. Breast feeding should be ceased if Paroxetine prescribed. Not for use in children.

Should be used with caution in mania, epilepsy and heart disease.

Should not be stopped suddenly, but dose should be slowly reduced over several days.

 Do not take if:
• taking MAOI antidepressants.

SIDE EFFECTS

Common: Generally minimal. Nausea, drowsiness, sweating, tremor, tiredness, dry mouth, sleeplessness, impotence.

Unusual: Headache, fever, palpitations, sweating, rash, blurred vision.

INTERACTIONS

Other drugs:

• MAOI

• Anticoagulants, Phenytoin, Tryptophan.

Other substances:

• Use of alcohol with Paroxetine is not advised.

PRESCRIPTION

Yes

PERMITTED IN SPORT

Yes

OVERDOSE

Symptoms may include nausea, tremor, dilated pupils, dry mouth and irritability. Death or serious effects have not occurred. Seek medical attention.

OTHER INFORMATION

One of the newer antidepressants released in the 1990s that has dramatically improved the treatment of depression because of its safety and lack of side effects. May take up to two weeks for patient to notice any improvement in depression.

Pectin

TRADE NAME

Orabase, Orahesive (with Carmellose and other ingredients).

Also found in some locally produced antidiarrhoeal medications.

DRUG CLASS

Fibre.

USES

Mild diarrhoea, mouth and other ulcers.

DOSAGE

 Apply to ulcer as required. Take as required to control diarrhoea.

FORMS

Powder, ointment, liquid.

PRECAUTIONS

Safe in pregnancy, breast feeding and children.

Use with caution in reduced intestinal absorption.

SIDE EFFECTS

Minimal.

INTERACTIONS

Other drugs:

• May affect absorption of some drugs (eg: digoxin) if swallowed.

PRESCRIPTION

No

PERMITTED IN SPORT

Yes

OVERDOSE

Not likely to be harmful if excess swallowed.

OTHER INFORMATION

Derived from apple fibre.

Penciclovir

TRADE NAME

Vectavir.

DRUG CLASS

Antiviral.

USES

Cold sores, Herpes simplex infections.

DOSAGE

 Apply every two hours from first sign of infection.

FORMS

Cream.

PRECAUTIONS

May be used in pregnancy (B1), breast feeding and children over 12 years.

Use with caution in infants.

Avoid contact with eyes, inside of mouth, nostrils and other moist membranes.

 Do not take if:

* suffering from immune deficiency.

SIDE EFFECTS

Minimal.

INTERACTIONS

None significant.

PRESCRIPTION

Yes

PERMITTED IN SPORT

Yes

Penicillamine

TRADE NAME

Distamine.

USES

Severe rheumatoid arthritis, Wilson's disease, cystinuria, heavy metal poisoning (eg: lead).

DOSAGE

 Rheumatoid disease: One or two tablets, one to three times a day. Other conditions: Up to 2000mg a day depending upon severity and response.

FORMS

Tablets (white) of 125mg. and 250mg.

PRECAUTIONS

Must not be used in pregnancy (D) unless essential for the life of the mother. Breast feeding should be ceased before use. May be used in children when medically indicated.

Use with caution in liver disease, brain disorders.

Avoid surgery if possible. Regular blood tests essential.

Regular checks of skin, eyes and temperature necessary.

Ensure adequate vitamin B intake.

Patient must be made aware of the adverse effects of this medication before use.

 Do not take if:

* using Gold or Chloroquine.

SIDE EFFECTS

Common: Rash, fever, joint pains, enlarged glands, itch.

Unusual: Hair loss, ringing noise in ears, abnormal blood tests, nausea, loss of appetite, vomiting, diarrhoea, blood clots, taste changes.

Severe but rare (stop medication, consult doctor): Significant rash, severe belly pain, yellow skin (jaundice), vision disturbances, unusual bleeding or bruising.

INTERACTIONS

Other drugs:

• Gold, Chloroquine, Isoniazid.

PRESCRIPTION

Yes

PERMITTED IN SPORT

Yes

OVERDOSE

May cause permanent organ damage. Administer activated charcoal or induce vomiting if medication taken recently. Seek medical attention.

OTHER INFORMATION

Although it has serious side effects, Penicillamine may give great relief to sufferers of severe rheumatoid arthritis, and may be life saving in heavy metal poisoning. Risks minimal if taken under close supervision of a competent physician.

PENICILLINS

See Amoxycillin, Ampicillin, Cloxacillin, Flucloxacillin, Penicillin G, Piperacillin, Pivmecillinam, Ticarcillin

Penicillin G

(Benzyl Penicillin)

TRADE NAME

Crystapen

DRUG CLASS

Penicillin antibiotic.

USES

Treatment of infections caused by susceptible bacteria.

DOSAGE

 Two to four injections a day, or by drip into a vein.

FORMS

Injection.

PRECAUTIONS

Safe in pregnancy (A), children and breast feeding.

Use with caution in kidney failure and leukaemia.

 Do not take if:

• allergic to Penicillin

• suffering from glandular fever

SIDE EFFECTS

Common: Mild diarrhoea, nausea, vomiting.

Unusual: Fever, headache, dizziness, hot flushes, tiredness, black tongue.

Severe but rare (stop medication, consult doctor): Itchy rash, hives, severe diarrhoea, yellow skin (jaundice), muscle pains, throat tightness.

INTERACTIONS

None significant

PRESCRIPTION

Yes

PERMITTED IN SPORT

Yes

OVERDOSE

Not life threatening unless allergic to Penicillin. Vomiting and diarrhoea only likely effects.

OTHER INFORMATION

One of the older types of Penicillin. Does not cause dependence or addiction.

Pentazocine

(Pentazocine hydrochloride and Pentazocine lactate)

TRADE NAMES

Fortral.

Fortagesic (with Paracetamol).

DRUG CLASS

Narcotic, Analgesic.

USES

Moderate to severe pain.

DOSAGE

 25 to 100mg. every three or four hours after food.

FORMS

Fortral: Tablets of 25mg. (white), capsules of 50mg. (yellow/grey), injection.

PRECAUTIONS

Not for use in pregnancy (C) unless medically necessary. May cause difficulty in breathing for the newborn if given in the few hours before birth. Use with caution in breast feeding. May be used in children over one year.

Use with caution in severe kidney disease, severe lung disease, severe liver disease, asthma, thyroid disease, pituitary disease, epilepsy, heart attack or head injury.

 Do not take if:

- Using machinery or driving a vehicle.

SIDE EFFECTS

Common: Nausea, dizziness, sedation, mood changes, headache, sweating.

Unusual: Vomiting, contracted pupils, hallucinations, rapid heart rate.

Severe but rare (stop medication, consult doctor): Difficulty in breathing.

INTERACTIONS

Other drugs:

- MAOI, Sedatives, Tetracycline, Phenytoin.

Other substances:

- Do not use alcohol while taking Pentazocine.

PRESCRIPTION

Yes (restricted).

PERMITTED IN SPORT

No

OVERDOSE

Serious. May cause convulsions, sedation, coma, difficulty in breathing and rarely death. Administer activated charcoal or induce vomiting if medication taken recently and patient alert. Seek urgent medical attention. Antidote available.

OTHER INFORMATION

May cause dependence or addiction if used inappropriately. Available since the late 1960s.

Peppermint oil

TRADE NAMES

Colpermin, Mintec.

Also found in numerous liniments, soothing creams and other medications for indigestion.

DRUG CLASS

Antispasmodic.

USES

Irritable bowel, excess bowel gas, passing excess wind.

DOSAGE

 Take three or four times a day 30 minutes before food as needed.

FORMS

Capsules, tablets.

PRECAUTIONS

Safe to use in pregnancy, breast feeding and children over six years.

SIDE EFFECTS

Common: Minimal.

Unusual: Heartburn, anal irritation, rash.

INTERACTIONS

None significant.

PRESCRIPTION

No

PERMITTED IN SPORT

Yes

OVERDOSE

Exacerbation of side effects likely.

OTHER INFORMATION

Very safe and effective ancient remedy.

Pergolide

TRADE NAME

Celance.

DRUG CLASS

Antiparkinsonian.

USES

Parkinson's disease.

DOSAGE

 Gradually increasing dose taken three times a day until dose adequate to control condition.

FORMS

Tablets of 0.05mg. (white), 0.25mg.(green) and 1mg. (pink).

PRECAUTIONS

Not to be used in pregnancy (C), breast feeding or children.

Use with care in irregular heart beat.

Should not be stopped suddenly, but dosage should be reduced slowly over some weeks.

SIDE EFFECTS

Common: Generalised pain, nausea, incoordination, runny nose, double vision, fainting.

Unusual: Belly pain, hallucinations, tiredness, sleeplessness, shortness of breath.

INTERACTIONS

Other drugs:

• Phenothiazines, Metoclopramide, medications to lower blood pressure.

PRESCRIPTION

Yes

PERMITTED IN SPORT

Yes

OVERDOSE

May cause vomiting, convulsions, fainting, agitation, hallucinations and twitching. Induce vomiting if medication taken recently. Seek medical assistance.

OTHER INFORMATION

Used only in combination with Levodopa compounds. Not addictive. Released in 1993.

Pericyazine

See PHENOTHIAZINES

Perindopril

See ACE INHIBITORS

Permethrin

TRADE NAME

Lyclear.

DRUG CLASS

Antiparasitic.

USES

Head lice, scabies.

DOSAGE

 Lotion: Apply to just washed hair. Leave for ten minutes then rinse out
Cream: Apply to whole body except head and face. Wash off 8 to 12 hours later. Reapply after one week.

FORMS

Cream, lotion

PRECAUTIONS

Use with caution in pregnancy (B2), breast feeding and children. Not for use under six months of age.

Avoid contact with eyes, nostrils, mouth, anus and vagina.

Use with caution in elderly.

SIDE EFFECTS

Common: Skin stinging and burning, itch.

INTERACTIONS

None significant.

PRESCRIPTION

No

PERMITTED IN SPORT

Yes

OVERDOSE

If swallowed may cause alcohol intoxication, belly pain, nausea and vomiting. Seek medical attention.

OTHER INFORMATION

Treat all members of family and other close contacts at same time. Use fine comb repeatedly on hair to remove egg cases. Repeat treatment in one week if necessary.

Perphenazine

See PHENOTHIAZINES

Pertussis Vaccine

See Whooping Cough Vaccine

Pethidine

TRADE NAMES

Pethidine.

Pamergan (with Promethazine).

DRUG CLASS

Narcotic, Analgesic.

USES

Severe pain.

DOSAGE

 As directed by doctor. One or two tablets every three to four hours.

FORMS

Tablets of 50mg., injection.

SIDE EFFECTS

Common: Sedation, constipation, confusion, sweating, nausea, vomiting, loss of appetite.

Unusual: Difficulty passing urine, flushing, dizziness, slow heart rate, irregular heart rate, fainting, mood changes.

Severe but rare (stop medication, consult doctor): Difficulty in breathing, convulsions.

INTERACTIONS

Other drugs:

• MAOI, Sedatives, Pentazocine, Barbiturates, Phenothiazines, Amphetamines, other Narcotics.

Other substances:

• Should not be used with alcohol.

PRECAUTIONS

Should only be used during the later stages of pregnancy (C) if medically essential as it may reduce the desire to breathe in newborn infants. Use with caution in breast feeding. May be used in children.

Use with caution in colic caused by gall stones, pancreatitis, ulcerative colitis, underactive thyroid gland, enlarged prostate gland, head injury and shock.

Do not stop medication suddenly, but reduce dosage slowly.

Lower doses necessary in elderly.

 Do not take if:

• suffering from heart failure, severe head injury, acute diabetes, severe liver disease, severe alcoholism, poor lung function or convulsions.

• operating machinery, driving a vehicle or undertaking tasks requiring concentration.

PRESCRIPTION

Yes (restricted).

PERMITTED IN SPORT

No

OVERDOSE

Serious. Sedation, convulsions, coma and death may occur. Administer activated charcoal or induce vomiting if medication taken recently and patient alert. Seek emergency medical assistance. Antidote available.

OTHER INFORMATION

Highly addictive if used inappropriately. Very effective and unlikely to cause addiction if used appropriately for severe pain. Patients with terminal diseases (eg: cancer) should use dose adequate to control pain, and not be concerned about possibility of addiction. Derived from opium poppy and closely related to morphine and heroin, but not as addictive.

Phenazocine

TRADE NAME

Narphen.

DRUG CLASS

Narcotic, Analgesic.

USES

Severe pain.

DOSAGE

 One or two swallowed or dissolved under tongue every four to six hours.

FORMS

Tablet (white) of 5mg.

PRECAUTIONS

Not for use in pregnancy (except during labour), breast feeding and children.

Use with caution in liver and kidney disease.

Reduce dose in elderly.

 Do not take if:

- suffering from difficulty in breathing, emphysema, alcoholic, a poorly controlled epileptic, underactive thyroid gland.

- comatose.

SIDE EFFECTS

Common: Dizziness, nausea, constipation.

Unusual: Tolerance to dose.

Severe but rare (stop medication, consult doctor): Difficulty in breathing.

INTERACTIONS

Other drugs:

- MAOI, sedatives.

Other substances:

- Alcohol.

PRESCRIPTION

Yes (restricted).

PERMITTED IN SPORT

No

OVERDOSE

Serious. Sedation, convulsions, coma and death may occur. Administer activated charcoal or induce vomiting if medication taken recently and patient alert. Seek emergency medical assistance. Antidote available.

OTHER INFORMATION

Highly addictive if used inappropriately. Very effective and unlikely to cause addiction if used appropriately for severe pain.

Phenelzine

See MAOI

Phenindione

TRADE NAME

Dindevan.

DRUG CLASS

Anticoagulant.

USES

Prevention and treatment of blood clots (thromboses).

DOSAGE

 Very strictly as directed by doctor. Usually higher dose on starting, then dose varies depending on results of regular blood tests.

FORMS

Tablets of 10mg. (white), 25mg. (green) and 50mg. (white).

SIDE EFFECTS

Common: Bloating, passing wind. Severe (consult doctor immediately): Blood in urine, blood in faeces, black sticky faeces, skin rash, diarrhoea, vomiting, fever, sore throat, mouth ulcers, bruising.

INTERACTIONS

Other drugs:

• Interacts adversely with a wide range of medication. Do not take any other medication (including Aspirin or cold mixtures) without medical permission.

Other substances:

• Alcohol may increase effect of medication.

• Avoid foods rich in vitamin K (eg: leafy greens, fish).

PRECAUTIONS

Not to be used if pregnant (D) or breast feeding.

Care required in patients with high blood pressure, liver disease, kidney disease, peptic ulcer or bowel bleeding.

It is essential that all doctors in contact with the patient know that the patient is on Phenindione.

No surgery can be performed unless Phenindione has been ceased for some days.

Do not undertake any activity that may result in falls, bruising or extreme exertion.

 Do not take if:

• Unless carefully monitored by a doctor.

PRESCRIPTION

Yes

PERMITTED IN SPORT

Yes, but not advised in vigorous sport.

OVERDOSE

Life threatening! Will cause severe bleeding internally, bleeding gums, blood in urine and faeces. Urgent transport to hospital required. Antidote available.

OTHER INFORMATION

Patients should read additional information provided by their doctor carefully. Wearing a bracelet or necklet with information about the medication is advised for anyone using phenindione long term. Very effective medication, but must be used with great care.

Phenobarbitone

See BARBITURATES

PHENOTHIAZINES

TRADE and GENERIC NAMES

Clozaril (Clozapine).

Fentazine (Perphenazine).

Largactil (Chlorpromazine).

Melleril (Thioridazine).

Modecate, Moditen (Fluphenazine).

Motipress, Motival (Fluphenazine with Nortriptyline).

Neulactil (Pericyazine).

Nozinan (Methotrimeprazine).

Piportil Depot (Pipothiazine).

Stelazine (Trifluoperazine).

Triptafen (Perphenazine with Amitriptyline).

NB: Phenothiazines are underlined.

DRUG CLASS

Antipsychotics, Antiemetics (Chlorpromazine and Perphenazine).

USES

Schizophrenia, mania, psychoses, senile agitation, severe agitation in children, intractable vomiting, intractable hiccups, severe anxiety, other psychiatric conditions, increasing the effect of pain killers.

DOSAGE

 One to three tablets or capsules, two or three times a day. Dosage varies widely from one form to another depending on length of action and potency. Follow doctors instructions carefully.

FORMS

Tablets, capsules, mixture, suppository, injection.

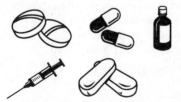

PRECAUTIONS

Should only be used in pregnancy (C) if medically necessary. High doses should be avoided late in pregnancy. Should be used with caution in breast feeding. Most forms may be used in children.

Should be used with caution in epilepsy, Parkinsonism, hypoparathyroidism, myasthenia gravis, low blood pressure, lung and kidney diseases.

Use with caution if operating machinery or driving a vehicle.

 ### Do not take if:

- suffering from depression, very poor circulation, phaeochromocytoma, liver disease or bone marrow disease.

- intoxicated with alcohol or Marijuana.

SIDE EFFECTS

Common: Drowsiness, reduced alertness, abnormal body temperature, low blood pressure, dermatitis, dry mouth, constipation, weight gain, blurred vision, stuffy nose.

Unusual: Itch, difficulty passing urine, confusion, dizziness, incoordination, tremor, slow breathing, irregular heart beat, skin pigmentation.

Severe but rare (stop medication, consult doctor): Yellow skin (jaundice), convulsions, repetitive unwanted movements, muscle rigidity, fever, coma.

INTERACTIONS

Other drugs:

• Adrenaline, Tricyclic Antidepressants, Guanethidine, Antacids, Barbiturates, Phenytoin, Lithium, Levodopa, Sedatives, Amphetamines, Beta Blockers, Hypoglycaemics, MAOI, Quinidine, Suxamethonium.

Other substances:

• Reacts adversely with alcohol and some foods.

PRESCRIPTION

Yes

PERMITTED IN SPORT

Yes

OVERDOSE

Very serious. Symptoms include drowsiness, confusion, restlessness, rapid heart rate, tremor, convulsions, difficulty in breathing and swallowing, coma and death. Administer activated charcoal or induce vomiting if taken recently and patient alert. Seek urgent medical attention.

OTHER INFORMATION

These drugs have revolutionised the lives of many psychiatric patients to the point where they can lead completely normal lives. First introduced in 1960s. Do not cause addiction or dependence.

See also Benperidol, Olanzapine, Prochlorperazine, Zotepine.

Phenylbutazone

See NSAID

Phenylephrine

TRADE NAMES

Minims Phenylephrine.

Betnovate Rectal (with Betamethasone, Lignocaine).

Isopto Frin (with Hypromellose).

Also found in numerous cold and flu preparations.

DRUG CLASS

Sympathomimetic (constricts blood vessels), Decongestant.

USES

Minor eye irritations, piles, nasal congestion.

DOSAGE

 Eye drops: One or two drops every three or four hours.

PRECAUTIONS

Safe to use in pregnancy (B2), breast feeding and children.

Use with caution in high blood pressure.

Do not use nasal sprays long term.

 Do not use eye drops if:

• suffering from glaucoma.

FORMS

Eye drops, ointment, nose sprays.

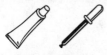

SIDE EFFECTS

Minimal.

INTERACTIONS

Other drugs:

• Antidepressants, Sedatives.

Other substances:

• Reacts with alcohol if taken by mouth.

PRESCRIPTION

No

PERMITTED IN SPORT

If taken by mouth: No
Other preparations: Yes

OVERDOSE

If taken by mouth may cause irritability, convulsions, palpitations, high blood pressure, angina and difficulty in passing urine. Administer activated charcoal or induce vomiting if medication taken recently. Seek urgent medical assistance. Nasal preparations if used excessively may cause rebound nasal stuffiness and congestion.

OTHER INFORMATION

Used widely in cold mixtures, eye drops and nasal sprays to ease irritation and congestion. Safe and effective if taken as directed, but do not take more than recommended dose or over use nose drops and sprays.

See also MYDRIATICS

Phenytoin

TRADE NAME

Epanutin.

DRUG CLASS

Anticonvulsant.

USES

Epilepsy, some forms of irregular heart beat.

DOSAGE

 One or two tablets, two or three times a day with water and food.

FORMS

Capsules, tablets, mixture, injection.

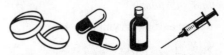

PRECAUTIONS

Not for use in pregnancy (D) unless absolutely essential, as the risk of foetal deformity is increased. Use with caution in breast feeding. May be used in children.

Lower doses required in elderly.

Use with caution in liver disease, heart disease, low blood pressure, porphyria.

Do not stop suddenly, but reduce dosage slowly over several weeks.

 Do not take if:

• suffering from some forms of heart disease.

SIDE EFFECTS

Common: Most side effects eased by slight reduction in dose. Slurred speech, incoordination, jerky eye movements, confusion.

Unusual: Dizziness, sleeplessness, nervous twitching, headache.

Severe but rare (stop medication, consult doctor): Enlarged glands in neck, groin or armpits.

INTERACTIONS

Other drugs:

- Wide range of medications can affect the blood levels of Phenytoin. Do not take any prescription medication without checking possible interactions with a doctor or pharmacist.

- Non-prescription medications that interact with Phenytoin include Aspirin, Antacids, Calcium, Vitamin D and Folic Acid.

- Oral contraceptive pill.

Other substances:

- Reacts adversely with alcohol.

PRESCRIPTION

Yes

PERMITTED IN SPORT

Yes

OVERDOSE

Doses of over 2000mg. to 5000mg. (depending on size, sex etc.) may be fatal. Symptoms include incoordination, incoherent speech, tremor, tiredness, vomiting, slow heart rate, coma, dilated pupils and death. Administer activated charcoal or induce vomiting if tablets taken recently and patient alert. Seek urgent medical assistance.

OTHER INFORMATION

For decades, Phenytoin has been the mainstay of epilepsy treatment world wide. Does not cause addiction or dependence.

Pholcodine

TRADE NAMES

Galenphol, Pavacol-D.

DRUG CLASS

Cough suppressant.

USES

Control of dry cough.

DOSAGE

 Take 5 to 15mls. four times a day.

FORMS

Mixture.

PRECAUTIONS

Safe to use in pregnancy (A), breast feeding and children.

SIDE EFFECTS

Common: Minimal.

Unusual: Nausea, drowsiness.

INTERACTIONS

None significant.

PRESCRIPTION

No

PERMITTED IN SPORT

Yes

OVERDOSE

Serious adverse effects unlikely.

OTHER INFORMATION

Very old medication. Widely used and very safe.

Phosphorus

TRADE NAME

Added to numerous non-prescription vitamin and mineral supplements.

DRUG CLASS

Mineral.

USES

Nutritional deficiency, hyperparathyroidism, multiple myeloma, some form of rickets, bone cancer.

DOSAGE

 Recommended daily dose 1000mg. Higher doses used in treating diseases listed above.

FORMS

Tablets, mixtures.

PRECAUTIONS

Safe to use in pregnancy, breast feeding and children.

Use with caution in kidney disease.

If high doses used, regular blood tests to check balance of all minerals in blood necessary.

SIDE EFFECTS

Common: Diarrhoea.

Unusual: Tissue calcium deposits, kidney stones.

INTERACTIONS

None significant.

PRESCRIPTION

No

PERMITTED IN SPORT

Yes

OVERDOSE

Unlikely to be serious.

OTHER INFORMATION

Phosphorus is a mineral found naturally in many foods including dairy foods, meat, fish, nuts, eggs and cereals. A natural deficiency is very unusual.

Phytomenadione

(Vitamin K)

TRADE NAME

Konakion.

DRUG CLASS

Haemostatic.

USES

Treatment and prevention of excessive bleeding (particularly in newborn infants), overdose of anticoagulants.

DOSAGE

 Depends on severity of bleeding.

FORMS

Tablets, injection.

PRECAUTIONS

Should be used with caution in pregnancy, breast feeding and children.

 Do not take if:

• suffering from severe allergy tendency.

SIDE EFFECTS

Common: Minimal

Severe but rare (stop medication, consult doctor): Yellow skin (jaundice), allergy reaction.

INTERACTIONS

None significant

PRESCRIPTION

No

PERMITTED IN SPORT

Yes

OVERDOSE

No serious effects, except in infants where anaemia may occur.

OTHER INFORMATION

Vitamin K is a fat soluble group of compounds essential for the formation of the factors that clot blood. It is found in most foods (particularly green leafy vegetables) and is also made by bacteria that live in the gut. The adequate daily allowance is 1mg. A lack of vitamin K is rare, but may occur if fat absorption from the gut is abnormal. Newborn infants can be low on Vitamin K and are often given Vitamin K at birth to prevent excessive bleeding.

See also Aminocaproic Acid, Tranexamic acid.

PILL, CONTRACEPTIVE

See ORAL CONTRACEPTIVES

Pilocarpine

TRADE NAMES

Minims Pilocarpine, Ocusert-Pilo, Pilogel, Salagen.

Isopto Carpine (with Hypromellose).

USES

Glaucoma, dry mouth, Sjögren syndrome.

DOSAGE

 Eye drops: Two drops three or four times a day.
Eye discs: Insert one a week.
Tablets: One or two three times a day after meals.

FORMS

Eye drops, eye gel, discs for eye insertion, tablets.

PRECAUTIONS

Safe to use in pregnancy, breast feeding and children.

 Do not take if:
• suffering from acute iritis.

SIDE EFFECTS

Common: Blurred vision.

INTERACTIONS

None significant.

PRESCRIPTION

Yes

PERMITTED IN SPORT

Yes

OVERDOSE

Seek medical advice. Unlikely to be serious.

OTHER INFORMATION

Commonly used medication for the treatment of glaucoma.

Pimozide

TRADE NAME

Orap.

DRUG CLASS

Antipsychotic.

USES

Chronic psychotic disorders.

DOSAGE

 One or more tablets once a day to a maximum of 20mg. a day.

FORMS

Tablet of 2mg. (white), 4mg. (green) and 10mg. (white).

PRECAUTIONS

Use with caution in pregnancy (B1), breast feeding and children.

Use with caution in heart disease, severe anxiety, aggressive behaviour, liver and kidney disease.

 Do not take if:

• suffering from active drug or alcohol abuse, depression, irregular heart beat, Parkinson's disease.

SIDE EFFECTS

Common: Tremor, excess salivation, muscle stiffness, dizziness.

Unusual: Difficulty in swallowing, disorientation, sleeplessness, rapid heart rate, restlessness, constipation, loss of appetite, menstrual irregularities.

Severe but rare (stop medication, consult doctor): Unwanted and uncontrolled muscle movements particularly of face, rigid muscles, fever.

INTERACTIONS

Other drugs:

• Anticonvulsants, Sedatives, Stimulants, Atropine, Antihypertensives, Antiarrhythmics, Levodopa, Phenothiazines, Tricyclic Antidepressants.

Other substances:

• Reacts adversely with alcohol.

PRESCRIPTION

Yes

PERMITTED IN SPORT

Yes

OVERDOSE

Relatively safe. Confusion and drowsiness most likely symptoms. Administer activated charcoal or induce vomiting if taken recently. Seek medical assistance.

Pindolol

See BETA BLOCKERS

Pine tar

See Tar

Piperacillin

TRADE NAME

Pipril.

Tazocin (with Tazobactam).

DRUG CLASS

Penicillin antibiotic.

USES

Treatment of infections caused by susceptible bacteria.

DOSAGE

 One injection every three to six hours or by continuous drip infusion.

FORMS

Injection.

PRECAUTIONS

May be used in pregnancy (B1), children and breast feeding when medically appropriate.

Use with caution in kidney failure, liver disease, meningitis, and venereal disease.

 ### Do not take if:

- allergic to Penicillin.
- suffering from glandular fever.

SIDE EFFECTS

Common: Pain at injection site, diarrhoea.

Unusual: Itch or rash, headache, nausea, dizziness, hot flushes, tiredness.

Severe but rare (stop medication, consult doctor): Itchy rash, hives, severe diarrhoea, yellow skin (jaundice), unusual bleeding or bruising.

INTERACTIONS

Other drugs:

- Vercuronium.

PRESCRIPTION

Yes

PERMITTED IN SPORT

Yes

OVERDOSE

Vomiting and diarrhoea likely.

OTHER INFORMATION

Used for more severe and unusual infections.

Piperazine

TRADE NAME

Pripsen.

DRUG CLASS

Anthelmintic.

USES

Threadworm and roundworm infestations of the gut.

DOSAGE

 One sachet, repeated after two weeks.

FORMS

Sachet of powder.

PRECAUTIONS

May be used in pregnancy and children over three months of age.

Use with caution in breast feeding.

Use with caution in brain disturbances.

 ### Do not take if:

- suffering from epilepsy, kidney and liver disease.

SIDE EFFECTS

Common: Minimal.

Unusual: Dizziness.

Severe but rare (stop medication, consult doctor): Visual disturbances.

INTERACTIONS

None significant.

PRESCRIPTION

No

PERMITTED IN SPORT

Yes

OVERDOSE

Unlikely to be serious.

Pipothiazine

See PHENOTHIAZINES

Piracetam

TRADE NAME

Nootropil.

DRUG CLASS

Anticonvulsant.

USES

Muscle spasms associated with seizures.

DOSAGE

 Slowly increase dosage as directed by doctor. Maximum 20g. a day.

FORMS

Tablets of 800 and 1200mg. (white), solution.

PRECAUTIONS

Not to be used in pregnancy, breast feeding and children.

Use with caution in all kidney disease.

Reduce dose in elderly.

Do not stop suddenly, but reduce dose slowly.

 Do not take if:
- suffering from severe kidney and liver disease.

SIDE EFFECTS

Common: Restlessness, sleeplessness, weight gain.

Unusual: Tiredness, nervousness, depression, diarrhoea, rash.

INTERACTIONS

Other drugs:

- Thyroid hormones.

Other substances:

- Alcohol.

PRESCRIPTION

Yes

PERMITTED IN SPORT

Yes

OTHER INFORMATION

Recently introduced medication that is almost invariably combined with other medications to control epilepsy.

Piroxicam

See NSAID

Pivmecillinam

TRADE NAME

Selexid.

DRUG CLASS

Penicillin antibiotic.

USES

Prevention or treatment of urinary infections.

DOSAGE

 Prevention: Two tablets, three or four times a day.
Treatment: Two tablets at once, then one tablet three times a day for three days.

FORMS

Tablets of 200mg. (white).

PRECAUTIONS

Use with caution in pregnancy.

May be used in breast feeding and children.

Use with caution in kidney disease.

 Do not take if:

- suffering from oesophageal strictures, intestinal obstruction.

- allergic to penicillin.

SIDE EFFECTS

Common: Nausea, diarrhoea.

Unusual: Rash.

INTERACTIONS

Other drugs:

- Methotrexate, Valproate.

PRESCRIPTION

Yes

PERMITTED IN SPORT

Yes

OVERDOSE

Exacerbation of side effects likely.

Pizotifen

TRADE NAME

Sanomigran.

DRUG CLASS

Antimigraine.

USES

Prevention of migraine.

DOSAGE

 0.5 to 3mg. a day as a single dose. Maximum 6mg. a day.

FORMS

Tablet of 0.5 and 1.5mg. (white).

PRECAUTIONS

Should be used with caution in pregnancy (B1), breast feeding and children.

Pizotifen has no effect on acute migraine attacks.

 Do not take if:

- suffering from glaucoma, difficulty in passing urine.

SIDE EFFECTS

Common: Sedation, increased appetite

Unusual: Dizziness, dry mouth, constipation, nervousness in children, swelling of tissues, headache, rash, muscle aches, tingling sensation, impotence.

INTERACTIONS

Other drugs:

• Increased sedation with sedatives, hypnotics and antihistamines.

Other substances:

• Reacts with alcohol to cause drowsiness.

PRESCRIPTION

Yes

PERMITTED IN SPORT

Yes

OVERDOSE

Serious. Administer activated charcoal or induce vomiting if taken recently. Symptoms include drowsiness, nausea, dizziness, reduced breathing, convulsions, coma. Seek urgent medical assistance.

OTHER INFORMATION

Older, widely used medication. Large doses often necessary. Increase dosage slowly.

Plague vaccine

See Yersinia pestis vaccine

Pneumococcal vaccine

TRADE NAMES

Pneumovax II, Pnu-Immune.

DRUG CLASS

Vaccine.

USES

Prevention of infections caused by Pneumococcal bacteria.

DOSAGE

 Single injection.

FORMS

Injection.

PRECAUTIONS

Not designed for use in pregnancy. May be used in breast feeding and children over two years.

Use with caution in heart and lung disease, reduced immunity, fever, current antibiotic treatment.

 Do not take if:

• receiving chemotherapy for Hodgkin's disease.

• previously vaccinated with this vaccine.

SIDE EFFECTS

Common: Local soreness and redness at site of injection.

Unusual: Rash, joint pain, fever.

INTERACTIONS

None significant.

PRESCRIPTION

Yes

PERMITTED IN SPORT

Yes

OVERDOSE

Significant adverse reactions and allergy reactions may occur if a second vaccination is given to an adult. Children may require a second vaccination.

OTHER INFORMATION

Not used routinely but restricted to patients who are elderly, have lung diseases, have (or are about to have) their spleen removed, who are chronically ill, or who are in an institution where the disease has occurred.

PODOPHYLLUMS

TRADE and GENERIC NAMES

Condyline, Warticon (Podophyllotoxin).

Posalfilin (Podophyllum resin with Salicylic acid).

USES

Warts.

DOSAGE

 Cream and ointment: Apply two or three times a week.
Paint: Apply once or twice a day.

FORMS

Cream, ointment, paint.

PRECAUTIONS

Not to be used in pregnancy or breast feeding. Not for use in infants. Use with caution in children.

Use with caution in diabetes and poor circulation.

Do not use on moles, birthmarks or unusual warts, but seek medical advice.

Use on only a limited number of warts at one time.

Avoid use on normal skin.

SIDE EFFECTS

Common: Burning, redness of skin.

Unusual: Skin pain.

INTERACTIONS

None significant.

PRESCRIPTION

Yes

PERMITTED IN SPORT

Yes

OTHER INFORMATION

Ancient and commonly used remedy for warts that is usually effective.

Podophyllotoxin

See PODOPHYLLUMS

Poliomyelitis vaccine

TRADE NAME

Polio Sabin.

DRUG CLASS

Vaccine.

USES

Prevention of poliomyelitis.

DOSAGE

 Three drops on a spoon or lump of sugar given three times at two monthly intervals. Booster dose at five years.

FORMS

Drops (must be carefully stored at 4°C).

SIDE EFFECTS

Common: Minimal.

Unusual: Headache, vomiting, diarrhoea.

INTERACTIONS

Other drugs:

• Other live vaccines.

PRECAUTIONS

Not designed to be used during pregnancy (B2), but inadvertent use unlikely to cause any serious effect. May be used during breast feeding, in children and infants.

Use with caution in diarrhoea, vomiting or infection.

 Do not take if:

• suffering from fever or reduced immunity.

PRESCRIPTION

Yes

PERMITTED IN SPORT

Yes

OVERDOSE

Unintentional additional dose is unlikely to have any serious effect.

OTHER INFORMATION

Poliomyelitis is a viral infection that causes muscle paralysis and sometimes death. It has been eradicated from Britain by vaccination, but is still widespread in many poorer countries.

Poloxamer 188

TRADE NAME

Codalax (with Danthron).

DRUG CLASS

Laxative.

USES

Constipation, particularly if caused by use of powerful pain killers.

DOSAGE

 5 to 10mLs. at night.

FORMS

Liquid.

PRECAUTIONS

Safe in pregnancy (A), breast feeding and children over three months.

Not for long term use. May cause intestinal dependence.

 Do not take if:

• suffering from suspected appendicitis, bleeding from anus, belly pain, obstructed gut.

SIDE EFFECTS

Common: Minimal.

Unusual: Colic, belly pain, diarrhoea.

INTERACTIONS

Other drugs:

• Other laxatives.

PRESCRIPTION

No

PERMITTED IN SPORT

Yes

OVERDOSE

Diarrhoea and belly cramps only likely effects.

Polyacrylic acid

See EYE LUBRICANTS

Polymyxin B

TRADE NAMES

Only available in combination with other medications.

Gregoderm (with Nystatin, Hydrocortisone).

Maxitrol (with Dexamethasone, Neomycin, Hypromellose).

Neosporin (with Neomycin, Gramicidin).

Otosporin (with Neomycin, Hydrocortisone).

Polyfax (with Bacitracin).

Polytrim (with Trimethoprim).

DRUG CLASS

Antibiotic.

USES

Bacterial infections of skin and eyes.

DOSAGE

 Eye drops and ointment: Insert every three to six hours.
Ear drops: Two drops, three times a day.
Skin ointment: Apply two or three times a day.

FORMS

Eye drops, eye ointment, ear drops, ointment.

PRECAUTIONS

Safe to use in pregnancy, breast feeding and children.

Not designed for long term regular use.

Do not use on large areas of skin.

SIDE EFFECTS

Common: Minimal.

Severe but rare (stop medication, consult doctor): Skin or eye irritation.

INTERACTIONS

None significant.

PRESCRIPTION

Yes

PERMITTED IN SPORT

Yes

Polystyrene sulfonate

See **Sodium polystyrene sulfonate**

Polyvinyl alcohol

See **EYE LUBRICANTS**

Potassium bicarbonate

See **ELECTROLYTES**

Potassium chloride

See **ELECTROLYTES**

Potassium clavulanate

See **Clavulanic acid**

Potassium clorazepate

See **ANXIOLYTICS**

Potassium hydroxyquinolone

TRADE NAMES

Quinocort (with Hydrocortisone).

Quinoderm, Quinoped (with Benzoyl peroxide).

DRUG CLASS

Antifungal, Antibiotic.

USES

Gel: Acne.

Cream: Mild fungal and bacterial skin infections combined with dermatitis.

DOSAGE

Gel: Massage into affected skin one to three times a day.
Cream: Apply two or three times a day.

FORMS

Cream, gel

PRECAUTIONS

Safe to use in pregnancy, breast feeding and children.

Avoid eyes, mouth and nostrils.

SIDE EFFECTS

Common: Minimal.

Unusual: Skin irritation.

INTERACTIONS

None significant.

PRESCRIPTION

No

PERMITTED IN SPORT

Yes

Potassium p-Aminobenzoate

(Aminobenzoic Acid)

TRADE NAME

Potaba

USES

Peyronie's disease (deformed erect penis), scleroderma.

DOSAGE

Six tablets or capsules, four times a day.

FORMS

Tablets and capsules of 500mg., powder in sachet.

PRECAUTIONS

Not to be used in pregnancy, breast feeding or children.

Do not take if:
• suffering from kidney disease.

SIDE EFFECTS

Common: Loss of appetite, nausea.

INTERACTIONS

Other drugs:

• Sulphonamide antibiotics.

PRESCRIPTION

No

PERMITTED IN SPORT

Yes

OVERDOSE

Seek medical advice. Vomiting likely.

Povidone

See EYE LUBRICANTS

Povidone-Iodine

See Iodine

Pramipexole

TRADE NAME

Mirapexin.

DRUG CLASS

Antiparkinsonian.

USES

Parkinson's disease.

DOSAGE

 Initially .125mg. three times a day. Dose slowly increased as directed by doctor. Maximum 4.5mg a day.

FORMS

Tablets (white) of .125, .25 and 1mg.

PRECAUTIONS

Not to be used in breast feeding and children.

Use with considerable caution in pregnancy.

Use with caution in kidney disease, psychoses, schizophrenia and severe heart disease.

Blood pressure must be checked regularly.

Eye checks must be performed regularly.

SIDE EFFECTS

Common: Nausea, constipation, sudden and unpredictable onset of sleep.

Unusual: Tiredness, incoordination, hallucinations.

Severe but rare (stop medication, consult doctor): High blood pressure, eye damage.

INTERACTIONS

Other drugs:

• Cimetidine, Diltiazem, Quinidine, Quinine, Ranitidine, Procainamide, Digoxin, Triamterene, Amantadine, Verapamil, Trimethoprim, Sedatives.

Other substances:

• Alcohol.

PRESCRIPTION

Yes

PERMITTED IN SPORT

Yes

OVERDOSE

May be serious. Seek urgent medical attention. Induce vomiting or give activated charcoal if taken recently.

OTHER INFORMATION

Almost invariably used in combination with Levodopa. Introduced 1999 for the management of more severe forms of Parkinson's disease.

Pravastatin

TRADE NAME

Lipostat.

DRUG CLASS

Hypolipidaemic.

USES

High blood levels of cholesterol.

DOSAGE

 10mg. to 40mg. taken at bedtime on an empty stomach.

FORMS

Tablets (yellow) of 10mg, 20mg. and 40mg.

PRECAUTIONS

Must not be taken in pregnancy (C) as Pravastatin may cause miscarriage or foetal abnormalities.

Adequate contraception must be used by all women of child bearing potential who are taking this medication. Not to be used in breast feeding or children.

Must be used with caution in elderly.

Do not take if:

- suffering from liver or kidney disease, alcoholism.

SIDE EFFECTS

Common: Muscle pains and weakness, rash, headache, nausea, diarrhoea, constipation, excess wind.

Unusual: Chest pain, vomiting, belly pains, heartburn, fatigue.

INTERACTIONS

Other drugs:

- Gemfibrizol.

Other substances:

- Reacts with alcohol

PRESCRIPTION

Yes

PERMITTED IN SPORT

Yes

OVERDOSE

No information available.

OTHER INFORMATION

Introduced in the early 1990's. Dangerous in pregnancy.

Prazosin

TRADE NAME

Hypovase.

DRUG CLASS

Antihypertensive, Alphablocker.

USES

High blood pressure, severe heart failure, Raynaud's phenomenon, enlargement of prostate gland.

DOSAGE

 Taken two or three times a day to a maximum of 20mg. per day.

FORMS

Tablets of 0.5mg. (white),1mg. (orange), and 2mg. (white).

PRECAUTIONS

Should be used with caution in pregnancy (B2) and breast feeding. Not designed to be used in children.

Always start at a very low dose and increase slowly.

Do not take if:

- suffering from phaeochromocytoma, low blood pressure on standing or poor liver function.

SIDE EFFECTS

Common: Headache, drowsiness, palpitations, swelling of tissue, nausea, nasal congestion, blurred vision, low blood pressure on standing.

Unusual: Vomiting, itchy skin.

Severe but rare (stop medication, consult doctor): Fainting.

INTERACTIONS

Other drugs:

• Additive effect from Diuretics.

PRESCRIPTION

Yes

PERMITTED IN SPORT

Yes

OVERDOSE

Drowsiness and depressed reflexes only effects.

OTHER INFORMATION

Very effective in high blood pressure. Found to temporarily reduce the size of the prostate gland and make it easier to pass urine. Delays prostate surgery, but does not remove long term necessity for surgery.

Prednisolone

TRADE NAMES

Deltacortril, Deltastab, Minims Prednisolone, Precortisyl Forte, Pred Forte, Predenema, Predfoam, Prednesol, Predsol (Prednisolone).

Predsol-N (with Neomycin).

Scheriproct (Prednisolone, Cinchocaine).

DRUG CLASS

Corticosteroid.

USES

Severe inflammation of skin (eczema, dermatitis etc.), anus (piles), rectum (ulcerative colitis), eyes and other tissues. Severe asthma, rheumatoid and other forms of severe arthritis, auto-immune diseases (eg: Sjøgren's syndrome), severe allergy reactions, and other severe and chronic inflammatory diseases.

DOSAGE

 Enema: Insert once a day for up to four weeks.
Suppositories: Insert twice a day for up to three weeks.
Eye and ear drops: Insert every two to four hours.
Tablets and mixture: As directed by doctor.

PRECAUTIONS

Should be used in pregnancy (C), breast feeding and children only on specific medical advice.

Eye preparations safe in pregnancy, breast feeding and children over three years.

Use with caution if under stress, and in patients with under active thyroid gland, liver disease, diverticulitis, high blood pressure, myasthenia gravis or kidney disease.

Avoid eyes with all forms except eye drops.

Use for shortest period of time possible.

Medication should not be ceased abruptly, but dosage should be slowly reduced.

 ### Do not use if:

• suffering from any form of infection, peptic ulcer or osteoporosis.

• having a vaccination.

FORMS

Ear drops, enema, eye drops, mixture, suppository, tablets, foam.

SIDE EFFECTS

Most significant side effects occur only with prolonged use of tablets or rectal preparations.

Common: May cause bloating, weight gain, rashes and intestinal disturbances. Eye and ear drops - Rarely cause adverse reactions away from eyes and ears.

Unusual: Biochemical disturbances of blood, muscle weakness, bone weakness, impaired wound healing, skin thinning, tendon weakness, peptic ulcers, gullet ulcers, bruising, increased sweating, loss of fat under skin, premature ageing, excess facial hair growth in women, pigmentation of skin and nails, acne, convulsions, headaches, dizziness, growth suppression in children, aggravation of diabetes, worsening of infections, cataracts, aggravation of glaucoma, blood clots in veins and sleeplessness.

Severe but rare (stop medication, consult doctor): Any significant side effect should be reported to a doctor immediately.

INTERACTIONS

Other drugs:

• Tablets and rectal preparations may be affected by Oral contraceptives, Barbiturates, Phenytoin and Rifampicin.

PRESCRIPTION

Yes

PERMITTED IN SPORT

Most: No.
Eye drops: Yes

OVERDOSE

Medical treatment is required. Serious effects and death rare.

OTHER INFORMATION

Extremely effective and useful medication if used correctly. Must be used with extreme care under strict medical supervision. Lowest dose and shortest possible course should be used. Not addictive.

Prilocaine

See ANAESTHETICS, LOCAL

Primidone

TRADE NAME

Mysoline.

DRUG CLASS

Anticonvulsant.

USES

Epilepsy.

DOSAGE

 Requires individual planning by a doctor, depending on nature and timing of convulsions.

FORMS

Tablets of 250mg. (white).

SIDE EFFECTS

Common: Usually minimal and dose related. Drowsiness.

Unusual: Nausea, headache, dizziness, vomiting, rash.

INTERACTIONS

Other drugs:

• Anticonvulsants, Anticoagulants, Oral contraceptive pill, Sedatives.

Other substances:

• Reacts adversely with alcohol.

PRECAUTIONS

Not to be used in pregnancy (D) unless absolutely necessary as it may cause bleeding problems in the newborn infant. Use with caution in breast feeding. May be used in children.

Use with caution in kidney, liver and lung disease.

Lower doses necessary in elderly.

Do not stop suddenly, but reduce dosage slowly.

Use with caution if operating machinery, driving a vehicle or undertaking tasks that require coordination and alertness.

 Do not take if:

• suffering from porphyria.

PRESCRIPTION

Yes

PERMITTED IN SPORT

Yes

OVERDOSE

Serious. Symptoms may include incoordination, reduced breathing and coma. Administer activated charcoal or induce vomiting if medication taken recently and patient alert. Seek urgent medical assistance.

Probenecid

TRADE NAME

Benemid.

DRUG CLASS

Uricosuric.

USES

Prevention of gout, reducing level of uric acid in blood, prolonging the effectiveness of Penicillins and Cephalosporins.

DOSAGE

 One or two tablets twice a day.

FORMS

Tablet (white) of 500mg.

PRECAUTIONS

Use with caution in pregnancy (B2). Safe for use in breast feeding and children over two years.

Use with caution in kidney disease, peptic ulcer and acute gout.

 Do not use if:

• suffering from kidney stones.

SIDE EFFECTS

Common: Headache, nausea, frequent urination, rash, fever, sore gums.

Unusual: Vomiting, diarrhoea, flushing, hair loss, dizziness.

INTERACTIONS

Other drugs:

• Aspirin, Pyrazinamide, Sulphonamides, Methotrexate.

Other substances:

• Alcohol may aggravate gout.

PRESCRIPTION

Yes

PERMITTED IN SPORT

No

OVERDOSE

Exacerbation of side effects likely.

OTHER INFORMATION

Does not cause addiction or dependence. May be used with Penicillin in the treatment of gonorrhoea to extend effect of Penicillin.

Procainamide

TRADE NAME

Pronestyl.

DRUG CLASS

Antiarrhythmic.

USES

Control and prevention of some types of heart beat irregularities.

DOSAGE

 One or two tablets, four to six times a day.

FORMS

Tablets of 250mg. (white), injection.

PRECAUTIONS

Should be used with caution in pregnancy (B2). Should not be used in breast feeding.

Should be used only if medically essential in children. Should be used with caution in kidney and liver disease.

Routine blood tests may be required with long term treatment to check on cell types and numbers.

 Do not take if:

• suffering from myasthenia gravis or atrio-ventricular heart conduction block.

SIDE EFFECTS

Common: Generally well tolerated. Low blood pressure, stomach upsets.

Unusual: Depression, dizziness, hallucinations, fever, rash, flush, shivering, itchy skin, mild arthritis, bad taste.

INTERACTIONS

Other drugs:

• Amiodarone, propranolol, other Antiarrhythmics, Cimetidine, Anticholinergics, Antihypertensives, Captopril, Sulphonamides, Trimethoprim.

Other substances:

• Alcohol.

PRESCRIPTION

Yes

PERMITTED IN SPORT

Yes

OVERDOSE

Rapid heart rate, vomiting and low blood pressure may occur. Administer activated charcoal or induce vomiting if tablets taken recently. Seek medical assistance.

Prochlorperazine

TRADE NAMES

Buccastem, Stemetil.

DRUG CLASS

Antiemetic, Antihistamine.

USES

Nausea, vomiting, dizziness, Meniere's disease.

DOSAGE

Tablets: One tablet two to four times a day.
Buccal tablets: Dissolve between upper lip and gum once or twice a day.
Suppository: One every six to eight hours as needed.

FORMS

Tablets (cream) of 5mg., buccal tablets (yellow), suppositories, granules in sachet, syrup, injection.

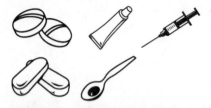

PRECAUTIONS

Should be used in pregnancy (C) only if medically essential. Use with caution in breast feeding. Not for use in children under two years or less than 10Kg.

Use with caution in epilepsy, Parkinson's disease, underactive thyroid gland, myasthenia gravis, Reye's syndrome, phaeochromocytoma, enlarged prostate gland, low calcium states, kidney or liver disease.

Lower doses necessary in elderly.

 Do not take if:

- suffering from shock, brain diseases, bone marrow disease.

SIDE EFFECTS

Common: Constipation, dry mouth, drowsiness, tremor, blurred vision.

Unusual: Swelling of tissues (oedema), low blood pressure, irregular heart beat, rash, difficulty in passing urine, headache, sleeplessness.

Severe but rare (stop medication, consult doctor): Yellow skin (jaundice), difficulty in breathing, convulsion.

INTERACTIONS

Other drugs:

- Sedatives, Desferrioxamine, Anticholinergics, Procarbazine, L-Dopa, Anticoagulants, Thiazides, Propranolol, Guanethidine.

Other substances:

- Reacts adversely with alcohol.

PRESCRIPTION

Yes

PERMITTED IN SPORT

Yes

OVERDOSE

Serious, particularly in children. Symptoms include confusion, restlessness, rapid heart rate, tremor, twitching, convulsions, difficulty breathing, coma and rarely death. Administer activated charcoal or induce vomiting if medication taken recently and patient alert. Seek urgent medical assistance.

OTHER INFORMATION

Widely used and effective. Available for over 30 years. Does not cause addiction or dependence. Related to the Phenothiazines.

Procyclidine

TRADE NAME

Arpicolin, Kemadrin.

DRUG CLASS

Antiparkinsonian.

USES

Parkinson's disease, other muscle movement disorders.

DOSAGE

 Half to two tablets three times a day.

FORMS

Tablet of 5mg. (white), syrup.

PRECAUTIONS

Safe for use in pregnancy (A). Use with caution in breast feeding and children.

Use with caution in glaucoma, intestinal obstruction, enlarged prostate gland and psychiatric conditions.

Use with caution in elderly.

SIDE EFFECTS

Common: Dry mouth, blurred vision, nausea.

Unusual: Vomiting, rash, dizziness, hallucinations.

PRESCRIPTION

Yes

PERMITTED IN SPORT

Yes

OVERDOSE

Unlikely to be serious. Seek medical advice.

OTHER INFORMATION

Does not cause addiction or dependence.

Progesterone

TRADE NAMES

Crinone, Cyclogest, Gestone.

DRUG CLASS

Sex hormone.

USES

Premenstrual tension (PMT), abnormal vaginal bleeding, adjunct to oestrogen in hormone replacement therapy, endometriosis, maintenance of early pregnancy, aid to infertility, postnatal depression.

DOSAGE

 Vaginal gel: Second daily for last two weeks of menstrual cycle for PMT.
Suppository: Insert rectally or vaginally once or twice a day for last two weeks of menstrual cycle for PMT.

FORMS

Vaginal gel, suppository, injection.

PRECAUTIONS

May be used with care in pregnancy and breast feeding.

Not for use in children.

Use with caution in diabetes, migraine, epilepsy, liver disease.

 Do not take if:

- suffering from breast cancer, liver disease, undiagnosed abnormal vaginal bleeding.

- history of blood clots.

SIDE EFFECTS

None significant.

INTERACTIONS

None significant.

PRESCRIPTION

Yes

PERMITTED IN SPORT

Yes

Proguanil

TRADE NAMES

Paludrine.

Malarone (with Atovaquone).

DRUG CLASS

Antimalarial

USES

Prevention or treatment of malaria.

DOSAGE

 Two tablets a day.

FORMS

Tablets.

PRECAUTIONS

Use with caution in pregnancy (B2) and breast feeding.

Use with caution in kidney disease.

SIDE EFFECTS

Common: Loss of appetite, nausea, diarrhoea, headache.

Unusual: Vomiting, rash, dizziness, hair loss.

INTERACTIONS

Other drugs:

• Magnesium salts (antacids).

PRESCRIPTION

Yes

PERMITTED IN SPORT

Yes

OVERDOSE

Very serious. May be fatal. Administer activated charcoal or induce vomiting if taken recently. Seek urgent medical attention.

OTHER INFORMATION

Not addictive or dependence forming.

PROKINETIC AGENTS

(Increase rate of stomach emptying)

See Cisapride

Promethazine

See ANTIHISTAMINES, SEDATING

Propafenone

TRADE NAME

Arythmol.

DRUG CLASS

Antiarrhythmic.

USES

Prevention and treatment of some forms of abnormal heart rhythm.

DOSAGE

 150 to 300mg., two or three times a day.

FORMS

Tablets (white) of 150 and 300mg.

SIDE EFFECTS

Common: Dizziness, nausea, bitter taste, irregular bowel habits, headache.

Unusual: Fatigue, vomiting, skin rashes, slow heart rate.

Severe but rare (stop medication, consult doctor): Worsening heart beat irregularities.

INTERACTIONS

Other drugs:

• Other antiarrhythmics, Digoxin, Cimetidine, Warfarin, Propranolol, Metopralol, Rifampicin, Tricyclic antidepressants, Cyclosporin, Theophylline.

Other substances:

• Alcohol.

PRECAUTIONS

Not to be used in pregnancy, breast feeding and children.

Use with caution in asthma, liver and kidney disease, heart structure abnormalities, and any type of heart failure.

Treatment should be started in hospital.

Use lower doses in elderly.

Use care if pacemaker present.

Do not take if:

• suffering from uncontrolled congestive cardiac failure, shock, very slow heart rate, blood electrolyte disturbances, severe lung diseases, very low blood pressure, myasthenia gravis, some types of irregular heart rhythm.

PRESCRIPTION

Yes

PERMITTED IN SPORT

Yes

OVERDOSE

Very serious. Seek urgent medical attention. Induce vomiting or give activated charcoal if swallowed recently.

OTHER INFORMATION

Used only for serious, difficult to control, heart beat rhythm abnormalities.

Propamidine isethionate

(Dibromopropamide isethionate)

TRADE NAME

Golden Eye Ointment

DRUG CLASS

Antiseptic.

USES

Mild eye infections.

DOSAGE

 Apply two or three times a day.

FORMS

Eye drops, eye ointment.

PRECAUTIONS

Safe to use in pregnancy, breast feeding and children.

Not to be used regularly for longer than one week.

SIDE EFFECTS

Minimal

INTERACTIONS

None significant.

PRESCRIPTION

No

PERMITTED IN SPORT

Yes

OTHER INFORMATION

Commonly used as first line treatment for conjunctivitis.

Propiverine

TRADE NAME

Detrunorm.

DRUG CLASS

Anticholinergic.

USES

Unstable bladder control, urinary incontinence, urinary urgency.

DOSAGE

 One tablet, two to four times a day.

FORMS

Tablets of 15mg. (pink).

SIDE EFFECTS

Common: Dry mouth, blurred vision, drowsiness.

Unusual: Nausea, diarrhoea, difficulty passing urine, tiredness.

Severe but rare (stop medication, consult doctor): Unable to pass urine.

INTERACTIONS

Other drugs:

• Tricyclic antidepressants, Tranquillisers, Anticholinergics, Amantadine, Salbutamol, Isoniazid, Sedatives.

PRECAUTIONS

Not to be used in pregnancy, breast feeding and children.

Use with caution in overactive thyroid gland, angina, coronary artery disease, heart failure, irregular heart beat rhythm, rapid heart rate, enlarged prostate, heartburn and hiatus hernia.

 Do not take if:

• suffering from bladder outflow obstruction, myasthenia gravis, bowel obstruction, severe ulcerative colitis, megacolon, glaucoma, severe liver or kidney disease.

PRESCRIPTION

Yes

PERMITTED IN SPORT

Yes

OVERDOSE

Exacerbation of side effects only likely effects.

Propranolol
See BETA BLOCKERS

Propyl salicylate
See SALICYLATES

Prostaglandin E1
See Alprostadil

Protamine zinc insulin

See INSULINS

PROTON PUMP INHIBITORS

TRADE AND GENERIC NAMES

Zoton (Lansoprazole).

Heliclear (Lansoprazole with Clarithromycin, Amoxycillin).

Losec (Omeprazole).

Pariet (Rabeprazole).

Protiun (Pantoprazole).

DRUG CLASS

Anti-ulcer.

USES

Severe peptic ulcers of the stomach and duodenum, ulcers of the oesophagus, over production of acid in stomach (eg: Zollinger Ellison syndrome).

DOSAGE

 One or two capsules once a day. Swallow capsule whole.

FORMS

Capsules, tablets.

PRECAUTIONS

Safe use in pregnancy (B3) and while breast feeding not proven, but may be used if essential.

SIDE EFFECTS

Common: Minimal

Unusual: Nausea, vomiting, diarrhoea, constipation, belly pains, passing wind, headache.

Severe but rare (stop medication, consult doctor): Skin rash, breast enlargement in both sexes.

INTERACTIONS

Other drugs:

• Diazepam (sedation).

• Phenytoin (increases effect of phenytoin).

• Warfarin (dosage of warfarin may need to be decreased).

PRESCRIPTION

Yes

PERMITTED IN SPORT

Yes

OVERDOSE

Unlikely to be serious.

OTHER INFORMATION

Expensive, effective and safe. Relatively new class of drug which reduces acid secretion in stomach to heal ulcers.

Protriptyline

See TRICYCLIC ANTIDEPRESSANTS

Proxymetacaine

See ANAESTHETICS, LOCAL

Pseudoephedrine

TRADE NAME

Galpseud, Sudafed.

Dimotane Plus (with Brompheniramine).

Galpseud Plus (with Chlorpheniramine).

Sudafed Plus (with Triprolidine).

DRUG CLASS

Decongestant.

USES

Congestion of nose and sinuses.

DOSAGE

 One tablet or capsule two to four times a day.

FORMS

Tablets, capsules, mixture, syrup.

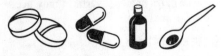

PRECAUTIONS

Use with caution in pregnancy (B2) and breast feeding. May be used in children.

Use with caution in high blood pressure, enlarged prostate gland and bladder problems.

SIDE EFFECTS

Common: Sleeplessness, rapid heart rate.

Unusual: Hallucinations, sweating, flushing, difficulty in passing urine.

Severe but rare (stop medication, consult doctor): Chest pain.

INTERACTIONS

Other drugs:

• Other Decongestants, MAOI, Furazolidone, medications used to treat high blood pressure.

PRESCRIPTION

No

PERMITTED IN SPORT

No

OVERDOSE

Serious. May cause irritability, convulsions, palpitations, high blood pressure, angina and difficulty in passing urine. Administer activated charcoal or induce vomiting if medication taken recently. Seek urgent medical assistance.

OTHER INFORMATION

Very widely used medication for colds and flu. Safe and effective if taken in recommended dose. Should not be used to combat drowsiness.

PSYCHOTROPICS

(Alter the functioning of the brain)

See ANTIDEPRESSANTS, ANTIPSYCHOTICS, ANXIOLYTICS, Marijuana

Psyllium

TRADE NAME

Used in some bulking agents and fibre supplements.

DRUG CLASS

Fibre.

USES

Constipation.

DOSAGE

 Take required amount with water two or three times a day.

FORMS

Granules, powder.

PRECAUTIONS

Safe in pregnancy and breast feeding.

 Do not take if:

• on a salt, potassium or sugar restricted diet

• suffering from severe constipation with impacted faeces.

• suffering from belly pain, nausea or vomiting.

SIDE EFFECTS

Common: Minimal

Unusual: Diarrhoea, belly discomfort

INTERACTIONS

None significant

PRESCRIPTION

No

PERMITTED IN SPORT

Yes

OVERDOSE

Take additional water. Belly discomfort and passing excess wind only effects.

OTHER INFORMATION

Widely used, natural fibre supplement.

Pyrazinamide

TRADE NAMES

Zinamide.

Rifater (with Isoniazid, Rifampicin).

USES

Tuberculosis.

DOSAGE

 One tablet three or four times a day in combination with other medication for the treatment of tuberculosis.

FORMS

Zinamide: Tablets (white) of 500mg.

PRECAUTIONS

Should be used in pregnancy only if medically essential. Breast feeding should be ceased before use. Use with caution in children.

Use with caution in gout, diabetes and kidney disease.

Regular blood tests to check liver function and blood count necessary.

 Do not take if:
- suffering from liver disease.

SIDE EFFECTS

Common: Fever, loss of appetite.

Unusual: Liver tenderness and enlargement, gout, nausea, vomiting.

Severe but rare (stop medication, consult doctor): Yellow skin (jaundice), severe joint pain.

INTERACTIONS

None significant.

PRESCRIPTION

Yes

PERMITTED IN SPORT

Yes

OVERDOSE

Attacks the brain to cause convulsions and coma. Administer activated charcoal or induce vomiting if medication taken recently. Seek urgent medical attention.

PYRIDOSTIGMINE

TRADE NAME

Mestinon.

DRUG CLASS

Anticholinesterase.

USES

Myasthenia gravis, inability to pass urine, paralysis of small intestine.

DOSAGE

 One to three tablets once or twice a day

FORMS

Tablets of 60mg. (white).

PRECAUTIONS

Should be used in pregnancy (C) only when medically essential. Safe for use in breast feeding. Use with caution in children.

Dosage must be carefully monitored by doctor.

Use with caution in epilepsy, slow heart rate, asthma, recent heart attack, irregular heart beat, overactive thyroid gland, and peptic ulcer.

 Do not take if:
- suffering from gut obstruction.

SIDE EFFECTS

Common: Slow heart rate, headache, nausea, diarrhoea, excess salivation, cough, wheeze, bowel noises.

Unusual: Confusion, slurred speech, vomiting, belly cramps, desire to pass urine, muscle cramps, contracted pupils.

Severe but rare (stop medication, consult doctor): Difficulty breathing, chest pain.

INTERACTIONS

Other drugs:
- Muscle relaxants, Atropine, Aminoglycosides, drugs used to treat irregular heart beat, some anaesthetics.

PRESCRIPTION

Yes

PERMITTED IN SPORT

Yes

OVERDOSE

Serious. May cause diarrhoea, vomiting, difficulty in breathing, weakness, low blood pressure, slow heart rate and heart attack. Seek urgent medical attention.

OTHER INFORMATION

Useful for the few patients with the distressing muscle disease of myasthenia gravis.

See also Donepezil

Pyridoxine

(Vitamin B6)

TRADE NAMES

A large number of non-prescription preparations include Pyridoxine (Vitamin B6) alone or in combination with other vitamins and minerals.

DRUG CLASS

Vitamin.

USES

Vitamin B deficiency, nervous tension, mouth ulcers, premenstrual tension, hardening of arteries.

DOSAGE

 Recommended daily allowance: Females - 0.9 to 1.4 mg. a day; Males - 1.3 to 1.9 mg a day.

FORMS

Tablets, capsules, mixture, drops, injection.

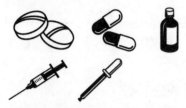

PRECAUTIONS

Safe in pregnancy, breast feeding and children.

Do not take in high doses or for prolonged periods of time.

Ensure adequate protein intake in diet.

SIDE EFFECTS

Common: Minimal.

Unusual: Sensory nerve damage.

INTERACTIONS

Other drugs:

• Oral contraceptives, L-dopa.

PRESCRIPTION

No

PERMITTED IN SPORT

Yes

OVERDOSE

May cause sensory nerve damage.

OTHER INFORMATION

Pyridoxine is a water soluble vitamin. It is essential for the metabolism of protein. Remember, vitamins are merely chemicals that are essential for the functioning of the body, and if taken to excess, act as a drug.

Pyrimethamine

TRADE NAME

Daraprim.

Fansidar (with Sulfadoxine).

Maloprim (with Dapsone).

DRUG CLASS

Antimalarial.

USES

Prevention and treatment of malaria, toxoplasmosis.

DOSAGE

Prevention: One tablet a week. Treatment: Two tablets at once, then one tablet a day.

FORMS

Tablets, injection.

PRECAUTIONS

Should not be used in pregnancy (B3) unless medically essential. May be used in breast feeding and children.

Use with caution in liver and kidney disease.

Ensure adequate fluid intake.

 Do not take if:
• suffering from folate deficiency.

SIDE EFFECTS

Common: Minimal.

Unusual: Rash, nausea, colic, vomiting, diarrhoea.

INTERACTIONS

Other drugs:

• Co-trimoxazole, Lorazepam.

PRESCRIPTION

Yes

PERMITTED IN SPORT

Yes

OVERDOSE

Serious. Induce vomiting if taken recently. Give additional fluids. Seek urgent medical assistance.

OTHER INFORMATION

Used in areas where chloroquine resistant malaria occurs (eg: New Guinea, Solomon Is., southeast Asia).

Pyrithione zinc

TRADE NAMES

Polytar AF (with Tars and other ingredients).

Numerous over the counter antiseptic and antidandruff shampoos contain Pyrithione zinc, usually combined with other ingredients.

DRUG CLASS

Antiseptic, antifungal.

USES

Dandruff

DOSAGE

 Apply once every day or two.

FORMS

Shampoo, cream.

PRECAUTIONS

Safe to use in pregnancy, breast feeding and children. Avoid eye contact.

SIDE EFFECTS

Minimal

INTERACTIONS

None

PRESCRIPTION

No

PERMITTED IN SPORT

Yes

Quetiapine

TRADE NAME

Seroquel.

DRUG CLASS

Antipsychotic.

USES

Treatment of schizophrenia.

DOSAGE

 Gradually increased from 25mg. twice a day to maximum dose of 350mg. twice a day.

FORMS

Tablets of 25mg (peach), 100mg (yellow), 150mg. (cream) and 200mg (white).

PRECAUTIONS

Use with caution in pregnancy (B3), breast feeding and children.

Use with caution in heart disease, poor brain circulation, recent strokes, low blood pressure.

SIDE EFFECTS

Common: Dizziness and light headedness from low blood pressure, tiredness, dry mouth, runny nose, indigestion and constipation. Side effects often settle after two weeks.

Unusual: Rapid heart rate, fainting.

Severe but rare (stop medication, consult doctor): Seizures.

INTERACTIONS

Other drugs:

• Sedatives, sleeping medication (benzodiazepines), thioridazine, phenytoin, barbiturates, rifampicin.

Other substances:

• Alcohol.

PRESCRIPTION

Yes

PERMITTED IN SPORT

Yes

OVERDOSE

Unlikely to have serious consequences other than worsening of side effects. Seek medical attention.

OTHER INFORMATION

Introduced in 2000 to treat previously uncontrolled patients with schizophrenia.

See also other medications listed under Antipsychotics

Quinagolide

TRADE NAME

Norprolac.

USES

Hyperprolactinaemia (overactive pituitary gland producing excess breast milk).

DOSAGE

 Start with 25ug. at night, increasing slowly to a maximum of 150ug. at night.

FORMS

Tablets of 25ug. (pink), 50ug (blue), 75ug (white) and 150ug. (white).

PRECAUTIONS

Not to be used in pregnancy, breast feeding and children.

Non-hormonal contraception must be used.

Use with caution if history of psychotic disorders.

Check blood pressure regularly.

 Do not take if:

- suffering from kidney or liver disease.

SIDE EFFECTS

Common: Nausea, diarrhoea, headache, dizziness.

Unusual: Tiredness, loss of appetite, sleeplessness, swelling of tissue, nasal congestion.

Severe but rare (stop medication, consult doctor): Low blood pressure, psychotic reactions.

INTERACTIONS

Other drugs:

- None significant.

Other substances:

- Alcohol.

PRESCRIPTION

Yes

PERMITTED IN SPORT

Yes

OVERDOSE

May be serious. Seek urgent medical attention. Induce vomiting or give activated charcoal if swallowed recently.

Quinalbarbitone

See BARBITURATES

Quinapril

See ACE INHIBITORS

Quinidine

TRADE NAME

Kinidin Durules.

DRUG CLASS

Antiarrhythmic.

USES

Prevents some types of irregular heart beats.

DOSAGE

 Two to five tablets twice a day..

FORMS

Tablets of 250mg. (white).

PRECAUTIONS

Should only be used in pregnancy (C) if medically essential. Should not be used in breast feeding or children.

 Do not take if:

- suffering from thrombocytopenia, low blood pressure, bowel obstruction or kidney failure.

SIDE EFFECTS

Common: Nausea, vomiting, loss of appetite, diarrhoea, dizziness, noises in ears, blurred vision, headache.

Unusual: Psychiatric disturbances, fever, rash, worsening of asthma, anaemia.

Severe but rare (stop medication, consult doctor): Unusual bleeding, yellow skin, asthma.

INTERACTIONS

Other drugs:

• Digoxin, Anticoagulants, Phenytoin, Barbiturates, Rifampicin, Procainamide, Propranolol, Verapamil, Amiodarone, Nifedipine.

• Absorption of Quinidine slowed by antacids.

PRESCRIPTION

Yes

PERMITTED IN SPORT

Yes

OVERDOSE

Very serious. Administer activated charcoal or induce vomiting if tablets taken recently. Seek urgent medical assistance. Symptoms include blurred vision, deafness, weakness, dizziness, headache, nausea, vomiting, low blood pressure, diarrhoea, irregular heart rate and death.

QUINOLONES

(Antibiotics)

See Cinoxacin, Ciprofloxacin, Levofloxacin, Norfloxacin, Ofloxacin

Rabeprazole

See PROTON PUMP INHIBITORS

Rabies vaccine

TRADE NAME

Rabies Vaccine.

DRUG CLASS

Vaccine.

USES

Prevention of rabies.

DOSAGE

 Prevention: Two injections one month apart, repeat annually.
After suspect animal bite: Series of frequent injections as determined by doctor.

FORMS

Injection

PRECAUTIONS

Not designed for use in pregnancy, but must be used if mother exposed to bite from rabid animal. May be used in breast feeding and children.

Use with caution in immune deficiency and history of allergy.

SIDE EFFECTS

Common: Local redness, soreness and hardness at injection site.

Unusual: Fever, muscle pains, nausea, diarrhoea.

INTERACTIONS

Other drugs:

• Corticosteroids.

PRESCRIPTION

Yes

PERMITTED IN SPORT

Yes

OVERDOSE

An inadvertent additional injection is unlikely to have any serious adverse effects.

OTHER INFORMATION

Routinely given only to veterinarians and others working with animals in areas affected by rabies. Given after any bite by an animal in an area affected by rabies. Once symptoms of rabies occur, it is inevitably fatal. Rabies does not occur in Britain, but is widespread in Europe.

Raloxifene

TRADE NAME

Evista

USES

Prevention and treatment of osteoporosis after the menopause.

DOSAGE

 One tablet a day.

FORMS

Tablet (white) of 60mg.

PRECAUTIONS

Must never be used in pregnancy (X)(causes deformities of foetus), breast feeding or children.

Use with caution in liver disease.

Abnormal uterine bleeding must be diagnosed before use.

 Do not take if:

- still menstruating. For use in post-menopausal women only.
- medical history of blood clots.
- male

SIDE EFFECTS

Common: Hot flushes, leg cramps, sinus congestion.

Severe but rare (stop medication, consult doctor): Blood clots.

INTERACTIONS

Other drugs:

- Oestrogen supplements, cholestyramine, ampicillin, warfarin.

PRESCRIPTION

Yes

PERMITTED IN SPORT

Yes

OVERDOSE

Unlikely to result in serious consequences. Exacerbation of side effects likely. Seek medical assistance.

OTHER INFORMATION

Released in 1999 to assist women who are unable to tolerate normal post-menopausal hormone replacement therapy.

See also Alendronate sodium, Disodium etidronate, Salcatonin

Ramipril

See ACE INHIBITORS

Ranitidine

TRADE NAMES

Zantac.

Pylorid (with Bismuth citrate).

DRUG CLASS

Antiulcerant, H2 receptor antagonist.

USES

Prevention and treatment of ulcers of the stomach, oesophagus (gullet) and duodenum (upper small intestine). Prevention of acid reflux into the oesophagus (heartburn).

DOSAGE

 Up to 600mg a day in one or two doses.

PRECAUTIONS

Care should be taken with use in pregnancy (B1) and breast feeding. Children under twelve may be treated at the discretion of the doctor.

 Do not take if:

- suffering from severe kidney disease or phenylketonuria.

FORMS

Tablets, effervescent tablets, syrup, injection.

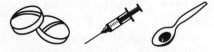

SIDE EFFECTS

Common: Headache, diarrhoea, rash.

Unusual: Tiredness, dizziness, sleeplessness, speeding or slowing of heart rate, constipation, joint pains, breast tenderness (both sexes).

Severe but rare (stop medication, consult doctor): Hepatitis (jaundice), pancreatitis (severe stomach pain).

INTERACTIONS

None significant

PRESCRIPTION

Yes

PERMITTED IN SPORT

Yes

OVERDOSE

No serious effects reported.

OTHER INFORMATION

Most widely used medication for the treatment of peptic ulcers. Very safe and effective.

See also Cimetidine, Famotidine, Nizatadine.

Reboxetine

TRADE NAME

Edronax.

DRUG CLASS

SSRI antidepressant.

USES

Depression.

DOSAGE

 One or two tablets twice a day.

FORMS

Tablet (white) of 4mg.

PRECAUTIONS

Should be used in pregnancy (B3) with considerable caution. Breast feeding should be ceased if prescribed. Not for use in children or elderly.

Should be used with caution in glaucoma, kidney and liver disease, urinary retention, mania, epilepsy and heart disease.

Should not be stopped suddenly, but dose should be slowly reduced over several days.

 Do not take if:
- taking MAOI antidepressants.

SIDE EFFECTS

Common: Generally minimal. Nausea, drowsiness, sweating, tremor, tiredness, dry mouth, sleeplessness, impotence, constipation, dizziness.

Unusual: Headache, fever, palpitations, sweating, rash, blurred vision, urinary retention.

INTERACTIONS

Other drugs:

- MAOI

- Anticoagulants, thiazide diuretics, some antifungals, macrolide antibiotics, Fluvoxamine, Antipsychotics, Tricyclic antidepressants, Cyclosporin.

Other substances:

• alcohol.

PRESCRIPTION

Yes

PERMITTED IN SPORT

Yes

OVERDOSE

Symptoms may include nausea, tremor, dilated pupils, dry mouth and irritability. Death or serious effects have not occurred. Seek medical attention.

OTHER INFORMATION

One of the newer antidepressants released in the late 1990s. May take up to two weeks for patient to notice any improvement in depression.

Repaglinide

TRADE NAME

Novonorm

DRUG CLASS

Hypoglycaemic.

USES

Complicated type two (maturity onset, non-insulin dependent) diabetes.

DOSAGE

 0.5 to 4mg before meals three times a day.

FORMS

Tablets of 0.5mg. (white), 1mg. (yellow) and 2 mg. (red).

PRECAUTIONS

Not to be used in pregnancy (C), breast feeding or children.

Only to be used when other treatments for type two diabetes are not controlling disease.

Use with caution in kidney and liver disease.

 Do not take if:

• suffering from type one (juvenile, insulin dependent) diabetes or ketoacidosis.

SIDE EFFECTS

Common: Nausea, dyspepsia, headache.

Unusual: Vomiting, pins and needles sensation, chest pain.

INTERACTIONS

Other drugs:

• Oral contraceptives, thiazides, corticosteroids, danazol, thyroid hormones, MAOI, beta-blockers, ACE inhibitors, salicylates, NSAID, octreotide, anabolic steroids.

Other substances:

• Alcohol.

PRESCRIPTION

Yes

PERMITTED IN SPORT

Yes

OVERDOSE

Low blood sugar with dizziness, headache, tremor, sweating and convulsions may occur. Give sweet drinks or injections of sugar. Seek medical assistance.

OTHER INFORMATION

Introduced in 2000 as an additional treatment for severe forms of type two diabetes. Normally used in combination with Metformin. Tolerance may gradually develop necessitating an increase in dosage.

See also other medications listed under HYPOGLYCAEMICS.

Reproterol

See BETA -2 AGONISTS

Resorcinol

TRADE NAME

Found in some locally produced acne and psoriasis preparations.

USES

Skin peeling agent, acne, psoriasis.

DOSAGE

 Varies between preparations. Follow directions on packaging.

FORMS

Gel, cream, solution, ointment.

PRECAUTIONS

Safe in pregnancy and breast feeding.

Not for use in infants.

Use with caution in children.

Avoid contact with eyes, mouth, nose, anus and vagina.

 Do not use on:

• inflamed or broken skin (cuts, grazes, burns etc.).

SIDE EFFECTS

Common: Skin inflammation.

INTERACTIONS

Other drugs:

• Other skin acne and psoriasis preparations.

PRESCRIPTION

No

PERMITTED IN SPORT

Yes

Retinols

(Vitamin A)

TRADE and GENERIC NAMES

Found in numerous vitamin and mineral preparations, as well as soothing and healing creams and lotions.

DRUG CLASS

Vitamin.

USES

Vitamin A deficiency, malnutrition, poor diet, soothing agent in creams for minor burns.

DOSAGE

 Recommended daily allowance: 2500 International Units a day.

FORMS

Capsules, tablets, mixture, lotion, cream.

PRECAUTIONS

Must not be used in pregnancy (D) as high doses may cause birth defects. May be used in breast feeding and with caution in children. Skin preparations safe in pregnancy.

Do not exceed recommended dose.

Use with caution in Vitamin K deficiency.

SIDE EFFECTS

Common: Minimal.

Severe but rare (stop medication, consult doctor): Yellow skin, particularly of palms and soles.

INTERACTIONS

None significant.

PRESCRIPTION

No

PERMITTED IN SPORT

Yes

OVERDOSE

Chronic overdosage will lead to carotenaemia in which excess Retinol is deposited in skin (causes it to turn yellow) and may cause damage to organs.

OTHER INFORMATION

Fat soluble vitamin. Dangerous in pregnancy and overdose. Remember, vitamins are merely chemicals that are essential for the functioning of the body, and if taken to excess, act as a drug.

See also Cod liver oil

REVERSIBLE INHIBITORS OF MONOAMINE OXIDASE (RIMA)

See Moclobemide

Riboflavine

(Vitamin B2)

TRADE and GENERIC NAMES

A large number of preparations include Riboflavine (Vitamin B2) alone or in combination with other vitamins and minerals.

DRUG CLASS

Vitamin.

USES

Vitamin B deficiency, arabinoflavinosis.

DOSAGE

 Recommended daily allowance: 1.0 to 1.7 mg a day.

FORMS

Tablets, capsules, mixture, drops.

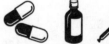

PRECAUTIONS

Safe in pregnancy, breast feeding and children.

SIDE EFFECTS

Minimal.

INTERACTIONS

None significant.

PRESCRIPTION

No

PERMITTED IN SPORT

Yes

OVERDOSE

Not harmful.

OTHER INFORMATION

Riboflavine is a water soluble vitamin found in dairy products, offal and green leafy vegetables. It is essential for the effective working of the lungs. Remember, vitamins are merely chemicals that are essential for the functioning of the body, and if taken to excess, act as a drug.

Rifabutin

TRADE NAME

Mycobutin.

USES

Tuberculosis (TB).

DOSAGE

 One or two capsules once a day.

FORMS

Capsule (red/brown) of 150mg.

PRECAUTIONS

Not to be used in pregnancy (C) unless medically essential. Breast feeding should be ceased before use. Not to be used in children.

Use with caution in liver and kidney disease and eye inflammation.

Regular blood tests to check white cells, platelets and liver function essential.

Soft contact lenses may be stained.

Check eyes regularly for inflammation.

SIDE EFFECTS

Common: Nausea, vomiting, yellow skin (jaundice), unusual bruising, anaemia, arthritis, fever, rash.

Unusual: Eye inflammation, asthma.

INTERACTIONS

Other drugs:

• Dapsone, Narcotics, Anticoagulants, Corticosteroids, Quinidine, Hypoglycaemics, Clarithromycin, Oral contraceptives.

PRESCRIPTION

Yes

PERMITTED IN SPORT

Yes

OVERDOSE

May be serious. Seek medical assistance.

OTHER INFORMATION

Introduced in 1994 to treat resistant forms of tuberculosis.

Rifampicin

TRADE NAMES

Rifadin, Rimactane.

Rifater (with Isoniazid, Pyrazinamide).

Rifinah, Rimactazid (with Isoniazid).

USES

Treatment of tuberculosis and leprosy, prevention of Meningococcal and Haemophilus bacterial infections.

DOSAGE

 450mg. to 600mg. a day as a single daily dose in combination with other treatments.

FORMS

Capsules, tablets, syrup, infusion.

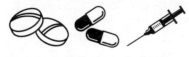

PRECAUTIONS

Should not be used in pregnancy (C) unless medically essential. Not to be used in breast feeding or infants. May be used with caution in children.

Use with caution in liver disease.

Designed to be used continuously long term.

 Do not take if:

- suffering from jaundice (yellow skin).

SIDE EFFECTS

Common: Heartburn, nausea, loss of appetite, intestinal cramps.

Unusual: Vomiting, headache, diarrhoea, drowsiness, fatigue, dizziness.

Severe but rare (stop medication, consult doctor): Yellow skin (jaundice).

INTERACTIONS

Other drugs:

- Anticoagulants, Corticosteroids, Cyclosporin, Digoxin, Quinidine, Hypoglycaemics, Dapsone, Narcotics, Oral contraceptives.

PRESCRIPTION

Yes

PERMITTED IN SPORT

Yes

OVERDOSE

Serious. Nausea, vomiting, drowsiness, brown stain to body fluids, convulsions, coma, jaundice and liver failure may occur. Administer activated charcoal or induce vomiting if medication taken recently. Seek urgent medical assistance.

Riluzole

TRADE NAME

Rilutek.

USES

Amyotrophic lateral sclerosis (Lou Gehrig disease), motor neurone disease.

DOSAGE

 One tablet twice a day.

FORMS

Tablets of 50mg. (white).

PRECAUTIONS

Not to be used in pregnancy, breast feeding or children.

Use with caution in liver and kidney disease.

Commence under specialist supervision.

Regular blood tests to check liver function and white blood cells necessary.

 Do not take if:

- suffering from severe liver disease.

SIDE EFFECTS

Common: Tiredness, nausea, vomiting, headache, belly pains, dizziness.

Unusual: Rapid heart rate, sleepiness, pins and needles around mouth.

Severe but rare (stop medication, consult doctor): Fever, low white cell count.

INTERACTIONS

Other drugs:

• Not known.

PRESCRIPTION

Yes

PERMITTED IN SPORT

Yes

OVERDOSE

Seek urgent medical attention. Induce vomiting or administer activated charcoal if swallowed recently.

RIMA (Reversible Inhibitor of Monoamine Oxidase Type A)

(Treat depression)

See Moclobemide

Rimexolone

TRADE NAME

Vexol.

DRUG CLASS

Corticosteroid.

USES

Eye inflammation after surgery, uveitis, inflamed conjunctiva.

DOSAGE

 One drop into eye four to twelve times a day.

FORMS

Eye drops.

PRECAUTIONS

May be used with caution in pregnancy and breast feeding. Not recommended in children.

Not for prolonged use.

Monitor eye pressure regularly.

 Do not take if:

• suffering from any form of eye infection.

SIDE EFFECTS

Common: Intermittent blurred vision.

Unusual: Eye discharge, eye discomfort or temporary pain, foreign body sensation.

Severe but rare (stop medication, consult doctor): Raised pressure in eye (haloes around objects, constantly blurred vision).

INTERACTIONS

Other drugs:

• Other eye preparations.

PRESCRIPTION

Yes

PERMITTED IN SPORT

Yes

OVERDOSE

Unlikely to be serious if swallowed.

Risedronate

TRADE NAME

Actonel.

DRUG CLASS

Bisphosphonate.

USES

Paget's disease of bone.

DOSAGE

 One tablet a day for two months. Swallow tablet whole in an upright position with water, at least half an hour before first food or drink of day, or at least two hours after eating.

FORMS

Tablets (white) of 30mg.

PRECAUTIONS

Not to be used in pregnancy, breast feeding or children.

Use with caution in kidney disease, oesophageal disease, mineral metabolism disorders.

Ensure adequate dietary calcium and vitamin D intake.

Do not take if:

- suffering from severe kidney disease, low blood calcium levels.

SIDE EFFECTS

Common: Nausea, diarrhoea, flu symptoms, chest pain, dizziness.

Unusual: Muscle pain, headache, rash, swelling of tissues, weight loss, shortness of breath, sinus congestion, eye irritation, dry eye, blurred vision, ringing in ears, passing urine at night.

INTERACTIONS

Other drugs:

- Antacids, calcium and magnesium supplements, iron.

PRESCRIPTION

Yes

PERMITTED IN SPORT

Yes

OVERDOSE

Serious. Symptoms include loss of appetite, tiredness, vomiting, diarrhoea, sweating, excess urine production, extreme thirst and headache. This may progress to high blood pressure and kidney failure. Administer activated charcoal or induce vomiting if taken recently. Seek medical assistance.

Risperidone

TRADE NAME

Risperdal.

DRUG CLASS

Antipsychotic

USES

Schizophrenia.

DOSAGE

 Start with low dose and gradually increase at direction of doctor. Maximum 8mg. twice a day.

FORMS

Tablets of 1mg. (white), 2mg. (orange), 3mg. (yellow), 4mg. (green) and 6mg. (yellow). Liquid.

SIDE EFFECTS

Common: Low blood pressure, sleeplessness, agitation, anxiety, headache.

Unusual: Tiredness, dizziness, constipation, nausea, poor concentration, weight gain, blurred vision, belly pain, impotence.

INTERACTIONS

Other drugs:

• Levodopa, Antihypertensives, Tricyclic antidepressants, Beta blockers.

PRECAUTIONS

Use with caution and only when necessary in pregnancy (B3) and breast feeding. Not for use in children under 15.

Use with caution in heart disease, low blood pressure, epilepsy or seizures, Parkinson's disease, liver or kidney disease.

Lower doses necessary in elderly.

PRESCRIPTION

Yes

PERMITTED IN SPORT

Yes

OVERDOSE

Drowsiness, sedation, rapid heart rate and low blood pressure may occur.Administer activated charcoal or induce vomiting if taken recently. Seek medical attention.

OTHER INFORMATION

Often very effective, but very expensive.

Ritodrine hydrochloride

TRADE NAME

Yutopar.

USES

Stops labour of pregnancy, reduces intensity of uterine contractions during labour.

DOSAGE

 Normally given by intravenous injection or infusion initially, then tablets are taken to continue effect.

FORMS

Injection, tablets (pale yellow) of 10mg.

PRECAUTIONS

Not to be used in any situation other than during premature or excessively severe labour of pregnancy.

Not to be used in pregnancy before 24 weeks.

Use with caution in heart disease, high blood pressure, diabetes, liver and kidney disease.

Close monitoring of mother and foetus essential.

 Do not take if:

• suffering from overactive thyroid gland, pre-eclampsia.

SIDE EFFECTS

Common: Rapid heart rate, lung congestion, palpitations, nausea, vomiting.

INTERACTIONS

Other drugs:

• Corticosteroids, Sympathomimetics, Beta-blockers, Digoxin, MAOI, Tricyclic antidepressants.

PRESCRIPTION

Yes

OVERDOSE

Exacerbation of side effects likely.

OTHER INFORMATION

Introduced in early 1980s, and has proved very useful in preventing premature births in some situations.

Ritonavir

TRADE NAME

Norvir.

DRUG CLASS

Antiviral.

USES

HIV infection, AIDS.

DOSAGE

 600mg. twice a day with food.

FORMS

Capsules of 100mg. (white), solution.

PRECAUTIONS

Use with considerable caution in pregnancy (B3), breast feeding and children.

Use with caution in liver disease.

SIDE EFFECTS

Common: Tiredness, raised triglyceride (fat) levels in blood, nausea, diarrhoea, abnormal pain, pins and needles sensation.

Unusual: Vomiting, dizziness, abnormal taste.

INTERACTIONS

Other drugs:

• Do NOT use with amiodarone, astemizole, benzodiazepines, cisapride, clonazepam, dextropropoxyphene, flecainide, quinidine, pethidine, piroxicam, rifabutin, terfenadine.

• Hypnotics, sedatives, oral contraceptives, other antivirals.

PRESCRIPTION

Yes

PERMITTED IN SPORT

Yes

OVERDOSE

May be serious. Induce vomiting or administer activated charcoal if medication taken recently. Seek immediate medical attention.

OTHER INFORMATION

Introduced in 1997.

Rivastigmine

TRADE NAME

Exelon.

DRUG CLASS

Anticholinesterase.

USES

Dementia of Alzheimer's disease.

DOSAGE

 Initially 1.5mg. twice a day, slowly increasing to a maximum of 6mg. twice a day.

FORMS

Capsules of 1.5mg. (yellow), 3mg. (orange), 4.5mg. (red) and 6mg. (orange/red).

PRECAUTIONS

Not to be used in pregnancy, breast feeding or children.

Treatment should be initiated by specialist.

Use with caution in heart disease, peptic ulcer history, asthma, emphysema, chronic bronchitis, enlarged prostate gland, and liver disease.

Monitor weight loss carefully.

 Do not take if:

- suffering from severe liver disease.

SIDE EFFECTS

Common: Tiredness, loss of appetite, dizziness, belly pains.

Unusual: Agitation, confusion, depression, diarrhoea, sweating, weight loss, tremor, headache, sleeplessness, respiratory and urinary infections.

Severe but rare (stop medication, consult doctor): Angina, bleeding from gut, fainting.

INTERACTIONS

Other drugs:

- Other anticholinergics.

PRESCRIPTION

Yes

PERMITTED IN SPORT

Yes

OVERDOSE

Serious. May cause diarrhoea, vomiting, difficulty in breathing, weakness, low blood pressure, slow heart rate and heart attack. Seek urgent medical attention.

OTHER INFORMATION

Introduced in 1999.

Rizatripan

TRADE NAME

Maxalt.

DRUG CLASS

Antimigraine.

USES

Treatment of some types of migraine.

DOSAGE

 10mg. swallowed or dissolved on tongue. Repeat after two hours if necessary.

PRECAUTIONS

Use with caution in pregnancy and breast feeding . Not recommended in children.

Patient must be carefully evaluated to exclude poor circulation to heart, brain and other organs before starting treatment.

Use with caution in kidney and liver disease, and phenylketonuria.

 Do not take if:

- suffering from severe kidney or liver disease, history of strokes or poor blood supply to brain, angina, significant heart disease, poor circulation, high blood pressure, paralysing migraine or other types of headache.

FORMS

Tablets (pink) of 5mg., soluble wafers of 10mg.

SIDE EFFECTS

Common: Dizziness, tiredness, muscle pains, chest and belly pains, palpitations.

Unusual: Rapid heart rate, nausea, diarrhoea, throat discomfort, shortness of breath, skin rash, blurred vision, hot flushes.

Severe but rare (stop medication, consult doctor): Angina, stroke, heart attack.

INTERACTIONS

Other drugs:

• MAOI, Ergotamine, Propranolol.

PRESCRIPTION

Yes

PERMITTED IN SPORT

Yes

OVERDOSE

Serious. Seek urgent medical attention.

OTHER INFORMATION

Introduced in 1999 to help patients with more serious and intractable cases of migraine.

Rofecoxib

TRADE NAME

Vioxx

DRUG CLASS

COX-2 Inhibitor.

USES

Osteoarthritis.

DOSAGE

 12.5 to 25mg. once a day.

FORMS

Tablets of 12.5mg. (white) and 25mg. (yellow).

PRECAUTIONS

Not for use in pregnancy (C). Use with caution in breast feeding and children.

Use with caution if history of peptic ulcer or intestinal bleeding. Use with caution in smokers, alcoholics, dehydration, asthma, high blood pressure, heart failure, infection, liver or kidney disease.

Use with care in elderly.

 Do not take if:

• suffering from active peptic ulcer, intestinal bleeding, active asthma, urticaria (hives).

SIDE EFFECTS

Common: Minimal.

Unusual: Intestinal upsets, allergy, anaemia, fluid retention.

Severe but rare (stop medication, consult doctor): Peptic ulcer.

INTERACTIONS

Other drugs:

• NSAID, Aspirin, Steroids, Anticoagulants, Rifampicin, Methotrexate, ACE Inhibitors, Lithium, Diuretics.

PRESCRIPTION

Yes

PERMITTED IN SPORT

Yes

OVERDOSE

Exacerbation of side effects likely. Induce vomiting or give activated charcoal if swallowed recently. Seek medical attention.

OTHER INFORMATION

Introduced 2000. Far less likely than other treatments for arthritis (eg. NSAIDs) to cause intestinal bleeding.

See also Celecoxib.

Ropinirole

TRADE NAME

Requip.

DRUG CLASS

Antiparkinsonian.

USES

Parkinson's disease.

DOSAGE

 Start with 0.25mg. three times a day. Increase each dose by 0.25mg. weekly as necessary, up to 3mg. three times a day. Maximum dose 24mg. a day.

FORMS

Tablets of 0.25mg. (white), 1mg. (green), 2mg. (pink) and 5mg. (blue).

PRECAUTIONS

Not to be used in pregnancy, breast feeding and children.

Use with caution in significant heart disease and psychoses.

Do not stop suddenly but withdraw slowly.

 Do not take if:
- suffering from severe liver or kidney disease.

SIDE EFFECTS

Common: Nausea, tiredness, leg swelling.

Unusual: Belly pain, fainting, vomiting, low blood pressure, slow heart rate.

INTERACTIONS

Other drugs:

- Blood pressure lowering medications, medications to control irregular heart beat, Oestrogens.

Other substances:

- Alcohol.

PRESCRIPTION

Yes

PERMITTED IN SPORT

Yes

OVERDOSE

Serious. Seek urgent medical attention. Induce vomiting or give activated charcoal if swallowed recently.

OTHER INFORMATION

Does not cause addiction or dependence.

Ropivacaine

See ANAESTHETICS, LOCAL

RU486

See Mifepristone

RUBEFACIENTS

(Liniments)

See Camphor, Menthol,
SALICYLATES

Rubella vaccine

TRADE NAMES

Erevax.

MMR II, Priorix (with Measles and
Mumps vaccines).

DRUG CLASS

Vaccine

USES

Prevention of rubella (German measles).

DOSAGE

 Single injection. Repeat in early
teen years if first dose given
under five years of age. Lifelong
protection usual.

PRECAUTIONS

Not to be used in pregnancy (B2),
but inadvertent use unlikely to have
serious effects. May be used in
breast feeding and children.

Use with caution if history of
convulsions.

 ## Do not take if:

• suffering from fever,
immune system
deficiency.

• blood transfusion within
three months.

FORMS

Injection.

SIDE EFFECTS

Common: Pain, soreness, redness,
firmness at site of injection.

Unusual: Fever, rash, headache, joint
pains, sore throat, tender glands.

INTERACTIONS

None significant

PRESCRIPTION

Yes

PERMITTED IN SPORT

Yes

OVERDOSE

No adverse effects likely from an
inadvertent additional dose.

OTHER INFORMATION

Rubella (German measles) is usually a
minor disease, although it may cause
significant arthritis, headache and fever,
but if caught by the mother during the
first three months of pregnancy it may
cause serious damage to the foetus.

RUTOSIDES

See Oxerutin

Sabin vaccine

See **Poliomyelitis vaccine**

Salbutamol

See **BETA-2 AGONISTS**

Salcatonin

TRADE NAMES

Calsynar, Miacalcic.

USES

Paget's disease of bone, excess blood calcium levels (hypercalcaemia).

DOSAGE

 By injection in a dose determined by doctor for each patient.

FORMS

Injection.

PRECAUTIONS

Not to be used in pregnancy, or breast feeding.

Use with great caution in children.

Not for long term use.

SIDE EFFECTS

Common: Nausea, vomiting, injection site inflammation.

INTERACTIONS

Other drugs:

• Digoxin.

PRESCRIPTION

Yes

PERMITTED IN SPORT

Yes

OTHER INFORMATION

Derived from a natural hormone found in salmon.

See also Calcitonin

SALICYLATES

TRADE and GENERIC NAMES

Acnisal, Occlusal, Verrugon (Salicylic acid)

Algesal (Diethylamine salicylate)

Aserbine (Salicylic acid with Malic acid, Benzoic acid and other ingredients)

Balmosa, Salonpas (Methyl salicylate with Menthol, Camphor and other ingredients)

Bonjela (Choline salicylate with Cetalkonium chloride)

Capasal (Salicylic acid with Coal tar and other ingredients)

Cocois (Salicylic acid with Coal tar, Coconut oil, and Sulphur)

Cuplex (Salicylic acid with Lactic acid and Copper)

Diprosalic (Salicylic acid with Betamethasone)

Duofilm (Salicylic acid with Lactic acid)

Gelcosal, Ionil T (Salicylic acid with Coal tar)

Meted (Salicylic acid with Sulphur)

Monophytol (<u>Methyl salicylate</u> , <u>Propyl salicylate</u>, <u>Salicylic acid</u> with Chlorbutol, Methyl undecenoate and other ingredients)

Movelat, Pyralvex (Salicylic acid with other ingredients)

Posalfilin (<u>Salicylic acid</u> with Podophyllum)

Pragmatar (<u>Salicylic acid</u> with Coal tar and Sulphur)

Psorin (<u>Salicylic acid</u> with Coal tar and Dithranol)

Radian B (<u>Methyl salicylate</u> with Menthol, Camphor, <u>Aspirin</u>)

Salactol, Salatac (<u>Salicylic acid</u> with Lactic acid)

Stiedex lotion (<u>Salicylic acid</u> with Desoxymethasone)

Numerous other ointments, creams and liniments contain various Salicylates

NB: Salicylates are underlined

Aspirin is also a Salicylate - see separate entry

DRUG CLASS

Rubefacient, Analgesic, Acid.

USES

Temporary relief of pain (eg: muscular, arthritic, gums). Relief of nasal congestion. Psoriasis, acne.

DOSAGE

 Muscle and joint pain: Massage liniments into clean dry skin two or three times a day. Nasal congestion: Inhale as required. Mouth ulcers: Apply gels every three hours. Psoriasis and acne: Apply to affected skin, leave for ten minutes, then wash off.

FORMS

Lotion, gel, cream, ointment, paint, shampoo, soap, spray, inhalation.

PRECAUTIONS

Safe in pregnancy and breast feeding.

Use with caution in children under 5 years.

Avoid contact with eyes, mouth, nose, anus and vagina.

Use sparingly on face, skin folds and thin skin.

May stain clothing.

 Do not use if:

• suffering from broken or infected skin.

SIDE EFFECTS

Minimal

INTERACTIONS

Other drugs:

• Aspirin interacts with mouth gels.

PRESCRIPTION

No.

If combined with steroids: Yes.

PERMITTED IN SPORT

Yes

OVERDOSE

May have serious effects in the unlikely event of the liniment being swallowed.

OTHER INFORMATION

Widely used and very safe.

See also Aspirin (Acetylsalicylic acid), Balsalazide and KERATOLYTICS.

Salicylic Acid

See **KERATOLYTICS, SALICYLATES**

Salmeterol

TRADE NAMES

Serevent.

Seretide (with Fluticasone).

DRUG CLASS

Bronchodilator.

USES

Long term control of asthma.

DOSAGE

 Two inhalations twice a day.

FORMS

Inhaler, accuhaler, diskhaler.

PRECAUTIONS

Use with caution in pregnancy (B3), breast feeding and children.

Do not exceed recommended dosage.

Use with caution in thyroid disease.

Not for treatment of acute asthma.

Regular checks of lung function advisable.

 Do not use if:

• under four years.

SIDE EFFECTS

Common: Tremor, rapid pulse, palpitations, headache.

Unusual: Temporary worsening of wheeze immediately after use.

INTERACTIONS

None significant.

PRESCRIPTION

Yes

PERMITTED IN SPORT

No

OVERDOSE

Dramatic worsening of side effects may occur. Seek medical assistance.

OTHER INFORMATION

Introduced in 1993 to assist in the control of severe chronic asthma. Does not cause addiction or dependence, but must be used under close medical supervision.

Salmonella typhi (Typhoid) vaccine

TRADE NAMES

Typherix, Typhim Vi.

DRUG CLASS

Vaccine

USES

Prevention of typhoid.

PRECAUTIONS

Not designed for use in pregnancy (B2), but unintentional use in pregnancy is unlikely to have any serious effects. Use with caution in breast feeding. Not for use in children under six years.

Use with caution in immune diseases.

 Do not take if:

• suffering from significant infection, diarrhoea (capsule only).

DOSAGE

Single injection gives three years protection.

FORMS

Injection.

SIDE EFFECTS

Common: Local pain, redness and swelling at injection site.

Unusual: Fever, nausea, diarrhoea, headache, tiredness.

INTERACTIONS

None significant.

PRESCRIPTION

Yes

PERMITTED IN SPORT

Yes

OVERDOSE

Inadvertent additional vaccination unlikely to cause any serious adverse effects.

OTHER INFORMATION

Not used routinely. Only given to persons travelling to or living in poorer countries where typhoid is widespread. Typhoid causes severe diarrhoea and vomiting and is caught from contaminated food or poor personal hygiene.

Salt (Sodium chloride)

See ELECTROLYTES

Saquinavir

TRADE NAMES

Fortovase, Invirase.

DRUG CLASS

Antiviral.

USES

AIDS, HIV infection.

DOSAGE

600mg. three times a day after a large meal and usually in combination with other antiviral agents.

FORMS

Capsule of 200mg.

PRECAUTIONS

Use with caution in pregnancy (B1), breast feeding and children.

Use with caution in diarrhoea, liver and kidney disease.

Use lower doses in elderly.

SIDE EFFECTS

Common: Tiredness, nausea, diarrhoea, abnormal pain, abnormal sensation.

Unusual: Vomiting, dizziness.

INTERACTIONS

Other drugs:

• Nifedipine, Clindamycin, Terfenadine, Astemizole, Cisapride, other drugs affecting liver function.

PRESCRIPTION

Yes

PERMITTED IN SPORT

Yes

OVERDOSE

No information available. Induce vomiting or administer activated charcoal if taken recently. Seek urgent medical attention.

SEDATIVES AND HYPNOTICS

(Sedate and induce sleep)

See BARBITURATES, Chloral hydrate, Chlormethiazole, Flunitrazepam, Midazolam, Nitrazepam, Temazepam, Zaleplon, Zolpidem, Zopiclone

SELECTIVE SEROTONIN REUPTAKE INHIBITORS (SSRI)

(Used for depression and excessive anxiety)

See Citalopram, Fluoxetine, Fluvoxamine, Paroxetine, Reboxetine, Sertraline, Venlafaxine

Selegiline

TRADE NAMES

Eldepryl, Zelapar.

DRUG CLASS

Antiparkinsonian.

USES

Advanced forms of Parkinson's disease.

DOSAGE

 One or two tablets once or twice a day.

FORMS

Tablets of 1.25, 5 and 10mg., syrup.

PRECAUTIONS

Use with caution in pregnancy (B2), breast feeding and children.

Use with caution in heart disease, peptic ulcer, high blood pressure, angina and psychiatric conditions.

 Do not take if:
• MAOI, Pethidine or Fluoxetine taken recently.

SIDE EFFECTS

Common: Tremor, dry mouth, nausea, slow urination, sweating.

Unusual: Restlessness, hallucinations, headache, irregular heart beat, vomiting, constipation, facial hair growth.

INTERACTIONS

Other drugs:

• MAOI, Pethidine, Fluoxetine.

PRESCRIPTION

Yes

PERMITTED IN SPORT

Yes

OVERDOSE

Very serious. Up to a 12 hour delay between taking overdose and onset of symptoms. May cause drowsiness, dizziness, headache, hallucinations, convulsions, coma, irregular heart beat and death. Administer activated charcoal or induce vomiting if medication taken recently. Seek urgent medical attention.

OTHER INFORMATION

Does not cause addiction or dependence. Often used in conjunction with Levodopa.

Selenium sulfide

TRADE NAME

Selsun.

DRUG CLASS

Antifungal.

USES

Dandruff, mild fungal infections of skin and scalp.

DOSAGE

 Apply to scalp for five minutes two or three times a week.

FORMS

Lotion.

PRECAUTIONS

Safe to use in pregnancy, breast feeding and children.

Avoid eyes.

 Do not use if:

- suffering from inflamed skin.
- permanent wave, tinting or bleaching of hair within two days.

SIDE EFFECTS

Common: Minimal

Severe but rare (stop medication, consult doctor): Skin irritation.

INTERACTIONS

None significant.

PRESCRIPTION

No

PERMITTED IN SPORT

Yes

OVERDOSE

Diarrhoea, nausea and vomiting may occur if swallowed.

OTHER INFORMATION

Simple and effective treatment for dandruff and pityriasis versicolor (a common fungal skin condition that shows up as white patches).

Senna

TRADE NAME

Senokot.

Manevac (with Ispaghula).

Pripsen (with Piperazine).

DRUG CLASS

Laxative.

USES

Constipation.

PRECAUTIONS

Safe in pregnancy (A) and breast feeding.

May be used in children over six years.

Do not use long term without medical advice.

 Do not take if:

- suffering from stomach pain or gut obstruction.

DOSAGE

 Tablets: Two to four tablets once (before going to bed) or twice a day.
Granules: One or two teaspoonfuls a day.

FORMS

Tablets, granules, syrup.

SIDE EFFECTS

Common: Minimal

Unusual: Belly discomfort.

Severe but rare (stop medication, consult doctor): Severe belly pain.

INTERACTIONS

None significant

PRESCRIPTION

No

PERMITTED IN SPORT

Yes

OVERDOSE

Diarrhoea and belly cramps only effects.

OTHER INFORMATION

Safe and widely used.

Sertraline

TRADE NAME

Lustral.

DRUG CLASS

SSRI antidepressant.

USES

Depression.

DOSAGE

 One to four tablets a day in morning with or without food.

FORMS

Tablet (white) of 50mg. and 100mg.

PRECAUTIONS

Should be used in pregnancy (B3) with considerable caution. Breastfeeding should be ceased if Paroxetine prescribed. Not for use in children.

Should be used with caution in mania, epilepsy, liver and kidney disease.

 Do not take if:

• taking MAOI antidepressants.

SIDE EFFECTS

Common: Generally minimal. Nausea, drowsiness, sweating, tremor, tiredness, dry mouth, sleeplessness, impotence.

Unusual: Headache, fever, palpitations, sweating, rash, blurred vision.

INTERACTIONS

Other drugs:

• MAOI

• Anticoagulants, Phenytoin, Tryptophan, Lithium, Tolbutamide.

Other substances:

• Use of alcohol is not advised.

PRESCRIPTION

Yes

PERMITTED IN SPORT

Yes

OVERDOSE

Symptoms may include nausea, tremor, dilated pupils, dry mouth and irritability. Death or serious effects unlikely. Seek medical attention.

Sevelamer

TRADE NAME

Renagel.

USES

Excess levels of phosphate in blood, usually caused by haemodialysis.

DOSAGE

 As determined by doctor after consulting blood test results.

FORMS

Capsules of 403mg. (white).

PRECAUTIONS

Use with caution in pregnancy, breast feeding and children.

Use with caution if swallowing is difficult, stomach retains food, or history of major bowel surgery.

Use with caution in inflammatory bowel disease.

Regular blood tests necessary to monitor electrolytes.

Vitamin supplements may be necessary.

 Do not take if:

• suffering from bowel obstruction.

SIDE EFFECTS

Unknown. Only released in 1999, and used by very few patients.

INTERACTIONS

Unknown. Only released in 1999, and used by very few patients.

PRESCRIPTION

Yes

PERMITTED IN SPORT

Yes

OVERDOSE

Unknown. Seek urgent medical attention.

SEX HORMONES

See Cyproterone acetate, Danazol, Etonogestrel, Hydroxyprogesterone hexanoate, Medroxyprogesterone acetate, MORNING AFTER PILL, Oestradiol, Oestriol, ORAL CONTRACEPTIVES, Stilboestrol, Testosterone

Sildenafil

TRADE NAME

Viagra

USES

Impotence, inability to obtain erection of the penis with appropriate stimulation.

DOSAGE

 25 to 100 mg. one to four hours before erection desired.

FORMS

Tablets (blue) of 25, 50 and 100 mg.

PRECAUTIONS

No for use in pregnancy (B1), breast feeding or by children.

Not recommended for use by women.

Use with caution in all heart diseases, abnormal anatomy of the penis (eg. Peyronie's disease), bleeding disorders, peptic ulcer disease, untreated diabetes and all diseases of the retina in the eye.

 ### Do not take if:

- taking medications containing nitrates (eg. anti-angina medication such as glyceryl trinitrate).
- suffering from angina, untreated high blood pressure or recent stroke
- inherited disorders of the retina.
- suffering from significant liver disease

SIDE EFFECTS

Common: Headache, flush, indigestion.

Unusual: Blue halos in vision, blurred vision.

Severe but rare (stop medication, consult doctor): Serious adverse effects on the heart and circulation of blood.

INTERACTIONS

Other drugs:

- Nitrate containing angina medications, other drugs for impotence, cimetidine, rifampicin, erythromycin, ketoconazole.

Other substances:

- Alcohol.

PRESCRIPTION

Yes (restricted on the NHS to men who have impotence due to prostate cancer, spinal injury, diabetes mellitus, kidney failure, multiple sclerosis, prostate surgery and a number of other specific conditions).

PERMITTED IN SPORT

Yes

OVERDOSE

May have adverse effects on the heart and circulation. Seek medical attention.

OTHER INFORMATION

Introduced in 1998. Very effective, and generally very safe if precautions followed.

See also Alprostadil

Silver nitrate
See KERATOLYTICS

Silver sulfadiazine (SSD)

TRADE NAME

Flamazine.

DRUG CLASS

Sulfonamide antibiotic.

USES

Burns, skin ulcers, sores, grazes.

PRECAUTIONS

Not to be used in pregnancy (C) or newborn infants. May be used in breast feeding (but not on breast) and older children.

Use with caution in liver and kidney disease.

 ### Do not use if:

- suffering from sulphur drug allergy.

DOSAGE

 Apply very thickly once every day or two.

FORMS

Cream.

SIDE EFFECTS

Minimal

INTERACTIONS

None significant.

PRESCRIPTION

Yes

PERMITTED IN SPORT

Yes

OTHER INFORMATION

Excellent cream for soothing serious burns and preventing or treating infection in burns and skin ulcers. Usually covered by a non-adhesive dressing over a thick (3 to 5 mm.) layer of cream.

Simethicone

See Dimethicone

Simvastatin

TRADE NAME

Zocor.

DRUG CLASS

Hypolipidaemic.

USES

Excess blood levels of cholesterol and triglycerides (fats).

DOSAGE

 10 to 80mg. a day at night t.

FORMS

Tablets of 10mg. (peach), 20mg. (tan), 40mg. (red) and 80mg. (red).

PRECAUTIONS

Should not be used in pregnancy (C) unless no alternative available. Not for use in breast feeding or children.

Regular blood tests to check blood fats and liver enzymes are necessary.

Use with caution in liver and kidney disease.

 Do not take if:

• suffering from severe liver disease, myopathy.

SIDE EFFECTS

Common: Constipation, diarrhoea, excess wind, nausea, headache.

Unusual: Vomiting, heartburn, back pain, muscle pain, dizziness, sleeplessness, cough, bronchitis, pins and needles sensation, rash, sinusitis, blurred vision, depression.

Severe but rare (stop medication, consult doctor): Yellow skin (jaundice).

INTERACTIONS

Other drugs:

• Anticoagulants, Niacin, Nicotinic acid, Digoxin.

• Immunosuppressive treatment.

PRESCRIPTION

Yes (restricted to severe high blood cholesterol levels not controlled by diet).

PERMITTED IN SPORT

Yes

OVERDOSE

Liver stress only likely effect.

OTHER INFORMATION

Drug released in the late 1980's that has improved the treatment of excess cholesterol. Very safe and generally well tolerated.

Sodium acid citrate

See ELECTROLYTES

Sodium acid phosphate

TRADE NAMES

Carbalax (with Sodium bicarbonate).

Fleet, Fletcher's Phosphate (with Sodium phosphate).

DRUG CLASS

Laxative.

USES

Constipation.

DOSAGE

 Suppositories: One or two a day.
Solution: 45mLs with water twice a day.

FORMS

Enema, solution, suppository.

PRECAUTIONS

Use with care in pregnancy, breast feeding and children.

Use with caution in colostomy, poor kidney function and any heart disease.

 Do not take if:

- suffering from heart failure, intestinal obstruction, megacolon, kidney failure, ulcerative colitis, diverticulitis, undiagnosed abdominal pain, vomiting.

SIDE EFFECTS

Common: Diarrhoea, nausea.

INTERACTIONS

Other drugs:

- Calcium channel blockers, Diuretics, Lithium, Oral contraceptives, Anticonvulsants, Antibiotics, Diabetic medication.

PRESCRIPTION

No

PERMITTED IN SPORT

Yes

OVERDOSE

Severe diarrhoea and electrolyte deficiencies likely.

OTHER INFORMATION

Usually used when other laxatives have failed.

See also Sodium Phosphate

Sodium aurothiomalate

See GOLD

Sodium bicarbonate

See ANTACIDS , ELECTROLYTES

Sodium cellulose phosphate

TRADE NAME

Calcisorb.

USES

Reduces level of calcium in blood stream, reduces risk of calcium stones in kidney, osteopetrosis.

DOSAGE

 One sachet three times a day with food or water.

FORMS

Powder in sachet.

PRECAUTIONS

Not to be used in pregnancy, breast feeding or children.

Regular blood tests to check on blood chemistry recommended.

 Do not take if:

- suffering from severe kidney disease, heart failure.

SIDE EFFECTS

Common: Diarrhoea

Unusual: Weight gain, arthritis.

INTERACTIONS

Other drugs:

- Mineral supplements.

PRESCRIPTION

Yes

PERMITTED IN SPORT

Yes

OVERDOSE

Severe diarrhoea only likely effect.

OTHER INFORMATION

Does not cause dependence or addiction.

Sodium chloride (Common Salt)

See ELECTROLYTES

Sodium clondronate

TRADE NAME

Bonefos.

USES

High levels of calcium in blood and bone pain due to bone tumours.

DOSAGE

 2400 to 3200mg. once a day initially, reducing to 1600mg. once a day. Do not take within two hours of food.

PRECAUTIONS

Use with considerable caution in pregnancy (B3), breast feeding and children.

Use with caution in dehydration and kidney disease.

Regular blood tests to check calcium levels necessary.

Maintain adequate fluid intake.

 Do not take if:

- suffering from severe intestinal inflammation.

FORMS

Capsules of 400mg. (yellow), tablets of 400mg. (white), infusion.

SIDE EFFECTS

Common: Low blood calcium, stomach upsets.

Severe but rare (stop medication, consult doctor): Blood chemistry disorders, kidney failure.

INTERACTIONS

Other drugs:

• Other medications affecting phosphorus or calcium levels.

• Estamustine, NSAIDs, Antacids.

PRESCRIPTION

Yes

PERMITTED IN SPORT

Yes

OVERDOSE

Serious blood chemistry disorders possible that may lead to major organ failure. Seek urgent medical attention. Induce vomiting or give activated charcoal if swallowed recently.

Sodium cromoglycate

(Cromolyn sodium, Disodium cromoglycate)

TRADE NAME

Hay-Crom, Opticrom. For use in eye.

Cromogen, Intal. For use in lungs.

Aerocrom (with Salbutamol). For use in lungs.

Rynacrom. For use in nose.

Nalcrom. For use in gut.

USES

Prevention (but not treatment) of asthma. Prevention (but not treatment) of hay fever. Prevention (but not treatment) of allergic reactions in the eye. Prevention (but not treatment) of food allergies.

DOSAGE

 Inhaler: Two inhalations up to four times a day.
Nasal spray: One spray to each nostril, two to four times a day.
Eye drops: One or two drops into eye, four to six times a day.
Capsules: Two capsules, four times a day before food.

FORMS

For use in eye: Drops (keep in door of refrigerator).
For use in lungs: Capsules for spinhaler (keep cool), metered aerosol, inhaler.
For use in nose: Nasal spray.
For use in gut: Capsules of 100mg. (clear).

PRECAUTIONS

Safe in pregnancy (A), children and breast feeding.

Do not stop suddenly from full dose, as recurrence of asthma or allergic condition may occur.

SIDE EFFECTS

Common: Hoarse voice and bad taste with inhaled forms.

Unusual: Headache, stuffy nose, nosebleed, throat irritation.

Severe but rare (stop medication, consult doctor): Rash, hives, increased wheezing, joint pain, muscle pain, palpitations.

INTERACTIONS

None significant

PRESCRIPTION

Yes

PERMITTED IN SPORT

Yes

OVERDOSE

No problems encountered other than increased likelihood of side effects.

Sodium fluoride

See Fluoride

Sodium fusidate and Fusidic acid

TRADE NAME

Fucidin, Fucithalmic.

Fucibet (with Betamethasone).

Fucidin H (with Hydrocortisone).

DRUG CLASS

Antibiotic

USES

Infections caused by susceptible bacteria, particularly lung, heart, eye and skin infections.

DOSAGE

 Tablets: Two tablets three times a day with meals.
Ointment: Apply two or three times a day for seven days.
Eye drops: One drop twice a day.

FORMS

Gel, cream, tablets, suspension, eye drops.

  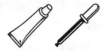

PRECAUTIONS

Should not be used in pregnancy (C) unless medically essential. Should be used with caution in breast feeding and infants. Safe for use in children.

Not designed for long term use.

Use with caution in liver disease.

SIDE EFFECTS

Common: Ointment - Skin irritation, skin pain.
Swallowed forms - Nausea, loss of appetite, diarrhoea.
Eye drops - Temporary irritation.

Unusual: Belly discomfort, vomiting, dizziness.

Severe but rare (stop medication, consult doctor): Yellow skin (jaundice).

INTERACTIONS

Other drugs:

• Lincomycin, Rifampicin.

PRESCRIPTION

Yes

PERMITTED IN SPORT

Yes

OVERDOSE

Belly pain and diarrhoea likely. Long term overdosage may cause liver damage.

OTHER INFORMATION

Used only for more severe and complex infections, particularly in cystic fibrosis.

Sodium iron edetate

See Iron

Sodium lauryl sulfoacetate

TRADE NAME

Relaxit (with Sodium Citrate, Sorbic acid, Glycerol and Sorbitol).

USES

Constipation.

DOSAGE

 One tube rectally at night.

FORMS

Rectal enema.

PRECAUTIONS

Safe in pregnacy, breast feeding and children.

Insert only half nozzle length in children under three years.

SIDE EFFECTS

Minimal

INTERACTIONS

None significant

PRESCRIPTION

No

PERMITTED IN SPORT

Yes

OVERDOSE

Diarrhoea only effect.

OTHER INFORMATION

Commonly used in elderly. Very safe and effective.

Sodium perborate

TRADE NAME

Bocasan.

DRUG CLASS

Antiseptic

USES

Mouth and gum inflammation and soreness.

DOSAGE

 One sachet dissolved in water and used as mouthwash four times a day after meals.

FORMS

Powder

PRECAUTIONS

Safe to use in pregnancy, breast feeding and children.

Do not swallow.

SIDE EFFECTS

Minimal

INTERACTIONS

None significant

PRESCRIPTION

No

PERMITTED IN SPORT

Yes

OVERDOSE

Diarrhoea and nausea only likely effects if swallowed in large quantities.

Sodium phosphate

TRADE NAME

Fleet Enema, Fleet Phospho-Soda, Fletchers Phosphate (with Sodium acid phosphate).

DRUG CLASS

Laxative.

USES

To clean bowel prior to surgery or colonoscopy, constipation.

DOSAGE

 Use enema once a day. 45mLs. solution with water twice a day.

FORMS

Solution, enema.

PRECAUTIONS

Use with caution in pregnancy and breast feeding.

Use with caution in diabetes, kidney disease, electrolyte disturbances, colostomy, belly pain, vomiting, people prone to dehydration.

Reduce dose in elderly.

Not for repeated use.

 Do not take if:

- suffering from bowel obstruction, bowel paralysis, impacted faeces, megacolon, ascites, poor kidney function, congestive heart failure, dehydration, ileostomy.

- under 12 years of age.

SIDE EFFECTS

Common: Dehydration, nausea, electrolyte imbalances.

Unusual: Vomiting, allergic reactions.

Severe but rare (stop medication, consult doctor): Rare and serious complications.

INTERACTIONS

Other drugs:

- Diuretics, Lithium.

- Will affect absorption of all swallowed medications, including contraceptive pill.

PRESCRIPTION

No

PERMITTED IN SPORT

Yes (guaranteed to cause failure in almost any sport!).

OVERDOSE

Severe diarrhoea and dehydration with significant electrolyte disturbances that may lead to organ damage and heart attack. Vomiting likely after overdose as side effect of medication.

OTHER INFORMATION

Normally only used as a preparation for a medical procedure on the large bowel in association with a strict diet.

Sodium picosulfate

TRADE NAME

Laxoberal.

Picolax (with Magnesium citrate).

DRUG CLASS

Laxative.

USES

Preparation of bowel for surgery or colonoscopy, constipation.

DOSAGE

 5 to 15mLs. of solution once a day at night. Powder in sachet dissolved in water once or twice a day.

FORMS

Powder for solution, liquid.

PRECAUTIONS

Not to be used in pregnancy (C) or children under 20 Kg.

Use with caution in breast feeding and children.

Use with caution in heart disease, phenylketonuria, dehydration, electrolyte disturbances, if prone to aspiration.

Reduce dose in elderly.

 ### Do not take if:

- suffering from bowel obstruction, bowel paralysis, belly pain, colitis, bowel inflammation.

SIDE EFFECTS

Common: Nausea, bloating, anal irritation, belly discomfort.

Unusual: Vomiting.

INTERACTIONS

Other drugs:

- Affects absorption of all swallowed medications, including contraceptive pill.

PRESCRIPTION

No

PERMITTED IN SPORT

Yes

OVERDOSE

Severe diarrhoea and dehydration with significant electrolyte disturbances that may lead to organ damage and heart attack. Vomiting likely after overdose as side effect of medication.

Sodium polystyrene sulfonate

TRADE NAME

Resonium A.

DRUG CLASS

Detoxifying agent.

USES

Reducing very high blood potassium levels.

DOSAGE

 15g. one to four times a day.

FORMS

Powder

PRECAUTIONS

May be used in pregnancy, breast feeding and children.

Use with caution in heart disease, high blood pressure and tissue swelling.

Regular blood tests to monitor effect on blood chemistry essential.

SIDE EFFECTS

Common: Loss of appetite, bowel discomfort, constipation, nausea, vomiting.

Unusual: Impaction of faeces.

INTERACTIONS

Other drugs:

• Digoxin, Antacids, Laxatives.

Other substances:

• Reacts with fruit juices.

PRESCRIPTION

Yes

PERMITTED IN SPORT

Yes

OVERDOSE

Severe constipation possible.

OTHER INFORMATION

Resonium A is not absorbed from the gut, but draws Potassium out of the body to pass out in the faeces.

Sodium valproate

TRADE NAME

Epilim.

DRUG CLASS

Anticonvulsant.

USES

Epilepsy

DOSAGE

 Dosage increased slowly until desired control achieved, usually between 1000mg. and 2000mg. a day taken in one or more doses with or after food.

FORMS

Tablets, coated tablets, syrup, injection.

PRECAUTIONS

Not to be taken in pregnancy (D) unless medically essential as the risk of foetal abnormality is significantly increased. Use with caution in breast feeding. May be used in children.

Use with caution in in kidney disease and during surgery (may increase bleeding).

Do not stop medication suddenly, but reduce dosage slowly.

 Do not take if:

• suffering from liver disease.

• family history of severe liver disease.

SIDE EFFECTS

Common: Usually reduced by using slow release form or reducing dosage. Nausea, belly cramps, loss of appetite, diarrhoea,

Unusual: Drowsiness, hair loss, rash, irregular menstrual periods, swelling of tissues.

Severe but rare (stop medication, consult doctor): Unusual bleeding or bruising, yellow skin (jaundice), severe belly pain.

INTERACTIONS

Other drugs:

• Other anticonvulsants, Sedatives, Clonazepam, Anticoagulants, Psychotropics, MAOI.

Other substances:

• Reacts adversely with alcohol.

PRESCRIPTION

Yes

PERMITTED IN SPORT

Yes

OVERDOSE

Death possible but rare. Symptoms include drowsiness, slow breathing, incoordination, confusion and coma. Administer activated charcoal or induce vomiting if taken recently and patient alert. Seek urgent medical attention.

OTHER INFORMATION

Very effective and relatively safe medication that has improved the life of many epileptics. Not addictive or dependence forming.

Somatropin

(Growth hormone)

TRADE NAME

Genotropin, Humatrope, Nordiject, Norditropin, Saizen, Zomacton.

DRUG CLASS

Hormone.

USES

Short stature due to growth hormone deficiency in children.

DOSAGE

 Administered weekly by injection.

FORMS

Injection, injector pen.

SIDE EFFECTS

Common: Irritation at injection site, allergy reaction, fluid retention, fat loss.

Unusual: Underactive thyroid gland, diabetes, slipped bony epiphysis.

Severe but rare (stop medication, consult doctor): Increased pressure of fluid within brain.

PRECAUTIONS

Not for use in pregnancy or breast feeding.

Use with caution in diabetes, ACTH deficiency, underactive thyroid gland, slipped epiphysis, increased pressure within brain.

Do not exceed recommended dose.

 Do not take if:

- Suffering from active tumour, cancer, brain growths.
- Adult.

INTERACTIONS

Other drugs:

- Steroids.

PRESCRIPTION

Yes

PERMITTED IN SPORT

No

OVERDOSE

Overgrowth of bones leading to pressure on nerves and brain (acromegaly), and imbalance in body's ability to deal with glucose.

OTHER INFORMATION

Used illegally by some sportsmen to aid body building.

Sorbide Nitrate

See Isosorbide

Sorbitol

TRADE NAMES

Glandosane (with Carboxymethylcellulose sodium).

Relaxit (with Glycerol, Sodium citrate and Sodium lauryl sulfoacetate).

DRUG CLASS

Laxative, Softening agent.

USES

Softening faeces in constipation, lubricant.

DOSAGE

 Enema: Once a day into rectum. Mouth spray: Spray as often as required for dry mouth.

FORMS

Mouth spray, suspension, enema, liquid.

PRECAUTIONS

Usually safe to use in pregnancy, breast feeding and children.

Not for prolonged use.

Use with caution in diabetes.

 Do not take if:

- suffering from appendicitis, undiagnosed abdominal pain.

- intolerant to fructose.

SIDE EFFECTS

Common: Passing excess wind, diarrhoea.

Severe but rare (stop medication, consult doctor): Disturbances to blood chemistry (electrolytes).

INTERACTIONS

Other drugs:

- Other laxatives, may interfere with absorption of any medication taken by mouth, including oral contraceptives.

Other substances:

- Fructose containing foods.

PRESCRIPTION

No

PERMITTED IN SPORT

Yes

OVERDOSE

Exacerbation of side effects likely. May cause serious blood chemistry disorders.

OTHER INFORMATION

Widely used and safe in correct dosage.

Sotalol

See BETA BLOCKERS

SPASMOLYTIC

(Eases intestinal spasms)

See Dicyclomine, Hyoscine

Spectinomycin

TRADE NAME

Trobicin.

DRUG CLASS

Antibiotic

USES

Severe or resistant gonorrhoea (venereal disease).

PRECAUTIONS

Use with caution in pregnancy (B1), breast feeding and infants. Safe to use in children.

DOSAGE

 Single injection.

FORMS

Injection.

SIDE EFFECTS

Common: Dizziness, nausea, chills, fever.

Unusual: Sleeplessness.

INTERACTIONS

None significant

PRESCRIPTION

Yes

PERMITTED IN SPORT

Yes

OTHER INFORMATION

Very effective and safe medication. Discontinued late 1999.

SPERMICIDES

See Nonoxynol-9

Spironolactone

TRADE NAME

Aldactone.

Aldactide (with Hydroflumethiazide).

Lasilactone (with Frusemide).

DRUG CLASS

Diuretic (aldosterone antagonist).

USES

High blood pressure, congestive cardiac failure, excess fluid retention, cirrhosis of liver, low blood potassium levels, excessive body and face hair in women, primary hyperaldosteronism.

DOSAGE

 Varies depending on usage from 25mg. to 400mg. a day in one or several doses.

FORMS

Tablets.

PRECAUTIONS

Should not be used in pregnancy (B3) unless medically essential. Should not be used in breast feeding or children.

Regular blood tests for level of blood chemicals (electrolytes) may be necessary.

 Do not take if:

• suffering from kidney failure.

SIDE EFFECTS

Common: Breast enlargement (both sexes), diarrhoea, gut cramps.

Unusual: Tiredness, headache, confusion, rash, fever, incoordination, impotence, irregular menstruation.

Severe but rare (stop medication, consult doctor): Unusual bleeding.

INTERACTIONS

Other drugs:

• Do not take with Potassium supplements, Amiloride or Triamterene.

• Reacts with Carbenoxolone, Digoxin.

PRESCRIPTION

Yes

PERMITTED IN SPORT

No

OVERDOSE

Large doses required for adverse effects. Pins and needles sensation, weakness, muscle spasms and paralysis are possible symptoms. Induce vomiting if tablets taken recently. Give extra fluids. Seek medical assistance.

OTHER INFORMATION

An old fashioned medication for removal of excess fluid from the body that has recently been given a new life because of its ability to reduce excess facial hair (hirsutism) in women. Must be taken for many months for this purpose.

SSD

See Silver sulfadiazine

SSRI (SELECTIVE SEROTONIN REUPTAKE INHIBITORS)

(Treat depression and abnormal anxiety)

See Citalopram, Fluoxetine, Fluvoxamine, Paroxetine, Reboxetine, Sertraline, Venlafaxine

Stanozolol

TRADE NAME

Stromba.

DRUG CLASS

Anabolic steroid.

USES

Blood vessel complications of Behçet's disease, hereditary angioedema.

DOSAGE

 2.5 to 10mg. a day.

FORMS

Tablets of 5mg. (white).

PRECAUTIONS

Not to be used in pregnancy and breast feeding.

May be used in children over one year of age.

Not for long term use in children.

Use with caution in fertile women. Adequate non-hormonal contraception essential.

Use with caution in kidney disease, heart disease and history of breast cancer.

Regular blood tests to check liver function necessary.

 Do not take if:
- suffering from prostate cancer, diabetes, porphyria or liver disease.

SIDE EFFECTS

Common: Rash, indigestion, cramps, headaches.

Unusual: Liver and thyroid gland damage.

INTERACTIONS

Other drugs:

- Anticoagulants (eg. warfarin), Hypoglycaemics (diabetes treatment).

PRESCRIPTION

Yes

PERMITTED IN SPORT

Yes

OVERDOSE

Likely to be very serious. Organ damage may result. Seek urgent medical assistance.

Stavudine

TRADE NAME

Zerit.

DRUG CLASS

Antiviral.

USES

HIV infection, AIDS.

DOSAGE

 Dosage as determined by doctor taken twice a day one hour before meals.

FORMS

Capsules of 15mg. (yellow/red), 20mg. (brown), 30mg. (light orange/dark orange), 40 mg. (dark orange), solution.

PRECAUTIONS

Use with caution in pregnancy (B3), breast feeding and children under 12 years.

Use with caution in peripheral neuropathy (nerve inflammation), pancreatitis, liver disease.

SIDE EFFECTS

Common: Nerve pain and inflammation, inflammation of pancreas.

Unusual: Liver damage.

INTERACTIONS

Other drugs:

• Zidovudine, Trimethoprim.

PRESCRIPTION

Yes

PERMITTED IN SPORT

Yes

OVERDOSE

No information available. Seek urgent medical attention. Induce vomiting or administer activated charcoal if taken recently.

OTHER INFORMATION

Introduced in 1997.

Sterculia

TRADE NAME

Normacol.

Normacol Plus (with Frangula).

Spasmonal Fibre (with Alverine Citrate).

DRUG CLASS

Fibre.

USES

Constipation, irritable bowel syndrome.

PRECAUTIONS

Safe in pregnancy and breast feeding.

Safe in children over six years.

 ## Do not take if:

• about to go to bed.

• suffering from ulcerative colitis.

DOSAGE

 Take one or two heaped teaspoons with water twice a day at least two hours before bed time.

FORMS

Granules.

SIDE EFFECTS

Common: Minimal

Unusual: Diarrhoea, belly discomfort.

INTERACTIONS

None significant.

PRESCRIPTION

No

PERMITTED IN SPORT

Yes

OVERDOSE

Take additional water. Belly discomfort and passing excess wind only effects.

OTHER INFORMATION

Widely used, natural fibre supplement.

STEROIDS (CORTICOSTEROIDS)

(Powerful reducers of inflammation)

See Beclomethasone, Betamethasone, Budesonide, Clobetasol, Clobetasone, Cortisone, Deflazacort, Desoxymethasone, Dexamethasone, Fludrocortisone, Flucinolone, Fluocortolone, Fluorometholone, Flurandrelone, Halcinonide, Hydrocortisone, Mometasone, Prednisolone, Rimexolone, Triamcinolone.

Stilboestrol

TRADE NAME

Tampovagan.

DRUG CLASS

Sex hormone.

USES

Female hormone replacement in menopause, vaginal dryness after menopause.

DOSAGE

 Insert one or two high into vagina at night.

FORMS

Vaginal pessary.

PRECAUTIONS

Not to be used in pregnancy (B1), breast feeding or children. Accidental usage in these situations unlikely to be harmful.

Use with caution in epilepsy, migraine, heart failure, high blood pressure, kidney disease, diabetes, porphyria or uterine disease.

Do not take if:

- suffering from liver disease, breast or genital cancer, blood clots.

SIDE EFFECTS

Common: Abnormal uterine bleeding, vaginal thrush, fluid retention, weight gain, breast tenderness.

Unusual: Rash, bloating, intestinal cramps.

Severe but rare (stop medication, consult doctor): Blood clots, calf or chest pain, yellow skin (jaundice).

INTERACTIONS

Other drugs:

• Other Sex hormones.

Other substances:

• Smoking increases risk of serious side effects.

PRESCRIPTION

Yes

PERMITTED IN SPORT

Yes

OVERDOSE

Vomiting and abnormal vaginal bleeding only likely effects if swallowed.

STIMULANTS

See Caffeine, Cocaine, Dexamphetamine, Methylphenidate, Nicotine

Streptodornase

See FIBRINOLYTICS

Streptokinase

See FIBRINOLYTICS

Sucralfate

TRADE NAME

Antepsin.

DRUG CLASS

Antiulcerant.

USES

Protects the lining of the stomach. Treats and prevents ulcers of the stomach and duodenum (upper small intestine).

DOSAGE

 One tablet three times a day one hour before meals, and a fourth tablet last thing at night before bed. Course usually limited to eight weeks.

FORMS

Tablets of 1g. (white), suspension.

PRECAUTIONS

Use with caution in pregnancy (B1). Safe in breast feeding. Not recommended for use in children.

 Do not take if:

• suffering from stomach cancer, bleeding ulcer or significant kidney disease.

SIDE EFFECTS

Common: Constipation, headache, itchy rash, nausea.

Unusual: Indigestion, dry mouth, diarrhoea, back pain, sleepiness, dizziness.

INTERACTIONS

Other drugs:

- Antacids should not be taken within half an hour.
- Tetracycline, Phenytoin, Digoxin, Norfloxacin, Ciprofloxacin, Warfarin and Cimetidine may have their effectiveness reduced while taking Sucralfate.

PRESCRIPTION

Yes

PERMITTED IN SPORT

Yes

OVERDOSE

Constipation and nausea only effects.

SUGAR

See Glucose

Sulconazole

See IMIDAZOLES

Sulfadoxine

TRADE NAME

Fansidar (with Pyrimethamine).

DRUG CLASS

Antimalarial.

USES

Prevention and treatment of malaria.

OTHER INFORMATION

Only available in combination with Pyrimethamine.

See Pyrimethamine for further information

Sulfametopyrazine

TRADE NAME

Kelfizine W.

DRUG CLASS

Sulphonamide antibiotic.

USES

Prevention of bronchitis and urinary infections.

DOSAGE

 One tablet a week.

FORMS

Tablets of 2g. (white).

PRECAUTIONS

Not for use in late pregnancy, breast feeding and children. Probably relatively safe in early and mid trimester pregnancy.

Use with caution in liver and kidney disease, and blood cell diseases.

Regular blood tests necessary to check for abnormal blood cells.

SIDE EFFECTS

Common: Nausea, diarrhoea, rashes, mouth soreness and inflammation.

Unusual: Vomiting.

Severe but rare (stop medication, consult doctor): Damage to blood cells, anaemia.

INTERACTIONS

Other drugs:

- Diabetes medications.

PRESCRIPTION

Yes

PERMITTED IN SPORT

Yes

OVERDOSE

Exacerbation of side effects likely. Administer activated charcoal or induce vomiting if tablets taken recently. Take as much fluid as possible. Kidney and blood cell damage possible. Seek medical assistance.

See also SULFONAMIDES

SULFONAMIDES (SULPHONAMIDES)

TRADE and GENERIC NAMES

Sultrin (Sulphathiazole, Sulphacetamide, Sulphabenzamide).

DRUG CLASS

Antibiotic.

USES

Treat bacterial vaginal infections.

DOSAGE

 One application once or twice a day into vagina.

FORMS

Vaginal cream.

PRECAUTIONS

Not to be used in pregnancy (C), breast feeding or infants. Safe for use in children.

Use with caution in liver or kidney disease.

SIDE EFFECTS

Common: Itch, redness, swelling.

Severe but rare (stop medication, consult doctor): Rash, severe belly pain, kidney damage.

INTERACTIONS

Other substances:

• Latex condoms and diaphragms.

PRESCRIPTION

Yes

PERMITTED IN SPORT

Yes

OTHER INFORMATION

Sulfonamides were the first antibiotics in the 1930s. Used less frequently now due to resistant forms of bacteria developing.Allergy to Sulfonamides a problem in some patients.

See also Silver sulfadiazine, Sulfadoxine, Sulfametapyrozine, Sulphamethoxazole, Sulphasalazine.

Sulindac
See NSAID

Sulphabenzamide
See SULFONAMIDES

Sulphacetamide
See SULFONAMIDES

Sulphamethoxazole

TRADE NAMES

Only available in combination with Trimethoprim - this combination is known as Co-trimoxazole.

Chemotrim, Septrin (with Trimethoprim).

DRUG CLASS

Sulfonamide antibiotic.

USES

Infections caused by susceptible bacteria, particularly infections of sinuses, lungs, urine and skin.

DOSAGE

 One or two tablets twice a day.

FORMS

Tablets, suspension, injection.

PRECAUTIONS

Should not be used in pregnancy (C). Use with caution in breast feeding. May be used in children over two years.

Use with caution in AIDS, blood disorders, asthma, allergic conditions, kidney and liver disease.

Not designed for long term use.

Lower doses and caution necessary in elderly.

Give additional fluids to dilute.

 Do not take if:

- suffering from severe liver disease, abnormal blood cells, bone marrow damage, severe kidney disease.

- under two years of age.

SIDE EFFECTS

Common: Nausea, loss of appetite, rash.

Unusual: Vomiting, diarrhoea.

Severe but rare (stop medication, consult doctor): Unusual bleeding or bruising, yellow skin (jaundice).

INTERACTIONS

Other drugs:

- Hypoglycaemics, Methotrexate, Urinary acidifiers, Anticoagulants, NSAID, Salicylates, Sulphinpyrazone, Phenytoin, Rifampicin, Cyclosporin, Thiazide diuretics, Pyrimethamine, Acetazolamide.

PRESCRIPTION

Yes

PERMITTED IN SPORT

Yes

OVERDOSE

Exacerbation of side effects likely. Administer activated charcoal or induce vomiting if tablets taken recently. Take as much fluid as possible. Kidney damage possible. Seek medical assistance.

OTHER INFORMATION

Widely used for two decades after its introduction in the mid 1960s, but now more effective and less toxic antibiotics tend to be used where possible.

See also Sulfonamides.

Sulphasalazine

TRADE NAME

Salazopyrin.

DRUG CLASS

Sulfonamide antibiotic.

USES

Ulcerative colitis, Crohn's disease, rheumatoid arthritis.

DOSAGE

 Tablets: 250mg to 2000mg up to four times a day with plenty of fluids.
Suppository: 500mg to 1000mg once or twice a day.

FORMS

Tablets of 500mg. (yellow), enteric coated tablets of 500mg. (yellow), suppositories of 500mg., enema, suspension.

PRECAUTIONS

Safe in pregnancy (A). Use with caution in breast feeding.

Blood and urine tests must be taken regularly during treatment to detect any adverse effects.

 Do not take if:

- suffering from allergy conditions or G6PD deficiency.

SIDE EFFECTS

Common: Nausea, vomiting, loss of appetite, fever, red skin, itchy skin, headache.

Unusual: Reversible infertility, belly pain, diarrhoea, pins and needles sensation, depression, dizziness, sleeplessness, cough.

Severe but rare (stop medication, consult doctor): Fever, bleeding, bruising, jaundice, sore throat. These symptoms may be signs of a severe blood disorder that may rarely occur with Sulfasalazine.

INTERACTIONS

Other drugs:

- Interacts with Anticoagulants, Methotrexate, Sulphonylureas.
- Increased effect of Sulfasalazine occurs if taken with Indomethacin, Phenylbutazone, Urinary acidifiers or Salicylates.

PRESCRIPTION

Yes

PERMITTED IN SPORT

Yes

OVERDOSE

Diarrhoea, bloody urine and kidney damage may occur. Seek urgent medical attention.

OTHER INFORMATION

Used for many years to successfully control intestinal inflammation. Found serendipitously to also control some forms of rheumatoid arthritis.

Sulphathiazole

See SULFONAMIDES

Sulphinpyrazone

TRADE NAME

Anturan.

DRUG CLASS

Uricosuric.

USES

Prevention of gout.

PRECAUTIONS

Use with caution in pregnancy (B2) and breast feeding. Not for use in children.

Use with caution in kidney stones, porphyria, kidney disease, heart failure, asthma.

Regular blood tests to check blood cells recommended.

Ensure adequate fluids are swallowed.

 Do not take if:

- suffering from acute gout, peptic ulcer, severe liver or kidney disease, hay fever, skin allergies.

DOSAGE

 One or two tablets two to four times a day with food or milk.

FORMS

Tablet (yellow) of 100 and 200mg.

SIDE EFFECTS

Common: Nausea, diarrhoea.

Unusual: Vomiting, stomach ulcer, rash.

Severe but rare (stop medication, consult doctor): Yellow skin (jaundice).

INTERACTIONS

Other drugs:

- Diuretics, Urinary alkalinisers, Anticoagulants, Aspirin, Penicillins, Sulfonamides, Sulfonylureas, Theophylline, Phenytoin.

Other substances:

- Alcohol may aggravate gout.

PRESCRIPTION

Yes

PERMITTED IN SPORT

Yes

OVERDOSE

Serious. May cause vomiting, diarrhoea, belly pains, irregular heart beat, low blood pressure, difficulty in breathing, convulsions, coma, liver and kidney failure and death. Administer activated charcoal or induce vomiting if medication taken recently and patient alert. Seek urgent medical attention.

OTHER INFORMATION

Does not cause addiction or dependence.

SULPHONAMIDES

(Sulphur containing antibiotics)

See Silver sulfadiazine, Sulfadoxine, Sulfametapyrozine, Sulphasalazine, Sulphamethoxazole, SULFONAMIDES

Sulphur

TRADE NAMES

Actinac (with Chloramphenicol, Hydrocortisone, Allantoin and other ingredients).

Cocois (with Coal tar, Salicylic acid, Coconut oil).

Meted (with Salicylic acid).

Pramatar (with Coal tar, Salicylic acid).

Also found in many other skin preparations.

USES

Acne, psoriasis.

DOSAGE

 Varies. Apply medication as directed on label.

PRECAUTIONS

Most forms safe in pregnancy and breast feeding.

Use with caution in children.

For external use only - do not swallow.

Avoid eyes, nostrils, mouth, ears, anus, vagina.

 Do not take if:

- skin broken, burnt or grazed.
- suffering from infected pustular acne or psoriasis.

FORMS

Cream, gel, lotion, ointment, shampoo.

SIDE EFFECTS

Common: Skin inflammation.

INTERACTIONS

Nil.

PRESCRIPTION

Most forms: No

Actinac: Yes.

PERMITTED IN SPORT

Yes

OTHER INFORMATION

Normally only available in combination with other medications.

Sulpride

TRADE NAMES

Dolmatil, Sulparex, Sulpitil.

DRUG CLASS

Antipsychotic.

USES

Schizophrenia.

DOSAGE

 Start with 200 to 400mg. twice a day, increasing slowly to a maximum of 1200mg. twice a day.

FORMS

Tablets of 200 and 400mg.

PRECAUTIONS

Use with caution in pregnancy and breast feeding.

Not for use in children under 14 years.

Use with caution in epilepsy, kidney disease and hypomania..

 Do not take if:

• suffering from phaeochromocytoma, severe liver or kidney disease, blood cell disorders.

SIDE EFFECTS

Common: Drowsiness, reduced alertness, abnormal body temperature, low blood pressure, dermatitis, dry mouth, constipation, weight gain, blurred vision, stuffy nose.

Unusual: Itch, difficulty passing urine, confusion, dizziness, incoordination, tremor, slow breathing, irregular heart beat, skin pigmentation.

Severe but rare (stop medication, consult doctor): Yellow skin (jaundice), convulsions, repetitive unwanted movements, muscle rigidity, fever, coma.

INTERACTIONS

Other drugs:

• Adrenaline, Tricyclic Antidepressants, Guanethidine, Antacids, Barbiturates, Phenytoin, Lithium, Levodopa, Sedatives, Amphetamines, Beta Blockers, Hypoglycaemics, MAOI, Quinidine, Suxamethonium.

Other substances:

• Reacts adversely with alcohol and some foods.

PRESCRIPTION

Yes

PERMITTED IN SPORT

Yes

OVERDOSE

Very serious. Symptoms include drowsiness, confusion, restlessness, rapid heart rate, tremor, convulsions, difficulty in breathing and swallowing, coma and death. Administer activated charcoal or induce vomiting if taken recently and patient alert. Seek urgent medical attention.

Sumatriptan

TRADE NAME

Imigran.

DRUG CLASS

Antimigraine.

USES

Treatment of acute migraine and cluster headache.

DOSAGE

 Tablets: One tablet immediately symptoms of migraine appear. Repeat if necessary. Maximum of three tablets a day.
Nasal spray: One spray into one nostril at onset of migraine. Repeat after two hours if necessary.
Injection: Self inject immediately symptoms of migraine appear. Repeat once in no less than one hour if necessary.

FORMS

Tablets of 50mg. (pink) and 100mg. (white), nasal spray, injection (auto-injector kit available).

PRECAUTIONS

Should not be used in pregnancy (B3) unless medically essential. Should be used with caution in breast feeding. Not for use in children.

Should be used with caution in liver and kidney disease, and in elderly.

Not to be used for prevention of migraine, only treatment of acute sattacks.

Must not be injected into a vein.

 Do not take if:

• suffering from angina, poor circulation to heart, recent heart attack, severe high blood pressure, recent stroke, irregular heart beat.

• Ergotamine used in previous 24 hours.

SIDE EFFECTS

Common: Chest pain, pain at injection site, tingling sensation, heat, heaviness, flushing, tightness, dizziness, weakness. Bitter taste with nasal spray.

Unusual: Fatigue, drowsiness, nausea, vomiting.

Severe but rare (stop medication, consult doctor): Significant chest pain (angina).

INTERACTIONS

Other drugs:

• Ergotamine.

Other substances:

• Does not interact with alcohol.

PRESCRIPTION

Yes

PERMITTED IN SPORT

Yes

OVERDOSE

Exacerbation of side effects only.

OTHER INFORMATION

Considered a wonder drug when introduced in the early 1990,s, Sumatriptan has given instant relief with minimal side effects to millions of migraine sufferers. Works far more effectively as an injection or nasal spray than if taken as tablets.

SYMPATHOMIMETICS (DECONGESTANTS)

See Ephedrine, Phenylephrine, Pseudoephedrine

T3, T4

See THYROID HORMONES

Tacalcitol

TRADE NAME

Curatoderm.

USES

Psoriasis plaques.

DOSAGE

 Apply sparingly to plaques once a day at bedtime.

FORMS

Ointment.

PRECAUTIONS

Use with care in pregnancy and breast feeding.

Not for use in children.

Use with caution in kidney disease, pustular and flaking psoriasis.

Do not use for more than 12 months.

 Do not take if:

- suffering from high blood calcium levels.
- under other circumstances

SIDE EFFECTS

Common: Local skin redness.

INTERACTIONS

None significant.

PRESCRIPTION

Yes

PERMITTED IN SPORT

Yes

Tacrolimus

TRADE NAME

Prograf.

DRUG CLASS

Immunosuppressant.

USES

Prevention of rejection of kidney and liver transplants.

PRECAUTIONS

Not to be used in pregnancy (C) except under exceptional circumstances.

Use with caution in breast feeding and children.

Careful monitoring of dosage and blood cells and body chemistry essential.

 Do not take if:

- suffering from certain conditions

DOSAGE

 Complex. Must be determined individually for each patient by doctor.

FORMS

Capsules of 1mg. (white) and 5mg. (grey/red), injection.

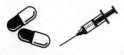

SIDE EFFECTS

Common: Tremor, headache, pins and needles sensation, nausea, diarrhoea.

Unusual: High blood pressure, excess sugar in blood, excess calcium in blood, skin rashes, wheeze.

Severe but rare (stop medication, consult doctor): Heart damage, diabetes, kidney and liver damage.

INTERACTIONS

Other drugs:

• Cyclosporin (serious interaction), Aminoglycosides, NSAIDs, Vancomycin, Amphoterecin B, Cotrimoxazole, Aciclovir, Ganciclovir, Potassium supplements, Amiloride, some vaccines, oral contraceptives.

Other substances:

• Grapefruit juice.

PRESCRIPTION

Yes

PERMITTED IN SPORT

Yes

OVERDOSE

Likely to be very serious. Induce vomiting or give activated charcoal if swallowed recently. Seek urgent medical attention.

Tamoxifen

TRADE NAMES

Nolvadex, Soltamox, Tamofen.

USES

Breast cancer, infertility.

DOSAGE

 10 to 20mg. once a day.

FORMS

Tablets.

PRECAUTIONS

Must not be used in pregnancy (D) unless mother's life is at risk as damage to foetus probable. Breast feeding must be ceased before use. Not for use in children.

Adequate contraception must be used by all fertile women during use of Tamoxifen.

SIDE EFFECTS

Common: Hot flushes, abnormal vaginal bleeding, itchy vulva, fluid retention, light headedness, nausea, vomiting, diarrhoea.

INTERACTIONS

Other drugs:

• Anticoagulants (eg. warfarin).

PRESCRIPTION

Yes

PERMITTED IN SPORT

Yes

OVERDOSE

Exacerbation of side effects likely.

OTHER INFORMATION

This medication has saved the lives of thousands of women with breast cancer, and has prevented recurrences in thousands more. Very useful and effective. Introduced in late 1980s.

Tamsulosin

TRADE NAME

Flomax

DRUG CLASS

Alpha one adrenergic blocker (alpha blocker).

USES

Reduces size of enlarged prostate gland.

DOSAGE

 One capsule a day, half hour before breakfast.

FORMS

Capsule of 400µg. (orange/brown).

SIDE EFFECTS

Common: Palpitations, dizziness, low blood pressure, inability to ejaculate during sexual intercourse.

Unusual: Itch, urinary tract infection, sleeplessness, diarrhoea.

Severe but rare (stop medication, consult doctor): Sudden drop in blood pressure with changes in position resulting in falls.

PRECAUTIONS

To be used only in males. If unintentionally taken during pregnancy (B2) or breast feeding, unlikely to be harmful.

Not for use in children.

Prostate cancer must be excluded before use.

Use with caution if heart attack within six previous months.

 Do not take if:

- suffering from low blood pressure, severe liver or kidney disease.

INTERACTIONS

Other drugs:

- Other alpha blockers, cimetidine, Diclofenac, warfarin, frusemide.

PRESCRIPTION

Yes

PERMITTED IN SPORT

Yes

OVERDOSE

Severe low blood pressure may occur. Give activated charcoal and seek medical attention.

OTHER INFORMATION

Introduced in 2000 as a more specifically targeted drug against the prostate gland. Other alpha blockers lower blood pressure as well as shrinking the prostate.

See also other medications listed under Alpha-Blockers

Tar

TRADE NAMES

Alphosyl (Coal tar with Allantoin).

Alphosyl HC (Coal tar with Hydrocortisone).

Carbo-Dome, Clinitar, Enorex, Gelcotar, Pentrax, PsoridermT Gel, Tar Band (Coal tar).

Capasal, Ionil T (Coal tar with Salicylic acid and other ingredients).

Cocois, Pragmatar (Coal tar with Sulphur, Salicylic acid and other ingredients).

Coltapaste (Coal tar with Zinc oxide).

Gelcosal (Coal tar with Salicylic acid).

Ionil T (Coal tar with Salicylic acid, Benzalkonium chloride).

Polytar (Coal tar with other ingredients).

Psorin (Coal tar with Dithranol, Salicylic acid).

Also found in numerous other skin preparations and soaps.

USES

Itchy skin, itchy anus, prickly heat, mild dermatitis, psoriasis, dandruff, skin ulcers.

DOSAGE

 Apply several times a day, or add to bath water.

FORMS

Lotion, cream, ointment, solution, bar, shampoo, bandage.

PRECAUTIONS

Safe to use in pregnancy, breast feeding and children.

SIDE EFFECTS

Common: Minimal.

Unusual: Skin irritation.

INTERACTIONS

None significant.

PRESCRIPTION

No, unless combined with a medication requiring a prescription.

PERMITTED IN SPORT

Yes

OTHER INFORMATION

The original dermatitis treatment, in use for thousands of years.

Tazarotene

TRADE NAME

Zorac

DRUG CLASS

Retinoid.

USES

Psoriasis with plaques.

DOSAGE

 Apply sparingly to plaques once a day in evening.

FORMS

Gel.

SIDE EFFECTS

Common: Skin itching, redness, burning and irritation.

Unusual: Skin pealing, rash, skin pain.

Severe but rare (stop medication, consult doctor): Blistering of skin.

INTERACTIONS

Other substances:

• Moisturisers, cosmetics.

PRESCRIPTION

Yes

PERMITTED IN SPORT

Yes

PRECAUTIONS

Never to be used in pregnancy (X), breast feeding and children.

Ensure adequate contraception during use.

Do not use for more than three months.

Avoid skin folds, face, scalp, eyes, genitals and inflamed skin.

Do not apply to normal skin.

Avoid excess exposure to sunlight of treated areas

Tazobactam

TRADE NAME

Tazocin (with Piperacillin).

DRUG CLASS

Antibiotic.

USES

Severe bacterial infections in hospital.

DOSAGE

 4.5grams every 8 hours by injection into muscle or slow infusion by a drip into a vein.

FORMS

Injection.

PRECAUTIONS

May be used with care in pregnancy (B1), breast feeding and children.

Use with caution in syphilis, kidney and liver disease.

Not for prolonged use.

Blood tests to check electrolyte balance, blood cells, kidney and liver function necessary.

SIDE EFFECTS

Common: Nausea, diarrhoea, rash, vein inflammation.

Unusual: Vomiting, blood clots.

Severe but rare (stop medication, consult doctor): Bloody diarrhoea, other abnormal bleeding..

INTERACTIONS

Other drugs:

• Heparin, anticoagulants (eg: warfarin), aminoglycosides.

PRESCRIPTION

Yes

PERMITTED IN SPORT

Yes See also Piperacillin.

TB vaccine

See BCG Vaccine

Telmisartan

See ANGIOTENSIN II RECEPTOR ANTAGONISTS

Temazepam

TRADE NAME

Temazepam.

DRUG CLASS

Hypnotic/Sedative, Benzodiazepine.

USES

Insomnia (sleeplessness).

DOSAGE

 5 to 20mg. 30 minutes before going to bed.

PRECAUTIONS

Should be used with caution in pregnancy (C), but not at all if delivery of infant imminent as it may decrease desire to breathe in newborn infant. Should be used with caution in breast feeding. Not for use in children.

Lower dose required in elderly.

Should be used intermittently and not constantly as dependency may develop.

Use with caution in glaucoma, myasthenia gravis, heart disease, kidney or liver disease, psychiatric conditions, depression and epilepsy.

 Do not take if:

- suffering from severe lung disease, confusion.
- tendency to addiction or dependence.
- operating machinery, driving a vehicle or undertaking tasks that require concentration and alertness.

FORMS

Tablets of 10mg. and 20mg., solution.

SIDE EFFECTS

Common: Confusion and falls in elderly, impaired alertness.

Unusual: Dizziness, incoordination, poor memory, headache, hangover in morning, slurred speech, nightmares.

INTERACTIONS

Other drugs:

- Other medications that reduce alertness (eg: Barbiturates, Antihistamines, Antianxiety drugs).
- Disulfiram, Anticonvulsants, Anticholinergics.

Other substances:

- Reacts with alcohol to cause excessive drowsiness.

PRESCRIPTION

Yes (restricted).

PERMITTED IN SPORT

Yes

OVERDOSE

Seldom life threatening. May cause drowsiness, confusion and coma. Induce vomiting if tablets taken recently. Seek medical assistance.

OTHER INFORMATION

Very safe, but dependency may develop. Often used to correct sleep pattern abnormalities induced by jet lag. Short half-life reduces morning hangover effect.

Temozolomide

TRADE NAME

Temodal.

DRUG CLASS

Cytotoxic.

USES

Brain cancers (glioma, astrocytoma).

DOSAGE

 Complex. As determined for each patient by doctor.

FORMS

Capsules (white) of 5, 20, 100 and 250mg.

PRECAUTIONS

Not to be used in pregnancy (D) and breast feeding.

Use with caution in children.

Partners of males using medication must not fall pregnant.

Use with caution in liver and kidney disease.

Regular blood tests essential.

Use lower dose in elderly.

 ### Do not take if:

• suffering from immunosuppression (eg. AIDS).

SIDE EFFECTS

Common: Nausea, diarrhoea, headache, tiredness.

Unusual: Vomiting, infertility.

INTERACTIONS

Other drugs:

• Other cancer treating drugs.

Other substances:

• Alcohol.

PRESCRIPTION

Yes

PERMITTED IN SPORT

Yes

OVERDOSE

Likely to cause serious organ damage. Seek urgent medical attention. Induce vomiting or give activated charcoal if swallowed recently.

OTHER INFORMATION

Introduced in 1998 for treatment of more resistant forms of brain cancer.

Tenoxicam

See NSAID

Terazosin hydrochloride

TRADE NAME

Hytrin.

USES

Benign enlargement of prostate gland, high blood pressure.

DOSAGE

 Slowly increasing dosage for three weeks to a maintenance level of 5mg. to 10mg. once a day in the morning.

PRECAUTIONS

Should be used with caution in pregnancy (B2), breast feeding.

Not recommended for children.

Use with caution if history of fainting.

FORMS

Tablets of 1mg. (white), 2mg. (yellow), 5mg. (brown), and 10mg. (blue).

SIDE EFFECTS

Common: Dizziness, light headedness, palpitations, blurred vision, tiredness.

Unusual: Low blood pressure, nasal congestion, faint, swelling of ankles, feet and hands.

INTERACTIONS

Other drugs:

• Other Antihypertensives, Diuretics, Beta-blockers.

PRESCRIPTION

Yes

PERMITTED IN SPORT

Yes

OVERDOSE

Severe low blood pressure could result.

OTHER INFORMATION

Does not cause addiction or dependence. Introduced in 1994.

Terbinafine

TRADE NAME

Lamisil.

DRUG CLASS

Antifungal.

USES

Fungal infections of skin (ringworm) and nails.

DOSAGE

 Tablets: One tablet a day for several weeks.
Cream: Apply once or twice a day to dry skin.

FORMS

Tablet (white) of 250mg., cream.

PRECAUTIONS

Use with caution in pregnancy (B1), breast feeding and children.

Use with caution in liver and kidney disease.

Avoid eye contact with cream.

 Do not take if:

• suffering from severe liver disease.

SIDE EFFECTS

Common: Cream - Redness, itching, stinging. Tablets - Nausea, diarrhoea, rash, itch, headache, dizziness.

Unusual: Vomiting, red skin, tiredness, chest pain, light headedness.

INTERACTIONS

Other drugs:

• Oral contraceptives, Cimetidine, Rifampicin.

Other substances:

• Reacts with alcohol.

PRESCRIPTION

Yes

PERMITTED IN SPORT

Yes

OVERDOSE

Unlikely to have serious effects. Seek medical advice.

OTHER INFORMATION

Introduced in 1993. Very effective and safe, but quite expensive.

Terbutaline

See BETA-2 AGONISTS

Testosterone

TRADE NAMES

Andropatch, Restandol, Sustanon, Testoderm, Viromone.

DRUG CLASS

Sex hormone

USES

Testosterone deficiency in males, male infertility, male osteoporosis, Klinefelter's syndrome. In combination with oestrogen used for menopause and after removal of ovaries in women.

Breast cancer in women.

Low libido in women (experimental).

DOSAGE

 Capsules: One to three capsules a day after food.
Patch: Apply one at night. Replace every 24 hours.

FORMS

Patches of 2.5, 5 and 6mg., capsules of 40mg. (brown), injection.

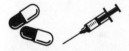

SIDE EFFECTS

Common: Unwanted penile erections, retention of fluid.

PRECAUTIONS

Not to be used in pregnancy (D), breast feeding or children.

Not to be used in women except in combination with Oestrogen.

Use with caution in heart disease, kidney disease, high blood pressure.

 Do not take if:
• suffering from prostate cancer, breast cancer.

INTERACTIONS

None significant.

PRESCRIPTION

Yes

PERMITTED IN SPORT

No

OVERDOSE

No specific problems short term. Long term inappropriate use may cause infertility, shrinking of testes, increased muscle bulk, high blood pressure, heart failure and increased risk of heart attack.

OTHER INFORMATION

Does not cause addiction or dependence. Sometimes used illegally and inappropriately by athletes and body builders with potentially serious consequences.

Tetanus vaccine

TRADE NAME

Clostet, Tetanus vaccine.

Terbutalin (Tetanus antitoxin).

ACT-HIB DTP, Infanrix-HIB (with Haemophilus influenzae B, Diphtheria and Whooping cough vaccines).

Diftavax, Dip/Tet, DTP (with Diphtheria Vaccine).

Infanrix (with Diphtheria and Whooping cough vaccines).

DRUG CLASS

Vaccine.

USES

Prevention of tetanus.

DOSAGE

 Three doses at monthly intervals, then three years later, then at 13 to 18 years of age, then every ten years throughout life.

FORMS

Injection.

PRECAUTIONS

Safe for use in pregnancy (A), breast feeding, children and infants.

 Do not take if:

- suffering from significant chest, throat, ear, nose or sinus infection.

- having treatment for some types of cancer and leukaemia.

SIDE EFFECTS

Common: Redness, swelling, soreness and lump at injection site.

Unusual: Fever, tiredness, allergic reaction.

INTERACTIONS

Other drugs:

- Chloramphenicol.

PRESCRIPTION

Yes

PERMITTED IN SPORT

Yes

OVERDOSE

An unintentional additional vaccination is unlikely to have any significant adverse effect.

OTHER INFORMATION

Tetanus is a world wide disease that is caught from spores in the soil entering a wound. This disease kills about half its victims, but it can be completely prevented by vaccination.

TETRACYCLIC ANTIDEPRESSANT

See Maprotiline

TETRACYCLINES

TRADE and GENERIC NAMES

Achromycin, Topicycline (Tetracycline hydrochloride).

Detelco (Tetracycline hydrochloride, Chlortetracycline, Demeclocycline).

Terramycin (Oxytetracycline).

Terra-Cortil (Oxytetracycline with Hydrocortisone).

Terra-Cortil Nystatin (Oxytetracycline with Nystatin, Hydrocortisone).

Trimovate (Oxytetracycline with Clobetasone, Nystatin).

DRUG CLASS

Tetracycline antibiotic.

USES

Infections caused by bacteria susceptible to Tetracyclines.

DOSAGE

 One or two capsules, three or four times a day.

FORMS

Capsules, tablets, solution.

PRECAUTIONS

Not to be used in pregnancy (D) or children under twelve years as Tetracyclines may cause permanent staining of teeth of foetus or child. Use with caution in breast feeding. Eye ointment safe to use in pregnancy, breast feeding and children.

Use capsules with caution in kidney disease.

Never use expired medication as it may become toxic.

 Do not take capsules if:

- suffering from severe kidney disease, systemic lupus erythematosus (SLE), Staphylococcal infection.

SIDE EFFECTS

Common: Loss of appetite, nausea, sore mouth, diarrhoea, difficulty in swallowing, inflamed colon.

Unusual: Vomiting, inflamed pancreas, rash, secondary fungal infection (thrush).

Severe but rare (stop medication, consult doctor): Severe belly pain, severe diarrhoea, tooth discolouration, significant skin rash.

INTERACTIONS

Other drugs:

- Anticoagulants, Penicillin, Antacids, Iron, Oral contraceptives.

Other substances:

- Milk may reduce absorption from gut.

PRESCRIPTION

Yes

PERMITTED IN SPORT

Yes

OVERDOSE

Exacerbation of side effects only likely effect.

OTHER INFORMATION

Used for a wide range of infections. Tetracycline has been superseded by more sophisticated antibiotics in the same group (eg: those listed below) in the last decade.

See also Chlortetracycline, Demeclocycline, Doxycycline, Lymecycline, Methacycline, Minocycline.

Theophylline

TRADE NAMES

Lasma, Nuelin, Slo-Phyllin, Theo-Dur, Uniphyllin.

Franol (with Ephedrine).

DRUG CLASS

Bronchodilator

USES

Asthma, emphysema, chronic bronchitis.

DOSAGE

 Liquid: 10mLs to 20mLs four times a day.
Tablets: One every six hours.
Sustained release capsules: One

twice a day.

FORMS

Tablets, sustained release tablets, capsules, liquid.

PRECAUTIONS

Safe to use in pregnancy (A), breast feeding and children.

Use with caution in infants.

Use with caution in heart disease, stomach ulcers, heartburn, kidney disease and liver disease.

Lower doses necessary in elderly and lighter patients.

Higher doses may be necessary in smokers.

Blood tests to monitor blood level of Theophylline may be necessary.

SIDE EFFECTS

Common: Nausea, vomiting, belly discomfort, rapid heart rate, tremor, palpitations.

Unusual: Irregular heart rate, convulsions, angina.

INTERACTIONS

Other drugs:

• Cimetidine, Erythromycin.

Other substances:

• Reacts with alcohol, caffeine and nicotine.

PRESCRIPTION

No

PERMITTED IN SPORT

Yes

OVERDOSE

Serious. May cause vomiting, headache, irritability, rapid heart rate, confusion, fever, delirium and convulsions. Seek urgent medical assistance.

OTHER INFORMATION

An early treatment for asthma that is still very useful. Dose must be finely adjusted to give adequate clinical response while avoiding side effects.

Thiabendazole

TRADE NAME

Mintezol.

DRUG CLASS

Anthelmintic.

USES

Tropical infestations such as strongyloidiasis (threadworms), dracunculiasis (guinea worm), larva migrans and trichinosis.

DOSAGE

 Must be individualised by doctor for each patient depending on disease, severity and weight of patient.

PRECAUTIONS

May be used in pregnancy (B3) if medically essential. Breast feeding should be ceased before use.

May be used in children weighing more than 15Kg.

Should not be used unless diagnosis definitely established.

Use with caution in liver and kidney disease, anaemia and malnutrition.

Ensure adequate fluid intake.

FORMS

Tablets (orange) of 500mg.

SIDE EFFECTS

Common: Nausea, vomiting, loss of appetite, dizziness.

Unusual: Diarrhoea, belly discomfort, itch, tiredness, giddiness, headache.

Severe but rare (stop medication, consult doctor): Fever, swelling of tissue.

INTERACTIONS

Other drugs:

• Theophylline.

PRESCRIPTION

Yes

PERMITTED IN SPORT

Yes

OVERDOSE

Exacerbation of side effects likely. Seek medical advice.

OTHER INFORMATION

In use for over forty years to control some of the more exotic tropical infestations.

Thiamine

(Vitamin B1)

TRADE NAME

Benerva.

A large number of other preparations include Thiamine (Vitamin B1) alone or in combination with other vitamins and minerals.

DRUG CLASS

Vitamin

USES

Vitamin B deficiency from fad diets, starvation and over cooked foods. Beriberi.

DOSAGE

 One tablet a day. Recommended daily allowance: Females - 0.8mg.; Males - 1.1mg.

FORMS

Tablets of 50mg.

PRECAUTIONS

Safe in pregnancy, breast feeding and children.

SIDE EFFECTS

Minimal.

INTERACTIONS

Other drugs:-

• Diuretics, some Laxatives.

PRESCRIPTION

No

PERMITTED IN SPORT

Yes

OVERDOSE

No serious effects.

OTHER INFORMATION

Thiamine is a water soluble vitamin found in liver, kidney, pork and whole grain. It is essential for the normal metabolism of carbohydrate foods. The symptoms of vitamin B deficiency include loss of appetite, muscle cramps, pins and needles sensation and ankle swelling. Remember, vitamins are merely chemicals that are essential for the functioning of the body, and if taken to excess, act as a drug.

THIAZIDE DIURETICS

TRADE and GENERIC NAMES

Accuretic (Hydrochlorthiazide with Quinapril).

Aldactide (Hydroflumethiazide with Spironolactone).

Amil-Co, Moducren, Moduret, Moduretic (Hydrochlorthiazide, Amiloride).

Aprinox, Neo-Naclex (Bendrofluazide).

Capozide (Hydrochlorthiazide with Captopril).

Carace Plus, Zestoretic (Hydrochlorthiazide with Lisinopril).

Co-Betaloc (Hydrochlorthiazide with Metoprolol).

Corgaretic (Bendrofluazide, Nadolol).

Cozaar-Comp (Hydrochlorthiazide with Losartan).

Diurexan (Xipamide - thiazide analogue diuretic)

Dyazide, Triam-Co (Hydrochlorthiazide with Triamterene).

Dytide (Benzthiazide, Triamterene).

Hydrosaluric (Hydrochlorthiazide).

Hygroton (Chlorthalidone - thiazide analogue diuretic).

Inderetic, Inderex (Bendrofluazide, Propranolol).

Innozide (Hydrochlorthiazide with Enalapril).

Kalspare (Chlorthalidone with Triamterene).

Kalten (Hydrochlorthiazide with Atenolol).

Metenix (Metolazone - thiazide analogue diuretic)

Monozide (Hydrochlorthiazide with Bisoprolol).

Navidrex (Cyclopenthiazide).

Navispare (Cyclopenthiazide with Amiloride).

Neo-Naclex K (Bendrofluazide, Potassium chloride).

Prestim (Bendrofluazide, Timolol).

Secadrex (Hydrochlorthiazide with Acebutolol).

Tenben (Bendrofluazide, Timolol).

Tenoret, Tenoretic (Chlorthalidone with Atenolol)

Trasidrex (Cyclopenthiazide with Oxprenolol).

Viskaldix (Clopamide, Pindolol).

NB: Thiazides are underlined.

Analogues are drugs that act like another drug.

DRUG CLASS

Diuretic (increases urine production).

USES

High blood pressure, tissue swelling, excess fluid states, heart failure.

DOSAGE

 One or two tablets in morning

PRECAUTIONS

Should not be used in pregnancy (C) unless medically essential. May reduce volume of milk in breast feeding, and is sometimes used for this purpose in women who wish to stop breast feeding.

Use with caution in kidney disease, liver disease, diabetes, SLE and asthma.

 Do not take if:

• suffering from complete kidney failure, gout.

FORMS

Tablets.

SIDE EFFECTS

Common: Increased urinary frequency.

Unusual: Nausea, vomiting, gut cramps, diarrhoea, dizziness, headache, rash.

Severe but rare (stop medication, consult doctor): Unusual bleeding, fainting.

INTERACTIONS

Other drugs:

• Lithium, Barbiturates, Digoxin, Insulin.

• Tablets for controlling maturity onset diabetes.

• Medications that lower blood pressure.

Other substances:

• Reacts with alcohol.

PRESCRIPTION

Yes

PERMITTED IN SPORT

No

OVERDOSE

Confusion, dizziness and gut spasms due to chemical (electrolyte) imbalances occur. Administer activated charcoal or induce vomiting if tablets taken recently, Give extra fluids. Seek medical assistance.

OTHER INFORMATION

Widely used for fluid problems for over forty years. Combined in low doses with many blood pressure medications to improve their effect.

See also Amiloride, Bumetanide, Diazoxide, Frusemide, Spironolactone, Triamterene.

Thioguanine

TRADE NAME

Lanvis.

USES

Leukaemia.

DOSAGE

 Must be individually determined by doctor for each patient depending on severity of disease, age and weight of patient.

FORMS

Tablets (yellow) of 40mg.

PRECAUTIONS

Must not be used in pregnancy (D) unless mother's life is at risk as damage to foetus may occur. Breast feeding must be ceased before use. May be used in children if medically essential.

Use with caution if infection present.

Regular blood tests to check blood cells and liver function essential.

 Do not take if:

• suffering from severe liver or kidney disease, significant viral infection, blood cell damage.

SIDE EFFECTS

Common: Nausea, vomiting, diarrhoea, mouth soreness.

Severe but rare (stop medication, consult doctor): Yellow skin (jaundice), unusual bleeding or bruising.

INTERACTIONS

None significant.

PRESCRIPTION

Yes

PERMITTED IN SPORT

Yes

OVERDOSE

Serious. Induce vomiting if medication taken recently. Seek urgent medical assistance.

Thioridazine

See PHENOTHIAZINES

Thymoxamine

TRADE NAME

Opilon.

DRUG CLASS

Alpha blocker.

USES

Raynaud's phenomenon (spasm of arteries causing poor circulation to fingers and toes).

DOSAGE

 One or two tablets, four times a day.

PRECAUTIONS

Not for use in pregnancy, breast feeding and children.

Use with caution in diabetes.

Not for long term use.

 Do not take if:

• suffering from active liver disease.

FORMS

Tablets of 40mg. (cream).

SIDE EFFECTS

Common: Nausea, diarrhoea, dizziness, headache.

Unusual: Facial flushing, rash.

Severe but rare (stop medication, consult doctor): Liver damage (jaundice - yellow skin).

INTERACTIONS

Other drugs:

• Tricyclic antidepressants, blood pressure medications.

PRESCRIPTION

Yes

PERMITTED IN SPORT

Yes

OVERDOSE

Low blood pressure, drowsiness and depressed reflexes only effects.

THYROID HORMONES

TRADE and GENERIC NAMES

Eltroxin (Thyroxine - T4).

Tertroxin (Liothyronine - T3).

USES

Under active thyroid gland, thyroiditis.

DOSAGE

 One or two tablets a day on an empty stomach. Start with low initial dose and slowly increase to a dose determined by doctor after regular blood tests.

FORMS

Tablets.

SIDE EFFECTS

Only occur with overdosage.

INTERACTIONS

Other drugs:

• Coumarin, Anticoagulants, Barbiturates, Narcotics, Catecholamines, Insulin, Tricyclic antidepressants, Digoxin, Corticosteroids, Colestipol, Phenytoin.

PRESCRIPTION

Yes

PERMITTED IN SPORT

Yes

OVERDOSE

Serious. May cause rapid heart rate, irregular heart beat, angina, restlessness, anxiety, tremor, headache, diarrhoea, vomiting, rapid breathing, fever, heart attack and death. Administer activated charcoal or induce vomiting if medication taken recently. Seek urgent medical assistance.

PRECAUTIONS

Safe to use in pregnancy (A), breast feeding and children.

Use with caution in heart disease and high blood pressure.

Do not take if:

• suffering from angina.

OTHER INFORMATION

Widely used to counter the slowly progressive effects of thyroid underactivity, a problem that is common in middle aged women. Does not cause addiction or dependence, but lifelong treatment usually necessary.

Thyroxine

See THYROID HORMONES

Tiagabine

TRADE NAME

Gabitril.

DRUG CLASS

Anticonvulsant.

USES

Some types of epilepsy causing partial seizures.

DOSAGE

 7.5mg. to 70mg. a day in three divided doses with meals, usually in combination with other anticonvulsants.

PRECAUTIONS

Use with caution in pregnancy (B3) and breast feeding. May be used in children.

Start with a very low dose and increase slowly.

Use with caution in elderly.

Do not stop suddenly, but reduce dose slowly.

Do not take if:

• suffering from severe liver disease.

FORMS

Tablets of 5mg., 10mg. and 15mg. (white).

SIDE EFFECTS

Common: Dizziness, tiredness, nervousness, tremor, diarrhoea.

Unusual: Depression, temperamental.

INTERACTIONS

Other drugs:

• Phenytoin, Carbamazepine, Primidone, Phenobarbitone.

Other substances:

• Alcohol.

PRESCRIPTION

Yes

PERMITTED IN SPORT

Yes

OVERDOSE

Tiredness, dizziness, incoordination, dazed appearance and coma may occur. Induce vomiting or give activated charcoal if tablets taken recently. Seek medical assistance.

OTHER INFORMATION

Introduced in 1998 for the management of more difficult and resistant cases of partial epilepsy.

Tiaprofenic acid

See NSAID

Tibolone

TRADE NAME

Livial.

USES

Symptoms of menopause, prevention of osteoporosis after menopause.

DOSAGE

 One tablet a day.

FORMS

Tablets of 2.5mg. (white).

PRECAUTIONS

Not to be used in pregnancy (D), breast feeding and children.

Use with caution in high cholesterol or triglycerides, liver disease or risk of blood clots (thromboses).

Do not commence in menopause until a year after last menstrual bleed.

 Do not take if:

• suffering from undiagnosed vaginal bleeding, hormone dependent tumours (eg. breast cancer), blood clots or severe liver disorders.

• male.

SIDE EFFECTS

Common: Weight gain, dizziness, headache, belly pain.

Unusual: Migraine, dermatitis, disturbed vision, skin irritation, nausea, constipation, breast pain, vaginal irritation.

Severe but rare (stop medication, consult doctor): Blood clots, liver damage, abnormal vaginal bleeding.

INTERACTIONS

Other drugs:

• Hormone replacement therapies used in menopause, anticoagulants, barbiturates, carbamazepine, rifampicin.

PRESCRIPTION

Yes

PERMITTED IN SPORT

Yes

OVERDOSE

Nausea and abnormal vaginal bleeding only likely effects.

OTHER INFORMATION

Released in 2000 as a completely new method of managing bone density loss after the menopause.

Ticarcillin sodium

TRADE NAME

Timentin (with Clavulanic acid).

DRUG CLASS

Penicillin antibiotic.

USES

Treatment of infections caused by susceptible bacteria.

DOSAGE

 Usually given by continuous drip infusion.

FORMS

Injection.

PRECAUTIONS

May be used in pregnancy (B1), children and breast feeding if clinically indicated.

Use with caution in kidney failure and heart disease.

 Do not take if:

• allergic to Penicillin

• suffering from glandular fever

SIDE EFFECTS

Common: Mild diarrhoea, nausea, vomiting.

Unusual: Itch, rash, headache, dizziness, hot flushes, tiredness.

Severe but rare (stop medication, consult doctor): Severe itchy rash, hives, severe diarrhoea, yellow skin (jaundice), unusual bruising or bleeding.

PRESCRIPTION

Yes

PERMITTED IN SPORT

Yes

OVERDOSE

Vomiting and diarrhoea likely.

OTHER INFORMATION

Used in more severe infections.

Ticlopidine

TRADE NAME

Ticlid.

DRUG CLASS

Anticoagulant.

USES

Prevention of blood clots, particularly in strokes and heart attacks.

DOSAGE

 One twice a day.

FORMS

Tablets of 250mg. (white).

PRECAUTIONS

Should be used with caution in pregnancy (B1), breast feeding and children.

Regular blood tests to monitor blood clotting time, liver function, blood cells and cholesterol required.

 Do not take if:

• suffering from severe liver or kidney disease, bleeding disorders, severe heart failure.

• due for surgery, including dental surgery.

SIDE EFFECTS

Common: Blood in faeces, black faeces, rash, headache, noises in ears.

Severe but rare (stop medication, consult doctor): Significant abnormal bleeding.

INTERACTIONS

Other drugs:

• Must not be used with other Anticoagulants or Aspirin.

• Theophylline, Cimetidine, Antacids, Phenytoin.

PRESCRIPTION

Yes

PERMITTED IN SPORT

Yes

OVERDOSE

Serious abnormal bleeding may occur. Seek urgent medical assistance.

Tiludronic acid

(Tiludronate disodium)

TRADE NAME

Skelid.

DRUG CLASS

Bisphosphonate.

USES

Paget's disease of bone.

DOSAGE

 Two tablets once a day two hours before or after food, with water, for three months. Do not reuse for six months.

FORMS

Tablets of 200mg. (white).

PRECAUTIONS

Use with caution in pregnancy (B2), breast feeding and children.

Ensure adequate calcium and vitamin D intake.

Use with caution in kidney disease.

 Do not take if:

• suffering from severe kidney disease.

SIDE EFFECTS

Common: Nausea, diarrhoea.

Unusual: Dizziness, giddiness, headache, tiredness, skin reaction.

INTERACTIONS

Other drugs:

• Indomethacin, antacids, mineral supplements.

Other substances:

• Food containing calcium.

PRESCRIPTION

Yes

PERMITTED IN SPORT

Yes

OVERDOSE

Serious. Symptoms include loss of appetite, tiredness, vomiting, diarrhoea, sweating, excess urine production, extreme thirst and headache.This may progress to high blood pressure and kidney failure. Administer activated charcoal or induce vomiting if taken recently. Seek medical assistance.

Timolol

See BETA BLOCKERS

Tinidazole

TRADE NAME

Fasigyn.

DRUG CLASS

Antibiotic.

USES

Infections caused by susceptible bacteria, particularly infections of gut and vagina.

DOSAGE

 Four tablets as a single dose.

FORMS

Tablets of 500mg. (white).

PRECAUTIONS

Should not be used in pregnancy (B3) or breast feeding.

Use with caution in children. Use with caution in kidney disease.

 Do not take if:

• suffering from brain disease, blood cell abnormalities.

SIDE EFFECTS

Common: Bad taste, nausea, loss of appetite, diarrhoea.

Unusual: Vomiting, headache, constipation, dizziness, rash.

INTERACTIONS

Other drugs:

• None significant.

Other substances:

• Reacts with alcohol.

PRESCRIPTION

Yes

PERMITTED IN SPORT

Yes

OVERDOSE

Exacerbation of side effects only likely effect.

OTHER INFORMATION

Introduced in the early 1980s as a rapid and effective form of treatment for Giardia of gut and Trichomonal infections of vagina.

Tioconazole

See **IMIDAZOLES**

Tizanidine

TRADE NAME

Zanaflex.

DRUG CLASS

Muscle relaxant.

USES

Muscle spasm caused by multiple sclerosis or spinal cord injury.

DOSAGE

 Increase dose very slowly to a maximum of 36mg. a day given in three or four doses.

FORMS

Tablets of 2 and 4mg. (white).

PRECAUTIONS

Use with caution in pregnancy, breast feeding and children.

Use with caution in kidney disease.

Regular blood tests to check liver function necessary.

Do not take if:

• suffering from liver disease.

SIDE EFFECTS

Common: Drowsiness, tiredness, dizziness, dry mouth.

Unusual: Nausea, diarrhoea, low blood pressure, sleeplessness, slow heart rate.

Severe but rare (stop medication, consult doctor): Hallucinations, liver damage (jaundice - yellow skin).

INTERACTIONS

Other drugs:

• Diuretics, Beta Blockers, blood pressure medications, Digoxin, Oral contraceptives, Sedatives.

Other substances:

• Alcohol.

PRESCRIPTION

Yes

PERMITTED IN SPORT

Yes

OVERDOSE

Seek medical attention. Liver damage likely. Give activated charcoal or induce vomiting if swallowed recently.

Tobramycin

TRADE NAME

Nebcin, TOBI.

DRUG CLASS

Aminoglycoside antibiotic.

USES

Severe infections, particularly meningitis, blood, eye and belly infections. Prevention and control of chronic lung infections.

DOSAGE

 Injection: Every eight hours, or by continuous drip infusion. Nebuliser: Use twice a day for a month, then stop for a month before restarting cycle.

FORMS

Injection, nebuliser solution.

SIDE EFFECTS

Common: Rash, nausea, headache.

Unusual: Ear and kidney damage (dose related), vomiting, delayed wound healing (eye).

Severe but rare (stop medication, consult doctor): Ear noises or deafness, unusual bleeding or bruising.

INTERACTIONS

Other drugs:

• Penicillin, Cephalosporins, Ethacrynic acid, Frusemide, Vitamin K.

PRESCRIPTION

Yes

PERMITTED IN SPORT

Yes

OVERDOSE

Ear and kidney damage possible. Give copious fluids to increase excretion through kidneys.

PRECAUTIONS

Not to be used in pregnancy (D) unless absolutely essential for mother's well being. Breast feeding must be ceased before use. Use with caution and only when essential in children.

Use with caution in kidney disease and muscle disorders.

Blood tests to check that correct dose is being administered are recommended.

Ensure adequate fluid intake during administration of medication.

OTHER INFORMATION

Very useful for the treatment of severe infections. Introduced in early 1980s.

Tocopherols
(Vitamin E)

TRADE NAMES

A large number of preparations include Tocopherols (Vitamin E) alone or in combination with other medications.

DRUG CLASS

Vitamin

USES

Used in many soothing and healing creams, red blood cell disorders, fat absorption disorders.

DOSAGE

 Recommended daily allowance: 8 to 10 mg a day.

FORMS

Tablets, capsules, mixture, cream.

PRECAUTIONS

Use with caution in pregnancy, breast feeding and children.

Do not take in high doses or for prolonged periods of time.

SIDE EFFECTS

Minimal.

INTERACTIONS

None significant.

PRESCRIPTION

No

PERMITTED IN SPORT

Yes

OVERDOSE

Dangerous. May cause blood clots, high blood pressure, breast lumps, headaches, vaginal bleeding, vision disturbances, muscle weakness and bowel disturbances if taken in high doses for a prolonged period of time.

OTHER INFORMATION

Tocopherol is a fat soluble vitamin found in polyunsaturated fatty acids in a wide variety of foods. Remember, vitamins are merely chemicals that are essential for the functioning of the body, and if taken to excess, act as a drug.

Tolfenamic acid

See NSAIDs

Tolnaftate

TRADE NAME

Tinaderm-M (with Nystatin).

DRUG CLASS

Antifungal.

USES

Fungal infections (tinea) of skin.

DOSAGE

 Apply two or three times a day.

FORMS

Cream.

SIDE EFFECTS

Common: Skin irritation.

INTERACTIONS

None significant

PRECAUTIONS

Safe to use in pregnancy, breast feeding and children.

Avoid eyes, nostrils, mouth, vagina and anus.

Seek medical advice if no improvement in ten days.

PRESCRIPTION

Yes

PERMITTED IN SPORT

Yes

OTHER INFORMATION

Very safe and generally effective.

Tolterodine

TRADE NAME

Detrusitol.

DRUG CLASS

Anticholinergic.

USES

Urgency and frequency of urination, urinary incontinence.

PRECAUTIONS

Not for use in pregnancy, breast feeding and children.

Use with caution in enlarged prostate, constipation, kidney and liver disease, hiatus hernia and some forms of neuropathy (nerve disease).

 Do not take if:

- suffering from urinary retention, uncontrolled glaucoma, myasthenia gravis, ulcerative colitis or megacolon.

DOSAGE

 2mg. twice a day.

FORMS

Tablets (white) of 1 and 2mg.

SIDE EFFECTS

Common: Dry mouth, nausea, constipation.

Unusual: Dry eyes, dry skin, tiredness, nervousness, pins and needles sensation.

INTERACTIONS

Other drugs:

- Some Antifungals, Macrolide antibiotics, other Anticholinergics, Cisapride, Metoclopramide.

PRESCRIPTION

Yes

PERMITTED IN SPORT

Yes

OVERDOSE

May be very serious, depending upon dose. Seek urgent medical advice.

Topiramate

TRADE NAME

Topamax.

DRUG CLASS

Anticonvulsant.

USES

Additional treatment for some forms of partial epilepsy.

DOSAGE

 25mg. to 200mg. twice a day. Increase dosage slowly.

FORMS

Tablets of 25mg. (white), 50mg. (cream), 100mg. (yellow), and 200mg. (pink), sprinkle.

PRECAUTIONS

Use with considerable caution in pregnancy (B3), breast feeding and children.

Use with caution in liver and kidney disease, psychiatric disorders.

Do not stop medication suddenly. Must be gradually withdrawn.

 Do not take if:
- suffering from kidney stones.

SIDE EFFECTS

Common: Drowsiness, dizziness, poor coordination, nausea, diarrhoea,

Unusual: Psychiatric disturbances, vomiting, low white blood cell count.

Severe but rare (stop medication, consult doctor): Kidney stones.

INTERACTIONS

Other drugs:

- Phenytoin, Carbamazepine, Digoxin, Sedatives, Hypnotics, low dose Oral contraceptives.

Other substances:

- Alcohol.

PRESCRIPTION

Yes

PERMITTED IN SPORT

Yes

OVERDOSE

No information available. Induce vomiting or administer activated charcoal if taken recently. Seek urgent medical attention.

OTHER INFORMATION

Introduced in 1997 to assist patient with poorly controlled epilepsy despite maximum use of existing medications. Not addictive.

Torasemide

TRADE NAME

Torem.

DRUG CLASS

Diuretic.

USES

Removing excess fluid from body in heart failure, kidney disease, lung disease and high blood pressure.

PRECAUTIONS

Not to be used in pregnancy, breast feeding and children.

Regular blood tests to check electrolyte levels and blood cells necessary.

Use with caution in gout and diabetes.

 Do not take if:

- suffering from severe kidney failure, severe liver disease, low blood pressure.
- sensitive to sulphas.

DOSAGE

 5 to 40mg. a day in morning.

FORMS

Tablets (white) of 2.5, 5 and 10mg.

SIDE EFFECTS

Common: Dry mouth, headache, dizziness.

Unusual: Muscle cramps, blood chemistry (electrolyte) disorders, nausea, diarrhoea, pins and needles sensation.

Severe but rare (stop medication, consult doctor): Blood cell damage.

INTERACTIONS

Other drugs:

- Digoxin, Corticosteroids, other blood pressure medications, Aminoglycoside antibiotics, Cephalosporin antibiotics, Lithium, ACE inhibitors, diabetes medications, Probenecid, NSAIDs, Cholestyramine, Theophylline and Cisplatin.

Other substances:

- Alcohol.

PRESCRIPTION

Yes

PERMITTED IN SPORT

No

OVERDOSE

Severe dehydration may result. Induce vomiting if tablets taken recently. Give extra fluids. Seek medical assistance.

Toremifene

TRADE NAME

Fareston.

DRUG CLASS

Antineoplastic.

USES

Some types of breast cancer in postmenopausal women.

DOSAGE

 One tablet a day.

FORMS

Tablets of 60mg. (white).

PRECAUTIONS

Not to be used in pregnancy (B3) unless essential for the health of the mother.

Not for use in breast feeding or children.

Use with caution in angina, heart disease, diabetes or history of recent blood clots.

Not for prolonged use.

 Do not take if:

- suffering severe liver disease or some conditions affecting the lining of the uterus.
- cancer of breast is oestrogen receptor negative.

SIDE EFFECTS

Common: Excess calcium in blood, hot flushes, sweating, dizziness, diarrhoea, nausea, vaginal discharge.

Unusual: Vomiting, unusual bleeding from vagina, swelling of tissue, muscle pain.

Severe but rare (stop medication, consult doctor): Blood clots.

INTERACTIONS

Other drugs:

- Phenytoin, Carbamazepine, Phenobarbitone, Thiazide diuretics, Warfarin, Ketoconazole, Macrolide antibiotics.

PRESCRIPTION

Yes

PERMITTED IN SPORT

Yes

OVERDOSE

Exacerbation of side effects likely. Induce vomiting or administer activated charcoal if tablets taken recently. Seek medical assistance.

OTHER INFORMATION

Released in 1998 as a new initial treatment for some types of breast cancer.

Tramadol

TRADE NAMES

Tramake, Zamadol, Zydol.

DRUG CLASS

Narcotic.

USES

Moderate to severe pain.

DOSAGE

 50 to 100mg. every six to twelve hours as needed. Maximum 600mg. a day.

FORMS

Capsules, tablets, powder in sachets, injection.

PRECAUTIONS

Use with considerable caution in pregnancy, breast feeding and children.

For short term use only.

Use with caution in undiagnosed abdominal pain, poor lung function, head injury, kidney and liver disease, and epilepsy.

 Do not take if:

- suffering from alcoholism.

- addicted to narcotics (eg. heroin).

SIDE EFFECTS

Common: Nausea, dizziness, constipation, sedation, sweating.

Unusual: Vomiting, convulsions, allergy reactions.

INTERACTIONS

Other drugs:

- Hypnotics, other Analgesics and Narcotics, Psychotropics, Sedatives, general anaesthetics, Buprenorphine, Pentazocine, drugs used for depression, Antipsychotics, MAOI, Carbamazepine, Quinidine, Ketoconazole, Erythromycin.

Other substances:

- Alcohol.

PRESCRIPTION

Yes

PERMITTED IN SPORT

Yes

OVERDOSE

Symptoms may include drowsiness, confusion, difficulty in breathing and coma. Induce vomiting if medication taken recently and patient alert. Seek urgent medical attention.

OTHER INFORMATION

May cause dependence and addiction. Introduced in 1999 for the short term control of severe pain.

Tramazoline

TRADE NAME

Dexa-Rhinaspray (with Dexamethasone).

DRUG CLASS

Vasoconstrictor.

USES

Congestion of nose, hay fever.

PRECAUTIONS

Use in pregnancy only if medically essential. Use with caution in breast feeding and children. Not for use in children under six years.

Use with caution in high blood pressure, glaucoma and thyroid disease.

Avoid eye contact.

Not to be used regularly long term.

DOSAGE

 One spray to each nostril three to six times a day.

FORMS

Nasal spray.

SIDE EFFECTS

Common: Tingling and burning of nose.

Unusual: Worsening of congestion in nose if used long term.

INTERACTIONS

Other drugs:

• None significant.

Other substances:

• Reacts with alcohol.

PRESCRIPTION

Yes

PERMITTED IN SPORT

Yes

OVERDOSE

Nasal congestion worsens if over used.

OTHER INFORMATION

Very effective medication in stuffy noses from any cause.

Trandolapril

See ACE INHIBITORS

Tranexamic acid

TRADE NAME

Cyklokapron.

DRUG CLASS

Haemostatic.

USES

Hereditary angioedema, severe heavy periods (menorrhagia), hyphaemia, control of bleeding during surgery.

DOSAGE

 As determined by doctor for each patient depending upon use.

FORMS

Tablets of 500mg. (white)., injection.

PRECAUTIONS

May be used with caution in pregnancy (B1), breast feeding and children.

Use with caution in kidney disease, blood in urine due to kidney disease, bleeding into body cavities.

 ## Do not take if:

• suffering from blood clots, recent history of blood clots, colour vision disturbances, bleeding around brain.

SIDE EFFECTS

Common: Nausea, diarrhoea.

Unusual: Impaired colour vision.

INTERACTIONS

None significant.

PRESCRIPTION

Yes

PERMITTED IN SPORT

Yes

OVERDOSE

Nausea and vomiting likely. See also HAEMOSTATIC AGENTS.

Tranylcypromine

See MAOI

Trazodone

TRADE NAME

Molipaxin.

DRUG CLASS

Antidepressant.

USES

Depression, abnormal anxiety.

DOSAGE

 50mg. to 300mg. once or twice a day. Most commonly 150mg. once a day.

FORMS

Tablets of 150mg. (pink), capsules of 50mg. (violet/green) and 100mg. (violet/fawn), slow release tablets of 150mg. (blue octagonal).

PRECAUTIONS

May be used with caution in pregnancy, breast feeding and children.

Use with caution in epilepsy, heart disease, liver and kidney disease.

SIDE EFFECTS

Common: Drowsiness, dizziness, headache.

Unusual: Nausea, light headedness, fainting.

Severe but rare (stop medication, consult doctor): Prolonged erection of penis, liver damage, blood cell damage.

INTERACTIONS

Other drugs:

• Muscle relaxants, MAOI, Phenytoin, Clonidine, Digoxin, Sedatives.

Other substances:

• Alcohol.

PRESCRIPTION

Yes

PERMITTED IN SPORT

Yes

OVERDOSE

Seek medical attention. Give activated charcoal or induce vomiting if swallowed recently.

Tretinoin

See KERATOLYTICS

Triamcinolone

TRADE and GENERIC NAMES

Adcortyl, Kenalog, Lederspan, Nasacort.

Adcortyl with Graneodin (with Neomycin, Gramicidin)

Audicort (with Neomycin).

Aureocort (with Chlortetracycline).

Nystadermal (with Nystatin).

Pevaryl TC (with Econazole).

Tri-Adcortyl (with Neomycin, Gramicidin, Nystatin).

DRUG CLASS

Corticosteroid.

USES

Severe inflammation of skin (eczema, dermatitis etc.), mouth and other tissues.

Severe rheumatoid and other forms of severe arthritis, auto-immune diseases, and other severe and chronic inflammatory diseases.

DOSAGE

 Skin preparations: Apply two or three times a day.
Ear drops: Insert two drops twice a day.
Injection: Limited number of injections to affected site or joint once or twice a week.

PRECAUTIONS

Should be used in pregnancy (C), breast feeding and children only on specific medical advice.

Skin and ear preparations safe in pregnancy, breast feeding and children.

Use injection with caution if under stress, and in patients with under active thyroid gland, liver disease, diverticulitis, high blood pressure, myasthenia gravis or kidney disease.

Avoid eyes with all forms.

Use for shortest period of time possible.

 Do not use: injection if:

- suffering from any form of infection, peptic ulcer, or osteoporosis.

- having a vaccination

FORMS

Cream, ointment, paste, ear drops, injection.

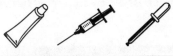

SIDE EFFECTS

Most significant side effects occur only with prolonged use.

Common: Injection - May cause bloating, weight gain, rashes and intestinal disturbances.
Ear drops and skin preparations - Rarely cause adverse reactions.

Unusual: Injection - Dose related effects. Biochemical disturbances of blood, muscle weakness, bone weakness, impaired wound healing, skin thinning, tendon weakness, peptic ulcers, gullet ulcers, bruising, increased sweating, loss of fat under skin, premature ageing, excess facial hair growth in women, pigmentation of skin and nails, acne, convulsions, headaches, dizziness, growth suppression in children, aggravation of diabetes, worsening of infections, cataracts, aggravation of glaucoma, blood clots in veins and sleeplessness.
Skin preparations - thinning of skin, scarring of skin, premature ageing of skin.

Severe but rare (stop medication, consult doctor): Any significant side effect should be reported to a doctor immediately.

INTERACTIONS

None significant.

PRESCRIPTION

Yes

PERMITTED IN SPORT

Yes

OVERDOSE

Exacerbation of side effects likely.

OTHER INFORMATION

Extremely effective and useful medication if used correctly. Lowest dose and shortest possible course should be used. Not addictive.

Triamterene

TRADE and GENERIC NAMES

Only available in combination with Hydrochlorthiazide.

Dyazide, Triam-Co (with Hydrochlorthiazide).

Dytide (with Benzthiazide).

Frusene (with Frusemide).

Kalspare (with Chlorthalidone).

DRUG CLASS

Potassium sparing diuretic.

USES

Excess fluid in body, conserving potassium stores in body.

DOSAGE

 One tablet, one to three times a day after meals.

FORMS

Tablets, capsules.

PRECAUTIONS

Should only be used in pregnancy if medically indicated. Not for use in breast feeding or children.

 Do not take if:

- suffering from liver or severe kidney disease.

SIDE EFFECTS

Common: Minimal.

Unusual: Nausea, vomiting, diarrhoea, weakness.

INTERACTIONS

Other drugs:

- ACE inhibitors, Lithium, Indomethacin.
- Medications used to treat high blood pressure.
- Should not be taken with Potassium supplements.

PRESCRIPTION

Yes

PERMITTED IN SPORT

No

OVERDOSE

No serious effects. If tablets taken recently induce vomiting. Seek medical assistance.

OTHER INFORMATION

Normally used in combination with a diuretic to prevent potassium being washed out of the body.

Tribavirin

TRADE NAMES

Rebetol, Virazole.

DRUG CLASS

Antiviral.

USES

Hepatitis C, severe bronchiolitis caused by the respiratory syncitial virus.

DOSAGE

 Complex. Individualised for each patient by doctor.

PRECAUTIONS

Absolutely forbidden in pregnancy (X) and breast feeding. Severe damage to foetus likely if taken during pregnancy.

Adequate contraception must be used for at least seven months after use of Tribavirin.

Female sexual partners of patients using Tribavirin must use adequate contraception as drug may pass to woman in semen.

Capsules not recommended in children. Nebuliser powder may be used in children.

Regular blood tests necessary to check blood cells, kidney and liver function when taking capsules.

An ECG to check heart function should be taken before and during treatment with capsules.

Use capsules with caution in heart failure, recent heart attack, liver disease, irregular heart beat, gout, mood disorders and thyroid disorders.

Nebuliser equipment must be monitored carefully to check for precipitation of powder in tubing.

 Do not take if:

- suffering from severe heart disease, thalassaemia, sickle cell anaemia, chronic kidney failure, history of significant psychiatric disturbances, severe liver disease (eg. cirrhosis), uncontrolled thyroid disease, and autoimmune disorders.

FORMS

Capsules of 200mg., nebuliser powder.

SIDE EFFECTS

CAPSULES

Damage to red blood cells, psychiatric disturbances, thyroid gland disorders, suicide, excess uric acid in blood, gout.

NEBULISER POWDER

Secondary bacterial infection, pneumonia, pneumothorax.

INTERACTIONS

Other drugs:

- Other antivirals.

PRESCRIPTION

Yes

PERMITTED IN SPORT

Yes

OVERDOSE

Very serious. Likely to cause severe organ damage. No further information available.

OTHER INFORMATION

Introduced 1999 to treat very specific severe and life threatening viral infections.

Triclosan

TRADE NAMES

Aquasept, Manusept, Ster-Zac Bath Concentrate.

Oilatum Plus (with Paraffin and Benzalkonium chloride).

DRUG CLASS

Antiseptic.

USES

Minor skin infections.

DOSAGE

 Depends on form. Usually once or twice a day, or as hand wash as required.

FORMS

Liquid.

PRECAUTIONS

Safe to use in pregnancy, breast feeding and children.

Avoid eyes.

Not for long term use.

SIDE EFFECTS

Minimal.

INTERACTIONS

None significant.

PRESCRIPTION

No

PERMITTED IN SPORT

Yes

OVERDOSE

Diarrhoea and vomiting only likely effects if swallowed.

OTHER INFORMATION

Very widely used and safe.

TRICYCLIC ANTIDEPRESSANTS

TRADE and GENERIC NAMES

Allegron (<u>Nortriptyline</u>).

Anafranil (<u>Clomipramine</u>).

Asendis (<u>Amoxapine</u>).

Concordin (Protriptyline).

Gamanil, Lomont (<u>Lofepramine</u>).

Lentizol (<u>Amitriptyline</u>).

Motipress, Motival (<u>Nortriptyline</u> with Fluphenazine).

Prothiaden (<u>Dothiepin</u>).

Sinequan (<u>Doxepin</u>).

Surmontil (<u>Trimipramine</u>).

Tofranil (<u>Imipramine</u>).

Triptafen (<u>Amitriptyline</u> with Perphenazine).

NB: Tricyclics are underlined.

DRUG CLASS

Antidepressants.

PRECAUTIONS

Should not be used in pregnancy (C) or breast feeding unless medically essential. May be used with caution in children.

Potentially suicidal patients should be watched carefully.

Use with caution in heart disease, kidney and liver disease.

Lower doses required in elderly.

Do not stop medication suddenly, but gradually reduce dosage over some days or weeks.

 Do not take if:
- suffering from glaucoma or difficulty in passing urine.

USES

Depression, sleeplessness (insomnia), bed wetting (Amitriptyline and Imipramine only).

DOSAGE

 One to four or more tablets or capsules usually taken in evening, but may be divided in equal or unequal doses through day when larger amount of medication taken.

FORMS

Tablets, capsules, mixture.

SIDE EFFECTS

Common: Drowsiness, dry mouth, dizziness, tremor, nausea, constipation, rapid heart rate.

Unusual: Confusion, difficulty in passing urine, decreased libido, vomiting, blurred vision, poor concentration, hallucinations, breast enlargement, intestinal cramps, rash.

Severe but rare (stop medication, consult doctor): Yellow skin (jaundice).

INTERACTIONS

Other drugs:

• Sedatives, MAOI, Anxiolytics, Cimetidine, Tolazamide, Barbiturates, Guanethidine, Antihistamines.

Other substances:

• Reacts with alcohol to cause drowsiness.

PRESCRIPTION

Yes

PERMITTED IN SPORT

Yes

OVERDOSE

May be very serious. Symptoms include blurred vision, inability to pass urine, delirium, agitation, incoordination, convulsions, reduced breathing, coma and death. Administer activated charcoal or induce vomiting if taken recently and patient alert. Seek urgent medical assistance. Patients with Tricyclic overdose are often observed in intensive care.

OTHER INFORMATION

Tricyclics are widely used and are the main medication for control of depression. Slow acting and may take two or more weeks for any positive effect to occur. In use for over 40 years.

Trifluoperazine

See PHENOTHIAZINES

Triglycerides

See Fatty acids

Trilostane

TRADE NAME

Modrenal.

USES

Breast cancer, hyperaldosteronism, excess activity of adrenal gland.

DOSAGE

 60 to 240mg. four times a day.

FORMS

Capsules of 60mg. (pink/black) and 120mg. (pink/yellow).

PRECAUTIONS

Must not to be used in pregnancy, breast feeding and children.

Non-hormonal contraception must be used by women.

Use with caution with physical stress, or any kidney or liver disease.

 Do not take if:

- suffering from severe kidney or liver disease.

SIDE EFFECTS

Common: Flushing, nausea, runny nose, diarrhoea.

Unusual: Vomiting.

INTERACTIONS

Other drugs:

- Potassium, Amiloride, Triamterene.

Other substances:

- High potassium foods (eg. bananas, apricots).

PRESCRIPTION

Yes

PERMITTED IN SPORT

Yes

Trimeprazine

See ANTIHISTAMINES, SEDATING

Trimethoprim

TRADE NAME

Monotrim, Trimopan.

Chemotrim, Septrin (with Sulphamethoxazole - this combination is known as Co-trimoxazole).

Polytrim (with Polymyxin B).

DRUG CLASS

Antibiotic.

USES

Urinary tract (bladder and kidney) infections, other bacterial infections.

DOSAGE

 One tablet twice a day.

FORMS

Tablets, suspension, drops, ointment.

PRECAUTIONS

Use in pregnancy (B3) only if medically essential. Not to be used in breast feeding, or in children under six years.

Use with caution in folate deficiency, liver and kidney disease.

Lower doses may be necessary in elderly.

 Do not take if:

- suffering from blood disorders, severe liver and kidney disease.

SIDE EFFECTS

Common: Itch, rash.

Unusual: Nausea, vomiting, fever.

Severe but rare (stop medication, consult doctor): Unusual bleeding or bruising.

INTERACTIONS

Other drugs:

• Anticoagulants, Pyrimethamine.

PRESCRIPTION

Yes

PERMITTED IN SPORT

Yes

OVERDOSE

Nausea, vomiting, dizziness, headache, depression, confusion and damage to bone marrow may occur. Administer activated charcoal or induce vomiting if medication taken recently. Seek medical assistance.

OTHER INFORMATION

Widely used for minor to moderate urinary infections. Synthetic antibiotic. Does not cause dependence or addiction.

Trimipramine

See TRICYCLIC ANTIDEPRESSANTS

Tripotassium dicitratobismuthate

See Bismuth

Triprolidine

See ANTIHISTAMINES, SEDATING

Tropicamide

See MYDRIATICS

Tropisetron

TRADE NAME

Navoban.

USES

Prevention of nausea and vomiting caused by cancer treatments and surgery.

DOSAGE

 One capsule in morning immediately on waking.

FORMS

Capsule (yellow/white) of 5mg., injection.

PRECAUTIONS

Should not be used in pregnancy (B3) or children unless medically essential. Breast feeding should be ceased before use.

Use caution if operating machinery or driving a vehicle.

Use with caution in high blood pressure, irregular heart rhythm, kidney and liver disease.

SIDE EFFECTS

Common: Tiredness, headache, dizziness, constipation.

Unusual: Diarrhoea, loss of appetite.

INTERACTIONS

Other drugs:

• Rifampicin, Barbiturates.

Other substances:

• Avoid food for one hour after taking capsule.

PRESCRIPTION

Yes

PERMITTED IN SPORT

Yes

OVERDOSE

Hallucinations and high blood pressure may occur. Seek medical assistance.

OTHER INFORMATION

Introduced in 1995.

Tryptophan

(L -Tryptophan)

TRADE NAME

Optimax.

DRUG CLASS

Antidepressant.

USES

Severe, prolonged, intractable depression.

DOSAGE

 Two to four tablets, three times a day.

FORMS

Tablets (white) of 500mg.

PRECAUTIONS

Use with caution in pregnancy, breast feeding and children.

Use with caution in kidney and liver disease.

Use lower doses in elderly.

 Do not take if:

• suffering from eosinophilia myalgia syndrome.

SIDE EFFECTS

Common: Drowsiness, nausea, headache.

Severe but rare (stop medication, consult doctor): Eosinophilia myalgia syndrome.

INTERACTIONS

Other drugs:

• MAOI, Phenothiazines, Diazepam and other Benzodiazepines.

PRESCRIPTION

Yes (restricted to specific doctors in some hospitals only).

PERMITTED IN SPORT

Yes

OVERDOSE

No specific information. Seek urgent medical attention.

Tuberculosis vaccine

See BCG vaccine

Typhoid vaccine

See Salmonella typhi vaccine

Tyrothricin

TRADE and GENERIC NAMES

Tyrozets (with Benzocaine).

DRUG CLASS

Antibiotic.

USES

Mild mouth and throat infections.

DOSAGE

 Dissolve one in mouth every three hours.

FORMS

Lozenge (pink).

PRECAUTIONS

Safe to use in pregnancy, breast feeding and children.

SIDE EFFECTS

Common: Minimal.

Unusual: Blackness or soreness of tongue.

Severe but rare (stop medication, consult doctor): Resistant bacterial infection.

INTERACTIONS

None significant.

PRESCRIPTION

No

PERMITTED IN SPORT

Yes

OVERDOSE

Nausea and diarrhoea only likely effects.

Ultralente insulin

See INSULINS

Undecenoic acid

TRADE NAMES

Ceanel (with Cetrimide and other ingredients).

Monophytol (with Salicylates and other ingredients).

DRUG CLASS

Antifungal.

USES

Psoriasis and dermatitis of scalp, tinea pedis (athlete's foot).

DOSAGE

 Use as shampoo two or three times a week. Paint feet twice daily until two weeks after apparent cure.

FORMS

Liquid, paint.

PRECAUTIONS

Safe to use in pregnancy, breast feeding and children.

Monophytol not to be used in pregnancy due to other ingredients.

Avoid eyes, nose and mouth.

Use with caution on broken skin.

SIDE EFFECTS

Minimal.

INTERACTIONS

None significant.

PRESCRIPTION

No.

PERMITTED IN SPORT

Yes.

OVERDOSE

Unlikely to have serious effects if swallowed.

Urea

TRADE NAMES

Aquadrate, Eucerin, Nutraplus.

Alphaderm (with Hydrocortisone).

Balneum Plus (with Lauromacrogols).

Calmurid (with Lactic acid).

Calmurid HC (with Lactic acid and Hydrocortisone).

Found in numerous other creams in combination with other medications.

USES

Skin moisturiser for dry skin, eczema, irritated skin.

PRECAUTIONS

Safe to use in pregnancy, breast feeding and children.

DOSAGE

 Apply as required. Use Hydrocortisone combinations twice a day.

FORMS

Cream.

SIDE EFFECTS

None

INTERACTIONS

None

PRESCRIPTION

No.

PERMITTED IN SPORT

Yes.

OTHER INFORMATION

Safe, simple, cheap and effective. In use for hundreds of years as a moisturiser.

Urea hydrogen peroxide

TRADE NAME

Exterol (with Glycerin).

USES

Softening hard ear wax.

DOSAGE

 Five drops twice a day for three to four days. Retain in ear.

FORMS

Ear drops.

PRECAUTIONS

Safe to use in pregnancy), breast feeding and children.

 Do not take if:
- suffering from perforated ear drum.

SIDE EFFECTS

Common: Effervescent sensation, discomfort.

INTERACTIONS

None in ear.

PRESCRIPTION

No.

PERMITTED IN SPORT

Yes.

OVERDOSE

Unlikely to have serious effects if swallowed.

URICOSURICS

(Reduce levels of uric acid in blood by increasing its loss in urine to prevent gout)

See Allopurinol, Probenecid, Sulphinpyrazone

URINARY ACIDIFIERS

(Make urine more acid)

See Ammonium chloride

URINARY ALKALINISERS

TRADE and GENERIC NAMES

Effercitrate, (Citric acid, Potassium citrate).

Mictral (Citric acid, Sodium bicarbonate and Sodium citrate with Nalidixic acid).

Optiflo G, Uriflex G, Uro-Tainer G
(Citric acid, Sodium bicarbonate,
Disodium edetate and other ingredients).

Optiflo R, Uriflex R, Uro-Tainer R
(Citric acid, Gluconolactone, Disodium
edetate and other ingredients).

Uro-Tainer Suby G (Sodium
bicarbonate with other ingredients).

USES

Bladder and kidney infection, excess
stomach acid.

DOSAGE

 One or two sachets dissolved in
water, three or four times a day.

FORMS

Powder in sachet, granules in sachet,
capsules, effervescent tablet, liquid.

PRECAUTIONS

Safe to use in pregnancy, breast
feeding and children.

Use with caution in heart disease.

 Do not take if:
- suffering from kidney
  failure.

SIDE EFFECTS

Common: Minimal

Unusual: Diarrhoea.

INTERACTIONS

Other drugs:
- Hexamine.

PRESCRIPTION

No.

PERMITTED IN SPORT

Yes.

OVERDOSE

Severe diarrhoea likely.

OTHER INFORMATION

Widely used to ease the symptoms of
urinary infections and prevent
recurrences. Does not cause addiction or
dependence.

URINARY ANTISEPTICS

(Prevent urine infection)

See Hexamine hippurate

Ursodeoxycholic acid

TRADE NAMES

Destolit, Urdox, Ursofalk

USES

Cirrhosis of liver, dissolving some types
of gall stones.

DOSAGE

 Complex. Must be determined
individually for each patient by
doctor.

PRECAUTIONS

Not for use in pregnancy and breast
feeding.

Use with caution in children.

Regular blood tests to check liver
function necessary.

 Do not take if:
- suffering from
  cholecystitis, bile duct
  inflammation, bile duct
  obstruction, inflamed
  bowel or peptic ulcer.

FORMS

Capsules of 150mg., 250mg. and 300mg.

SIDE EFFECTS

Common: Minimal.

Unusual: Diarrhoea, itchy skin, nausea, vomiting, sleep disturbances.

Severe but rare (stop medication, consult doctor): Worsening liver disease.

INTERACTIONS

Other drugs:

• Ciprofloxacin, Cyclosporin, Cholestyramine, Charcoal, Colestipol, Antacids, Oral contraceptives, Oestrogen.

PRESCRIPTION

Yes.

PERMITTED IN SPORT

Yes.

OVERDOSE

No information available. Seek medical attention.

VACCINES

(Prevent disease by stimulating immune system)

See BCG (TB) vaccine, Diphtheria vaccine, Haemophilus influenzae B (HiB) vaccine, Hepatitis A vaccine, Hepatitis B vaccine, Influenza vaccine, Measles vaccine, Mumps vaccine, Neisseria meningitidis vaccine, Poliomyelitis (Sabin) vaccine, Pneumococcal vaccine, Rabies vaccine, Rubella (German measles) vaccine, Salmonella typhi (typhoid) vaccine, Tetanus vaccine, Whooping cough vaccine, Yellow fever vaccine, Yersinia (plague) vaccine

Valaciclovir

TRADE NAME

Valtrex

DRUG CLASS

Antiviral.

USES

Shingles, genital herpes, herpes infection of eye.

DOSAGE

 Shingles: Two tablets three times a day for a week. Must be started within 72 hours of first sign of rash

Herpes: One tablet twice a day.

FORMS

Tablets of 500mg. (white).

PRECAUTIONS

Use with considerable caution in pregnancy (B3). Use with caution in breast feeding. Safe in children.

Use with caution in dehydration, kidney disease and immunosuppression.

SIDE EFFECTS

Common: Headache, nausea.

INTERACTIONS

Other drugs:

• Diuretics, Probenecid.

PRESCRIPTION

Yes.

PERMITTED IN SPORT

Yes.

OVERDOSE

Exacerbation of side effects only likely problem.

OTHER INFORMATION

Introduced in 1997 as a very effective antiviral.

See also Aciclovir, Famciclovir.

Valproate

See Sodium valproate, Valproic acid

Valproic acid

TRADE NAME

Convulex

DRUG CLASS

Anticonvulsant.

USES

Epilepsy.

DOSAGE

 300 to 1000mg. twice a day.

FORMS

Capsules of 150, 300 and 500mg.

PRECAUTIONS

Use with caution in pregnancy, breast feeding and children.

Use with caution in elderly.

Regular blood tests to check liver function necessary.

 Do not take if:
  • suffering from liver disease.

SIDE EFFECTS

Common: Standard urine tests show false positive for ketones (not a serious effect), nausea, diarrhoea.

Unusual: Liver damage, abnormal bleeding, dizziness.

Severe but rare (stop medication, consult doctor): Jaundice (yellow skin).

INTERACTIONS

Other drugs:

• Barbiturates, Antidepressants, Muscle relaxants.

Other substances:

• Alcohol.

PRESCRIPTION

Yes.

PERMITTED IN SPORT

Yes

OVERDOSE

Severe liver damage may occur. Induce vomiting or give activated charcoal if swallowed recently. Seek urgent medical attention.

See also Sodium valproate

Valsartan

See ANGIOTENSIN II RECEPTOR ANTAGONISTS

Vancomycin

TRADE NAME

Vancocin

DRUG CLASS

Antibiotic.

PRECAUTIONS

Use with caution in pregnancy (B2) and breast feeding. May be used when appropriate in children.

Use with caution in kidney disease, bowel inflammation and hearing loss.

Lower doses necessary in elderly. Not designed for long term use.

USES

Capsules: Severe intestinal infections. Injection, infusion: Very severe infections of heart, bone, lungs, blood and soft tissue.

DOSAGE

 One capsule every six hours.

FORMS

Capsules of 125mg. (peach/blue) and 250mg. (grey/blue), injection, infusion.

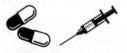

SIDE EFFECTS

Common: Indigestion, nausea, chills, diarrhoea.

Unusual: Vomiting, hearing loss, rash, muscle pain.

Severe but rare (stop medication, consult doctor): Noises in ears or reduced hearing.

INTERACTIONS

Other drugs:

• Aspirin.

PRESCRIPTION

Yes.

PERMITTED IN SPORT

Yes.

OVERDOSE

May cause kidney damage. Seek medical assistance.

OTHER INFORMATION

Very potent and effective antibiotic when used appropriately.

VASOCONSTRICTORS

(Constrict blood vessels)

See Antazoline, Xylometazoline

VASODILATORS

(Dilate blood vessels)

See Betahistine, Diazoxide, Naftidrofuryl oxalate, Nicotinic acid

Vasopressin

(Antidiuretic hormone)

TRADE NAME

Pitressin

DRUG CLASS

Antidiuretic

USES

Diabetes insipidus, some investigations.

DOSAGE

 May be given by injection, or soaked onto cotton buds which are inserted into nose.

FORMS

Injection.

PRECAUTIONS

Use with caution in pregnancy (B2), breast feeding and children.

Must not be given by intravenous injection.

Use with caution in artery disease, heart disease, angina, kidney disease, epilepsy, migraine, asthma, goitre, heart attack, blood clots, hardening of arteries.

SIDE EFFECTS

Common: Minimal.

Unusual: Sweating, tremor, dizziness, fainting, headache, nausea, gut cramps.

INTERACTIONS

None significant.

PRESCRIPTION

Yes.

PERMITTED IN SPORT

Yes.

OVERDOSE

Unlikely to cause serious effects.

OTHER INFORMATION

One of the few effective treatments for the rare disease diabetes insipidus, which is completely unrelated to sugar diabetes (diabetes mellitus).

Venlafaxine

TRADE NAME

Efexor

DRUG CLASS

Antidepressant.

USES

Depression.

DOSAGE

 Tablets: 37.5mg to 75mg twice a day. Increase dose slowly
Capsules: One a day with food.

FORMS

Tablets (peach) of 37.5mg. , 50mg. and 75mg., sustained release capsules (peach) of 75mg. and 150mg.

PRECAUTIONS

Use with caution in pregnancy (B2), breast feeding and children.

Use with caution in higher doses.

Check blood pressure regularly.

Use with caution in epilepsy, other psychiatric conditions, liver and kidney diseases.

Watch patient carefully if suicidal.

Do not stop suddenly, but reduce dose slowly.

 Do not take if:
• taking MAOI.

SIDE EFFECTS

Common: Dizziness, sleeplessness, nervousness, nausea, diarrhoea, dry mouth.

Unusual: Tiredness, vomiting, excess sweating, impotence, general tiredness.

Severe but rare (stop medication, consult doctor): High blood pressure.

INTERACTIONS

Other drugs:

• MAOI may cause very serious effects.

• Other antidepressants.

PRESCRIPTION

Yes.

PERMITTED IN SPORT

Yes.

OVERDOSE

May be serious. Induce vomiting or give activated charcoal if taken recently. Seek urgent medical attention.

OTHER INFORMATION

Introduced in 1997 for the management of more difficult cases.

See also SSRI.

Verapamil

See **CALCIUM CHANNEL BLOCKERS**

Vigabatrin

TRADE NAME

Sabril

DRUG CLASS

Anticonvulsant

USES

Epilepsy, particularly difficult to control epilepsy.

DOSAGE

 One or two tablets twice a day.

FORMS

Tablets (white) of 500mg., powder in sachet.

PRECAUTIONS

Not to be used in pregnancy (D) or breast feeding.

Use with care in psychiatric conditions and kidney disease.

Response to medication must be checked regularly by a doctor.

Use with caution in elderly.

Medication should not be stopped suddenly.

SIDE EFFECTS

Common: Drowsiness, weight gain, nausea, diarrhoea.

Unusual: Disturbed brain function, disturbed bowel function, vomiting, reduced alertness.

INTERACTIONS

Other drugs:

• Phenytoin

PRESCRIPTION

Yes.

PERMITTED IN SPORT

Yes.

OTHER INFORMATION

Released in 1994. Not addictive or dependence forming.

Vinblastine

See **VINCA ALKALOIDS**

VINCA ALKALOIDS

TRADE and GENERIC NAMES

Eldisine (Vindesine sulfate).

Navelbine (Virorelbine).

Oncovin (Vincristine sulfate).

Velbe (Vinblastine sulfate).

USES

Leukaemia, some lung cancers, blood disorders, Hodgkin's disease, advanced breast cancer, some other forms of cancer.

DOSAGE

 Must be individualised for each patient by doctor depending on disease, severity, response and weight of patient.

FORMS

Injection, infusion.

SIDE EFFECTS

Common: Loss of all body hair, pins and needles, nerve pain, muscle weakness, nausea, vomiting.

Unusual: Paralysis of some muscles, convulsions, constipation or diarrhoea, depression, headache, rash, fever, anaemia, jaw pain.

Severe but rare (stop medication, consult doctor): Unusual bleeding or bruising, yellow skin (jaundice).

INTERACTIONS

Other drugs:

• Phenytoin.

Other substances:

• Alcohol should be avoided during treatment.

PRESCRIPTION

Yes.

OVERDOSE

Frequently fatal.

PRECAUTIONS

Must not be used in pregnancy (D) unless mother's life is at risk as foetus may be damaged. Breast feeding must be ceased before use. May be used with caution in children.

Adequate contraception must be used by all women during treatment.

Regular blood and marrow tests to check blood and marrow cells and liver function essential.

Use with caution in nerve, muscle and lung disease.

 Do not take if:

• suffering from serious infection, nerve damage, severe liver disease.

OTHER INFORMATION

Despite significant side effects, these drugs may save the life of patients with leukaemia and other cancers.

Vincristine

See VINCA ALKALOIDS

Vindesine

See VINCA ALKALOIDS

Vinorelbine

See VINCA ALKALOIDS

VITAMINS

(Essential nutrients)

See Ascorbic acid (Vitamin C); Biotin (Vitamin H); Cholecalciferol, Calcitriol and Ergocalciferol (Vitamin D); Cyanocobalamin, Hydroxocobalamin (Vitamin B12); Nicotinic Acid (Vitamin B3); Pantothenic acid (Vitamin B5); Phytomenadione (Vitamin K); Pyridoxine (Vitamin B6); Retinols (Vitamin A); Riboflavine (Vitamin B2); Thiamine (Vitamin B1); Tocopherols (Vitamin E).

Vitamin A

See Retinol

Vitamin B1

See Thiamine

Vitamin B12

See Cyanocobalamin, Hydroxocobalamin

Vitamin B2

See Riboflavine

Vitamin B3

See Nicotinic acid

Vitamin B5

(Pantothenic acid).

See Panthenol

Vitamin B6

See Pyridoxine

Vitamin C

See Ascorbic acid

Vitamin D

See Cholecalciferol, Calcitriol and Ergocalciferol

Vitamin E

See Tocopherols

Vitamin H

See Biotin

Vitamin K

See Phytomenadione

Warfarin

TRADE NAME

Marevan.

DRUG CLASS

Anticoagulant.

USES

Prevention and treatment of blood clots (eg: lung clots, heart clots).

DOSAGE

 Precise dose as directed by doctor once a day at the same time.

FORMS

Tablets of 0.5mg. (white),1mg.(brown), 3mg. (blue) and 5mg. (pink).

SIDE EFFECTS

Common: Bruising, nose bleeds.

Unusual: Hair loss, itch, rash, fever, nausea, diarrhoea, belly pains.

Severe but rare (stop medication, consult doctor): Significant bleeding, blood in urine, blood in faeces, vomiting blood, black patch of skin.

INTERACTIONS

Other drugs:

• Interacts with a very wide range of medications. Do not take any medication (including cold mixtures, vitamins, and other chemist and supermarket lines) without checking with a doctor.

• Never take Aspirin or arthritis (NSAID) drugs with Warfarin.

Other substances:

• Reacts with alcohol and caffeine.

• Reacts with many foods. Do not alter diet without discussing with a doctor.

• Eat a constant amount of green leafy vegetables, meat and dairy products as a variation may affect the effect of Warfarin.

• Do not diet or binge eat without discussing with a doctor.

PRECAUTIONS

Must not be used in pregnancy (D) as it may cause foetal damage and death. Breast feeding should be ceased if use is medically necessary. May be used with caution in children.

Regular blood tests to check blood clotting time essential.

Other illnesses (eg: infection) may require an adjustment of Warfarin dosage.

Read literature accompanying medication very carefully. Ask questions of doctor about anything you do not understand.

Do not undertake any activity that may result in falls, bruising or extreme exertion.

 Do not take if:

• suffering from bleeding tendency, peptic ulcer, dementia, mental diseases, severe high blood pressure.

• due to have essential surgery, including dental surgery.

PRESCRIPTION

Yes

PERMITTED IN SPORT

Yes, but not recommended in active sport. Body contact sport forbidden.

OVERDOSE

Extremely serious. Administer activated charcoal or induce vomiting only if tablets taken very recently. Seek emergency medical assistance. Massive internal bleeding may cause sudden death. Antidote (Vitamin K) available. Blood transfusion may be necessary.

OTHER INFORMATION

Warfarin is the active ingredient of many rat poisons. If used correctly and carefully, Warfarin can save and prolong life with minimal or no side effects. Slightest variation of dose may cause adverse effects. Wearing a bracelet or charm with information about the medication is advised for anyone using Warfarin long term.

Whooping cough (Pertussis) vaccine

TRADE NAMES

Only available in combination with other vaccines.

DTP, Infanrix (with Tetanus and Diphtheria vaccines).

Act-Hib DTP, Infanrix-HiB (with HiB, Diphtheria and Tetanus vaccines).

DRUG CLASS

Vaccine.

USES

Prevention of whooping cough.

DOSAGE

 Three injections at monthly intervals starting at two months of age.

FORMS

Injection.

PRECAUTIONS

Not designed for use over two years of age.

Use with caution if history of brain disease or convulsions.

 Do not take if:

- suffering from acute illness, significant fever or epilepsy.
- previously infected with whooping cough.

SIDE EFFECTS

Common: Local redness and tenderness at injection site, persistent lump, fever.

Unusual: Tiredness, irritability, faint.

Severe but rare: Convulsion, brain inflammation.

INTERACTIONS

Vaccines other than poliomyelitis (Sabin) vaccine.

PRESCRIPTION

Yes

PERMITTED IN SPORT

Yes

OVERDOSE

An unintentional additional dose is unlikely to have any serious effect.

Xipamide

See **THIAZIDE DIURETICS**

Xylometazoline

TRADE NAMES

Otrivin.

Otrivin-Anthistin (with Antazoline).

Rynacrom Co (with Sodium cromoglycate).

DRUG CLASS

Vasoconstrictor.

USES

Nasal congestion, hay fever, eye inflammation, eye allergy.

DOSAGE

 Nose: Use in each nostril one to four times a day.
Eye: One or two drops two or three times a day.

FORMS

Nose drops and spray, eye drops.

SIDE EFFECTS

Common: Eye drops - temporary blurred vision, stinging. Nose drops - burning, stinging, sneezing, dry nose.

Unusual: Nose drops - worsening nasal congestion if over used, sleeplessness, light headedness, palpitations, headache.

PRECAUTIONS

Safe to use in pregnancy, breast feeding and children. Ensure children strength and not adult strength nose preparations used in children. Use eye drops with caution in children. Not to be used in nose long term.

 ### Do not take any form if:

- suffering from glaucoma or serious eye disease.

 ### Do not use eye drops if:

- using contact lenses.

INTERACTIONS

Other drugs:

- MAOI

Other substances:

- Reacts with alcohol

PRESCRIPTION

No

PERMITTED IN SPORT

Yes

OVERDOSE

If used excessively, nasal congestion rather than relief may occur. If swallowed, sedation, high blood pressure, rapid irregular heart rate and coma may occur. Seek medical assistance.

OTHER INFORMATION

Ensure instructions are followed and medication is not over used.

Y

Yellow fever vaccine

TRADE NAME

Arilvax.

DRUG CLASS

Vaccine

USES

Prevention of yellow fever.

DOSAGE

 Single injection gives ten years protection.

FORMS

Injection.

PRECAUTIONS

Not to be used in pregnancy. May be used with caution in breast feeding and children over one year.

 Do not take if:

- suffering from significant illness, cancer or immune disease.

- allergic to poultry or eggs.

SIDE EFFECTS

Common: Fever, tiredness, joint pains.

INTERACTIONS

None significant.

PRESCRIPTION

Yes (only available from specifically registered centres).

PERMITTED IN SPORT

Yes

OVERDOSE

An inadvertent additional vaccination is unlikely to have any serious consequences.

OTHER INFORMATION

Not routinely used. Only given to persons travelling to, or resident in, countries of tropical Africa and South America where yellow fever occurs. The disease is spread by mosquitoes.

Yersinia pestis (Plague) vaccine

TRADE NAME

Plague Vaccine

DRUG CLASS

Vaccine

USES

Prevention of plague (black death).

PRECAUTIONS

Use with caution in pregnancy. May be used in breast feeding and children.

Use with caution in fever from infection.

DOSAGE

Two injections at an interval of one to four weeks. Third injection necessary for children under twelve. Additional booster doses required every six months.

FORMS

Injection.

SIDE EFFECTS

Minimal.

INTERACTIONS

Other drugs:

• Other vaccines.

PRESCRIPTION

Yes

PERMITTED IN SPORT

Yes

OVERDOSE

Additional inadvertent vaccination unlikely to have any serious consequences.

OTHER INFORMATION

Not a routine travel vaccination. Only given to residents and visitors to an area where plague occurs.

Z

Zafirlukast

TRADE NAME

Accolate

DRUG CLASS

Leukotrene receptor antagonist.

USES

Prevention and treatment of asthma.

DOSAGE

 One or two tablets twice a day.

FORMS

Tablets (white) of 20mg.

PRECAUTIONS

May be used with caution in pregnancy (B1) and breast feeding. Use with caution in children.

Use with caution in unstable and sudden onset asthma.

Do not stop medication suddenly.

Use with caution if withdrawing from steroids.

Use with caution in liver disease.

SIDE EFFECTS

Common: Chest infection.

Unusual: Abnormal bleeding.

Severe but rare (stop medication, consult doctor): Liver and white blood cell damage.

INTERACTIONS

Other drugs:

• Warfarin, theophylline, erythromycin, terfenadine, aspirin.

PRESCRIPTION

Yes

PERMITTED IN SPORT

Yes

OVERDOSE

May cause damage to liver and blood cells. Induce vomiting or give activated charcoal if taken recently. Seek urgent medical attention.

OTHER INFORMATION

Expensive medication introduced in 1999 to assist asthmatics who are not adequately controlled by other medications.

Zalcitabine

TRADE NAME

Hivid.

DRUG CLASS

Antiviral.

USES

AIDS, HIV infection.

DOSAGE

 One or two tablets three times a day. Often used in combination with Zidovudine.

FORMS

Tablets of 0.375mg. (beige) and 0.75mg. (grey).

PRECAUTIONS

Must not be used in pregnancy (D). Use with caution in breast feeding and children.

Use with caution in peripheral neuropathy, pancreatitis, kidney and liver disease.

Regular blood tests to check liver and kidney function, and blood cells, are necessary.

SIDE EFFECTS

Common: Mouth ulcers, nausea, rash, itch, headache, muscle pain, tiredness.

Unusual: Pain on swallowing, loss of appetite, vomiting, dizziness, throat inflammation.

Severe but rare (stop medication, consult doctor): Belly pain (pancreatitis), numbness and burning in hands and feet (neuropathy).

INTERACTIONS

Other drugs:

• Aminoglycosides, Amphotericin, Foscarnet, Chloramphenicol, Cisplatinum, Dapsone, Didanosine, Disulfram, Ethionamide, Glutethamide, Hydralazine, Iodoquinol, Isoniazid, Nitrofurantoin, Phenytoin, Ribavrin, Vincristine.

PRESCRIPTION

Yes

PERMITTED IN SPORT

Yes

OVERDOSE

No information available. Induce vomiting or administer activated charcoal if taken recently. Seek urgent medical attention.

OTHER INFORMATION

Usually combined with other medications used to treat HIV infections.

Zaleplon

TRADE NAME

Sonata.

DRUG CLASS

Hypnotic.

USES

Severe insomnia resistant to other forms of treatment.

DOSAGE

 5 to 10mg. at bedtime.

PRECAUTIONS

Not to be used in pregnancy, breast feeding and children.

Not to be used for more than two weeks.

Use with caution in liver disease, depression and poor lung function.

Use with caution if history of alcohol or drug abuse.

 Do not take if:

• suffering from severe liver disease, sleep apnoea, myasthenia gravis, severe lung disease, psychiatric disturbances.

• history or suspicion of suicide.

FORMS

Capsules of 5mg. (whit/light brown with pink band) and 10mg. (white with pink band).

SIDE EFFECTS

Common: Rebound anxiety and insomnia when medication finished, dependence upon drug, loss of memory, headache, tiredness, drowsiness.

Unusual: Dizziness, poor reactions.

Severe but rare (stop medication, consult doctor): Psychiatric disturbances, liver damage.

INTERACTIONS

Other drugs:

• Antipsychotics, Hypnotics, Sedatives, Narcotics, Antidepressants, Antihistamines, Anticonvulsants, Ketoconazole, Cimetidine, Erythromycin, Barbiturates, Rifampicin and Carbamazepine.

Other substances:

• Alcohol, marijuana, heroin.

PRESCRIPTION

Yes

PERMITTED IN SPORT

Yes

OVERDOSE

May be very serious. Induce vomiting or give activated charcoal if swallowed recently. Seek urgent medical attention.

OTHER INFORMATION

May be addictive if used for more than a couple of weeks.

Zanamivir

TRADE NAME

Relenza

DRUG CLASS

Antiviral.

USES

Treatment of influenza. Must be started within 48 hours of first symptoms of influenza appearing.

DOSAGE

Two inhalations twice daily for five days.

FORMS

Disc inhaler.

PRECAUTIONS

Use with caution in pregnancy (B1) and breast feeding.

Use with caution in severe asthma.

SIDE EFFECTS

Common: Minimal.

Unusual: Dizziness, diarrhoea.

Severe but rare (stop medication, consult doctor): Asthma.

INTERACTIONS

None significant.

PRESCRIPTION

Yes

PERMITTED IN SPORT

Yes

OVERDOSE

Additional inhalations unlikely to have any serious effects.

OTHER INFORMATION

Released in 1999 as the first medication for the treatment of influenza. Developed in Australia.

Zidovudine

(Azidothymidine)

TRADE NAMES

Retrovir.

Combivir (with Lamivudine).

DRUG CLASS

Antiviral.

USES

AIDS (Acquired Immune Deficiency Syndrome), HIV (Human Immunodeficiency Virus) positive patients.

PRECAUTIONS

Not to be used in pregnancy (B3) unless medically essential. Breast feeding should be ceased before use. Not to be used in children unless medically essential.

Regular blood tests to check for organ and blood cell damage essential.

Patients must be fully informed of risks associated with this treatment by their doctor.

 ## Do not take if:

- not suffering from HIV/AIDS.
- planning to father children.

DOSAGE

 Retrovir: 500 to 600mg a day in divided doses.
Combivir: One twice a day.

FORMS

Retrovir: Capsules of 100mg. (white) and 250mg. (white/blue), tablets of 300mg. (white), syrup. Combivir: Tablets (white).

SIDE EFFECTS

Many side effects of Zidovudine may be caused by the disease (AIDS) it is treating. *Common:* Tiredness, fever, headache, loss of appetite, nausea, vomiting, muscle aches, sleeplessness, rash, blood cell damage.

Unusual: Belly discomfort, dizziness, pins and needles, shortness of breath.

Severe but rare: Impairs fertility, may cause cancer.

INTERACTIONS

Other drugs:

- Paracetamol, Probenecid, Phenytoin, Stavudine, Tribavirin, many other drugs and natural remedies.

PRESCRIPTION

Yes

PERMITTED IN SPORT

Yes

OVERDOSE

Causes vomiting. Uneventful recovery likely.

OTHER INFORMATION

Introduced in early 1990s in an attempt to slow the progress of HIV/AIDS, but does not cure the disease. Normally used in combination with other antivirals.

Zinc oxide

TRADE and GENERIC NAMES

Viscopaste, Zipzoc.

Anugesic-HC (with Hydrocortisone, Pramoxine, Benzyl benzoate and other ingredients).

Anusol (with Benzyl benzoate, Bismuth and other ingredients).

Anusol HC (with Hydrocortisone, Benzyl benzoate, Bismuth and other ingredients).

Coltapaste (with Coal tar).

E45 Sun (with Titanium oxide).

Hemocane (with Lignocaine, Bismuth oxide, Benzoic acid and other ingredients).

Hewletts Cream (with Lanolin).

Morhulin (with Cod liver oil).

Sprilon (with Dimethicone).

Sudocrem (with Wool fat, Benzyl benzoate and other ingredients).

Vasogen (with Dimethicone and Calamine).

Xyloproct (with Hydrocortisone, Aluminium Acetate, Lignocaine).

Also found in numerous other locally produced barrier creams.

DRUG CLASS

Mineral

USES

Skin protection, skin inflammation, mild fungal infections of skin, piles, skin ulcers, aid to healing.

DOSAGE

 Applied to affected area as needed.

FORMS

Cream, ointment, lotion, suppository, impregnated bandage, stockinette.

PRECAUTIONS

Safe in pregnancy, breast feeding and children of all ages.

SIDE EFFECTS

Common: Minimal.

Unusual: Sensitivity reactions.

INTERACTIONS

Other drugs:

• May prevent other creams from reaching skin and acting on skin if zinc oxide is applied first.

PRESCRIPTION

Most forms: No

Combined with Hydrocortisone: Yes.

PERMITTED IN SPORT

Yes

OTHER INFORMATION

Zinc oxide has been used for centuries to protect skin from injury, and to sooth irritation.

Zinc pyrithione

See Pyrithione zinc

Zinc sulphate

TRADE NAMES

Solvazinc, Z Span.

Efalith (with Lithium succinate).

Zinc sulphate is also found in numerous other locally produced mineral and vitamin supplements.

DRUG CLASS

Mineral.

USES

Mineral supplement, dermatitis, acne.

DOSAGE

 Recommended daily intake 12mg. per day. Apply ointment twice a day.

FORMS

Tablets, capsules, ointment.

PRECAUTIONS

Use tablets with caution in pregnancy and children. May be used in breast feeding.

Do not exceed recommended dose.

Do not take tablets constantly, but suspend medication intermittently.

Ensure adequate intake of fibre while taking tablets.

SIDE EFFECTS

Minimal.

INTERACTIONS

None significant.

PRESCRIPTION

No

PERMITTED IN SPORT

Yes

OVERDOSE

Constipation only likely serious effect.

OTHER INFORMATION

Low levels of zinc in the blood may reduce the body's ability to repair damage. May improve acne healing.

Zolmitriptan

TRADE NAME

Zomig.

DRUG CLASS

Antimigraine.

USES

Treatment of acute migraine.

DOSAGE

 One tablet at onset of migraine. Repeat after two hours if necessary.

PRECAUTIONS

Use with considerable caution in pregnancy (B3), breast feeding and children.

Use with caution in irregular heart rhythm and liver disease.

 Do not take if:

- suffering from angina, serious heart disease, poor circulation, significant high blood pressure, poor kidney function.

- history of recent heart attack, stroke or transient ischaemic attack.

FORMS

Tablets of 2.5mg. (yellow).

SIDE EFFECTS

Common: Tiredness, nausea, dizziness, warm sensation, pins and needles sensation.

Unusual: Dry mouth, throat pressure, muscle aches.

Severe but rare (stop medication, consult doctor): Chest pain.

INTERACTIONS

Other drugs:

• Ergotamine, MAOI, Cimetidine, Fluvoxamine, Quinolone antibiotics.

PRESCRIPTION

Yes

PERMITTED IN SPORT

Yes

OVERDOSE

Sedation only likely effect.

OTHER INFORMATION

Very effective medication, particularly if taken immediately migraine starts.

See also Sumatriptan

Zolpidem

TRADE NAME

Stilnoct.

DRUG CLASS

Hypnotic.

USES

Insomnia.

DOSAGE

 5 or 10 mg. at bedtime.

FORMS

Tablets (white) of 5 and 10mg.

PRECAUTIONS

Use with caution in pregnancy and breast feeding.

Not recommended in children.

Not to be used long term.

Use with caution in lung and liver diseases, depression.

 Do not take if:

• suffering from sleep apnoea, myasthenia gravis, severe lung or liver disease, psychiatric disturbances.

• history of drug abuse.

SIDE EFFECTS

Common: Rebound inability to sleep when medication ceased, nausea, diarrhoea, dizziness, tiredness.

Unusual: Headache.

Severe but rare (stop medication, consult doctor): Memory loss, confusion, depression, tremor, hallucinations.

INTERACTIONS

Other drugs:

• Other Sedatives and Hypnotics.

Other substances:

• Alcohol, heroin, marijuana.

PRESCRIPTION

Yes

PERMITTED IN SPORT

Yes

OVERDOSE

May be serious, but rarely life threatening. Induce vomiting or give activated charcoal if swallowed recently. Seek urgent medical attention.

OTHER INFORMATION

May cause dependence and addiction if used excessively.

See also Zaleplon.

Zopiclone

TRADE NAME

Imovane

DRUG CLASS

Sedative/Hypnotic.

USES

Insomnia (sleeplessness).

DOSAGE

 One tablet 30 minutes before bedtime.

FORMS

Tablet of 7.5mg. (white).

SIDE EFFECTS

Common: Drowsiness, headache, fatigue, taste disturbances, dry mouth.

Unusual: Dependency on medication.

PRECAUTIONS

Should not be used in pregnancy (C), breast feeding or children.

Designed for short term use only.

Use with caution in severe kidney and liver disease, poor thyroid function, depression and epilepsy.

Lower doses needed in elderly.

Dependence possible.

 Do not take if:

- suffering from myasthenia gravis, severe lung disease, sleep apnoea, recent stroke.

- operating machinery, driving a vehicle or undertaking tasks that require concentration and alertness.

INTERACTIONS

Other drugs:

- Other sedatives.

Other substances:

- Reacts with alcohol to increase sedation.

PRESCRIPTION

Yes

PERMITTED IN SPORT

Yes

OVERDOSE

Seldom life threatening. May cause drowsiness, confusion and coma. Induce vomiting if tablets taken recently. Seek medical assistance.

OTHER INFORMATION

Introduced in 1993 as an alternative to Temazepam. Very safe and effective. May cause dependence.

Zotepine

TRADE NAME

Zoleptil.

DRUG CLASS

Antipsychotic.

USES

Schizophrenia.

DOSAGE

 25 to 100mg. three times a day. Increase dosage slowly.

FORMS

Tablets of 25mg. (white), 50mg. (yellow) and 100mg. (pink).

PRECAUTIONS

May be used with considerable caution in pregnancy. Not to be used in breast feeding or children.

Use with caution in epilepsy, heart disease, low blood pressure, kidney and liver disease, prostate gland enlargement, difficulty in passing urine, glaucoma, Parkinson's disease and adrenal tumours.

Check blood pressure and blood chemistry regularly.

 Do not take if:

- suffering from acute gout, alcoholism.
- intoxicated.

SIDE EFFECTS

Common: Tiredness, fever, headache.

Unusual: Infections, unusual pains, low blood pressure, fainting, altered appetite, tissue swelling, excess thirst, blurred vision, conjunctivitis, impotence, urinary incontinence.

Severe but rare (stop medication, consult doctor): Liver damage (jaundice - yellow skin).

INTERACTIONS

Other drugs:

- Sedatives, other Antipsychotics, Fluoxetine, Diazepam, Anaesthetics.

Other substances:

- Alcohol.

PRESCRIPTION

Yes

PERMITTED IN SPORT

Yes

OVERDOSE

Very serious. Symptoms include drowsiness, confusion, restlessness, rapid heart rate, tremor, convulsions, difficulty in breathing and swallowing, coma and death. Administer activated charcoal or induce vomiting if taken recently and patient alert. Seek urgent medical attention.

OTHER INFORMATION

Introduced in 1999 to help more serious cases of schizophrenia.

See also PHENOTHIAZINES

Zuclopenthixol

TRADE NAME

Clopixol.

DRUG CLASS

Antipsychotic.

USES

Schizophrenia, severe psychoses, mania.

DOSAGE

 Capsules: 10mg to 50mg a day in divided doses.
Depot injection: One injection every two to four weeks
Injection: One injection every two to four days.

FORMS

Tablets of 2mg. (pink)10mg. (light brown), 25mg. (brown). Injection, depot injection.

SIDE EFFECTS

Common: Drowsiness, twitching, dry mouth, constipation.

Unusual: Uncontrolled movements, liver damage, blood cell damage, inability to vomit.

Severe but rare (stop medication, consult doctor): High fever, jaundice (yellow skin).

INTERACTIONS

Other drugs:

• Anticholinergics, Sedatives, Hypnotics, Tricyclic antidepressants, Metoclopramide, Piperazine.

Other substances:

• Alcohol.

• Organophosphate insecticides.

PRESCRIPTION

Yes

PERMITTED IN SPORT

Yes

OVERDOSE

Tiredness, convulsions, coma, low blood pressure and altered temperature may occur. Induce vomiting or give activated charcoal if capsules taken recently. Seek urgent medical attention.

PRECAUTIONS

Use only as a last resort in pregnancy (C). Use with caution in breast feeding and children.

Use with caution in Parkinsonism, epilepsy, glaucoma, poor blood supply to brain, severe hardening of arteries and heart disease, kidney and liver disease.

Use with caution in high temperatures.

Regular blood tests to check liver and blood cell function recommended.

Consider options carefully before using for prolonged period.

 Do not take if:

• suffering from coma, brain injury, abnormal blood cells in past or present, phaeochromocytoma.

• alcohol, narcotics or barbiturates recently consumed.

OTHER INFORMATION

Introduced in 1996 to control more difficult cases of schizophrenia and other psychiatric conditions. Does not cause addiction or dependence.

INDEX

All trade (brand) names, generic names and drug classes in this book are listed. Drug classes are shown in CAPITAL LETTERS.